Free DVD  Free DVD

Essential Test Tips Video from Trivium Test Prep

Dear Customer,

Thank you for purchasing from Trivium Test Prep! Whether you're looking to join the military, get into college, or advance your career, we're honored to be a part of your journey.

To show our appreciation (and to help you relieve a little of that test-prep stress), we're offering a **FREE NCLEX *Essential Test Tips* Video** by Trivium Test Prep. Our video includes 35 test preparation strategies that will help keep you calm and collected before and during your big exam. All we ask is that you email us your feedback and describe your experience with our product. Amazing, awful, or just so-so: we want to hear what you have to say!

To receive your **FREE NCLEX *Essential Test Tips* Video**, please email us at 5star@ triviumtestprep.com. Include "Free 5 Star" in the subject line and the following information in your email:

1. The title of the product you purchased.

2. Your rating from 1 – 5 (with 5 being the best).

3. Your feedback about the product, including how our materials helped you meet your goals and ways in which we can improve our products.

4. Your full name and shipping address so we can send your **FREE NCLEX *Essential Test Tips* Video**.

If you have any questions or concerns please feel free to contact us directly at 5star@triviumtestprep.com.

Thank you, and good luck with your studies!

NCLEX-RN PRACTICE TESTS 2022-2023:

Review Book with 1000+ Assessment Questions with Answer Rationales for the National Council Licensure Nursing Examination

E. M. Falgout

ABOUT THE AUTHORS

Roma Lightsey, MSN, BSN, RN has been a registered nurse since 2003 and specializes in critical care. She has written content for online nursing programs, NCLEX preparation materials, and peer-reviewed nursing journals. Lightsey has also worked as a national clinical nurse educator.

Rochelle Santopoalo, PhD, RN has been a registered nurse since 1977. She has more than four decades of experience in both nursing and higher education. Santopoalo has served in leadership roles at multiple rehabilitation-focused health care organizations and has taught at several universities.

TABLE OF CONTENTS

INTRODUCTION

Congratulations on choosing to take the NCLEX-RN! Passing the NCLEX-RN is an important step in obtaining your nursing licensure and embarking on an enriching and in-demand health care career.

In the following pages, you will find information about the NCLEX-RN, what to expect on test day, how to use this book, and the content covered on the exam. We also encourage you to visit the website of the National Council of State Boards of Nursing (https://www.ncsbn.org) to register for the exam and find the most current information on the NCLEX-RN.

Test Profile

The **National Council Licensure Examination (NCLEX)** is developed by the **National Council of State Boards of Nursing (NCSBN)** as part of licensure for nurses. The NCLEX measures nursing skills at the entry level. That is, an entry-level nurse should be able to pass the exam.

There are actually two separate NCLEX exams: the National Council Licensure Examination for Licensed Registered Nurses, or **NCLEX-RN**, and the National Council Licensure Examination for Licensed Practical/Vocational Nurses, or **NCLEX-PN**. This book prepares readers for the NCLEX-RN.

The NCSBN defines an **entry-level nurse** as a nurse with a maximum of six months' nursing experience. For the NCLEX-RN, as of April 1, 2019, the NCSBN will define *entry-level nurse* as a nurse with a maximum of 12 months' experience.

Applicants become eligible to take the NCLEX-RN after applying for licensure/registration to the regulatory body or board of nursing in the state where they wish to become licensed. Then, they may register for the NCLEX with **Pearson VUE**, which administers the exam. More details on exam administration and test day are found later in this chapter in *Exam Administration*.

Computer Adaptive Testing (CAT)

The NCLEX-RN is a computer-administered exam. It uses **Computer Adaptive Testing (CAT)**, an interactive form of examination. In CAT, the computer adapts to the examinee's abilities, selecting questions based on the examinee's responses. When the examinee answers a question correctly, the next question the computer presents is more difficult than the last. If the examinee answers a question incorrectly, the computer offers a question of lesser difficulty.

Remember: because CAT adapts to your abilities, once you submit an answer, you CANNOT go back to change your answer to a previous question.

Number of Questions

The NCLEX-RN is 265 questions long. To pass the exam, the examinee must answer a minimum of 75 questions out of 265.

Of the 75 questions, only 60 are scored questions; 15 are unscored, or *pretest* questions. These questions are not differentiated, so you must answer at least the first 75 questions of the exam and ideally as many questions as possible for the highest chances of passing.

Passing the NCLEX

There are three routes to passing the NCLEX-RN.

+ **The 95% Confidence Interval Rule:** When the computer is 95% certain the examinee is clearly above or below the passing standard, it stops administering questions and ends the exam.
+ **The Maximum-Length Exam:** The computer considers the final ability estimate of the examinee. If it is above the passing standard, the examinee passes.
+ **The Run-Out-Of-Time-Rule (R.O.O.T.):** This rule applies when the examinee runs out of time and the computer cannot apply the 95% Confidence Interval Rule. The computer estimates the examinee's ability on the last 60 questions. If their ability is above the passing standard, the examinee passes. If it is below the passing standard, or if the examinee did not complete the minimum required questions, the examinee fails.

Timing and Breaks

You will have six hours total to test. This time includes sample questions, tutorial, all breaks, and the post-exam questionnaire.

You are entitled to two optional breaks: one after two hours, and another after 3.5 hours.

Question Types

Most of the questions on the NCLEX-RN are **multiple-choice**, with four to six answer choices. However, some questions follow *alternate formats*.

Hot-spot questions ask you to move your cursor to label a place on a diagram or figure (for instance, an injection point on an image of a muscle). **Fill-in-the-blank questions** ask you to answer a question in your own words or to complete a calculation. **Ordered-response questions** may ask you to arrange a list of steps in a process, for example.

Guessing

The NCLEX-RN has **no guess penalty**. That is, if you answer a question incorrectly, no points are deducted from your score; you simply do not get credit for that question. Therefore, you should always guess if you do not know the answer to a question.

For multiple-choice questions, eliminate any answer choices you are sure are incorrect, and then guess from the remaining answer choices. If you are absolutely not sure which answer choices may be incorrect, guess anyway. The answer you choose just may be the correct one!

The Exam Process

Exam Administration

As mentioned above, the NCLEX-RN is administered by Pearson VUE at testing centers around the nation. Register online for the exam with Pearson VUE *after* applying for licensure with the regulatory body or board of nursing in your area. Please check the NCSBN website (www.ncsbn.org) for details on registration.

Arrive at least 30 minutes before the exam. Bring proper ID and your Authorization to Test (ATT) email, which you will receive after you register. Prepare to submit to biometric scanning (as of 2018, expect a palm vein scan).

Acceptable ID must be government issued, include a recent photograph and signature, and match the name on your Authorization to Test (ATT) email. If you do not have proper ID, you will not be allowed to take the test.

You will not be allowed to bring any personal items into the testing room, such as calculators or phones. You may not bring pens, pencils, or scratch paper. Prohibited items also include hats, scarves, and coats. You may wear religious garments, however. Most testing centers provide lockers for valuables.

You will be provided with an on-screen calculator and an erasable note board and marker by the testing center.

Obtaining Your Results

In some states, **unofficial results** or *Quick Results* are available two days after the exam. However, your **official results** will be released six weeks after the exam. Check with the board of nursing in your state for details.

Body of Knowledge

The NCLEX-RN covers four **Client Needs Categories**: Safe and Effective Care Environment, Health Promotion and Maintenance, Psychosocial Integrity, and Physiological Integrity.

Safe and Effective Care Environment is further broken down into two subcategories: Management of Care and Safety and Infection Control.

Likewise, Physiological Integrity is broken down into four subcategories: Basic Care and Comfort, Pharmacological and Parenteral Therapies, Reduction of Risk Potential, and Physiological Adaptation.

Each question on the NCLEX-RN falls into one of these categories or subcategories. However, questions, or *items*, are not divided by type on the NCLEX-RN. That is, they are not marked by category or subcategory.

Client Needs Content			
Client Needs Category/Subcategory			**Percentage of Items on the NCLEX-RN**
I.	Safe and Effective Care Environment		
	A.	Management of Care	17 – 23%
	B.	Safety and Infection Control	9 – 15%
II.	Health Promotion and Maintenance		6 – 12%
III.	Psychosocial Integrity		6 – 12%
IV.	Physiological Integrity		
	A.	Basic Care and Comfort	6 – 12%
	B.	Pharmacological and Parenteral Therapies	12 – 18%
	C.	Reduction of Risk Potential	9 – 15%
	D.	Physiological Adaptation	11 – 17%

Safe and Effective Care Environment

Questions under the **Safe and Effective Care Environment** category address how nurses relate to clients and health care professionals in the care delivery setting. This category is broken down into two subcategories: Management of Care, and Safety and Infection Control.

Safe and Effective Care Environment – Management of Care questions compose 17 to 23 percent of the exam. Content addressed in these questions focuses on nursing that improves the care delivery setting. More specifically, these questions may test your knowledge of client rights and nursing team collaboration and management. Expect questions on advocacy, self-determination, informed consent, advance directives and life planning, continuity of care, organ donation, referrals, and confidentiality, including information technology and security. Questions will also cover interdisciplinary team collaboration, management, delegating, supervision, ethical practice, general legal issues, performance and quality improvement, setting priorities, and other related issues.

Safe and Effective Care Environment – Safety and Infection Control questions make up 9 to 15 percent of the exam. These questions address creating a nonhazardous environment for health care workers and clients. Prepare to demonstrate your knowledge of safe equipment use, proper handling of infectious and hazardous materials, appropriate reporting of accidents or irregular incidents, preventing injuries, ergonomic principles, standard precautions to prevent surgical asepsis, proper use of restraints and safety devices, and more. Expect questions on implementing emergency response plans and security plans.

HEALTH PROMOTION AND MAINTENANCE

Health Promotion and Maintenance items compose 6 to 12 percent of the NCLEX-RN. These questions will test your ability to direct nursing care that promotes good health, and early detection and prevention of health problems. You will also be expected to demonstrate your knowledge of general human growth and development. More specifically, content will address developmental stages, the aging process, and ante/intra/postpartum and newborn care. Prepare for questions on self-care, including high risk behaviors and lifestyle choices. You are also likely to encounter items on physical assessment techniques, health screening, disease prevention, and general health promotion.

PSYCHOSOCIAL INTEGRITY

Psychosocial Integrity questions make up 6 to 12 percent of the exam. These questions examine your knowledge of how nurses support clients' mental, emotional, and social well-being. Questions also address mental illness. Expect content on coping mechanisms, therapeutic communication and environment, behavioral interventions, crisis intervention, abuse and neglect, end-of-life care, client support systems, and family dynamics. Questions may also address specific mental health concepts like sensory and perceptual alterations, grief and loss, and substance use disorder. In addition, prepare to consider religious, spiritual and cultural influences on health, and cultural awareness in nursing generally.

PHYSIOLOGICAL INTEGRITY

Questions under the Client Needs Category of **Physiological Integrity** fall into four separate subcategories. In general, these items address your knowledge of nursing from the physical perspective; that is, how nurses promote physical health.

Physiological Integrity – Basic Care and Comfort questions compose 6 to 12 percent of the NCLEX-RN. These questions test your knowledge of assisting clients in daily living activities, and may address issues like personal hygiene, oral hydration, nutrition, elimination, assistive devices, mobility, sleep, and non-pharmacological comfort interventions.

Physiological Integrity – Pharmacological and Parenteral Therapies questions compose 12 to 18 percent of the exam. Content mainly addresses administering medications and pharmacological interventions. Questions may include calculations. You may encounter specific questions about pharmacological pain management, side effects and contraindications of medications, blood and blood products, parenteral/intravenous therapies, and total parenteral nutrition.

Physiological Integrity – Reduction of Risk Potential questions compose 9 to 15 percent of the exam. These questions ask about creating a health care environment that lowers the risk of clients developing complications or health problems due to treatments, conditions, or procedures. Be alert for topics like diagnostic tests and their potential for complications, therapeutic procedures, complications from surgical procedures, laboratory values, the potential for alterations in body systems, and changes and abnormalities in vital signs.

Physiological Integrity – Physiological Adaptation questions compose 11 to 17 percent of the NCLEX-RN. This content relates to provision and management of care for patients with acute, chronic, or life-threatening conditions. Prepare for specific questions about medical emergencies, pathophysiology, hemodynamics, fluid and electrolyte imbalances, alterations in body systems, and unexpected responses to therapies.

INTEGRATED PROCESSES

Expect to encounter and show your knowledge of certain processes throughout the exam content. These **Integrated Processes** are at the heart of nursing; the NCLEX-RN *integrates* these concepts into the content of the test. Integrated processes mainly address nursing care and aspects of the nurse-client relationship.

The **nursing process** describes the approach to nursing care. Nurses take a clinical and scientific approach to client care. They use assessment, analysis, planning, implementation, and evaluation.

Caring describes how nurses interact with clients. Nurses should nurture an atmosphere of mutual respect and trust, offering encouragement, support, and compassion.

Communication and documentation refer to all interactions between the nurse and the client, the client's significant others, and the entire health care team. These include verbal and nonverbal interactions. Client care activities and related events are recorded in writing or electronically. These records must adhere to standards of practice and accountability.

Teaching and learning refer to the nurse promoting ongoing acquisition of skills and knowledge that promote behavioral change in the client.

Sensitivity to **culture and spirituality** is addressed throughout the exam. Communication and interaction between the nurse, the client, and the client's significant others should recognize and take into account the client's individual preferences.

Using This Book

In this book, you will find **one diagnostic test** of 100 questions. Questions are broken down by category and subcategory. Taking the diagnostic test will allow you to determine your strengths and weaknesses.

We have also provided **four practice tests** of 150 questions each modeled after the NCLEX-RN. These questions, like the exam itself, are scrambled; in other words, items are NOT broken down by category or subcategory.

Following the practice tests in this book, you will find a **question bank** broken down by category and subcategory. You can use this section to focus on question types where you desire more practice.

There are a total of 1,000 questions in the entire book. In our **answer keys**, every answer is explained in depth, including wrong answer choices. That way, you can learn from your mistakes.

We suggest you begin by taking the diagnostic test. Note your strengths and weaknesses. If you are particularly weak in a category or subcategory, you may wish to focus on the questions devoted to that area in the question bank before taking the first practice test. Otherwise, go on to take the first practice test.

Remember, on exam day, you will be judged by the first 60 scored questions of the first 75 questions you answer. Since scored and unscored items are not differentiated, those first 75 questions are important. Our practice tests are 150 questions long to help you will focus on 75 questions at a time, even while becoming accustomed to taking a longer test.

As on the NCLEX-RN, our book features mainly multiple-choice questions. However, we also provide hot-spot, fill-in-the-blank, ordered-response, and other unique alternate question types, just like the actual exam does. You will find these question formats scattered throughout the diagnostic and practice tests and in the question bank to give you an experience as close as possible to what you will see on exam day.

Ascencia Test Prep

With fields such as nursing, pharmacy, emergency care, and physical therapy becoming the fastest-growing industries in the United States, individuals looking to enter the health care industry or rise in their field need high quality, reliable resources. Ascencia Test Prep's study guides and test preparation materials are developed by credentialed industry professionals with years of experience in their respective fields. Ascencia recognizes that health care professionals nurture bodies and spirits, and save lives. Ascencia Test Prep's mission is to help health care workers grow.

Diagnostic Test

SAFE AND EFFECTIVE CARE ENVIRONMENT— MANAGEMENT OF CARE

1. The nurse is delegating tasks to an unlicensed assistive personnel (UAP). Which client task should the nurse delegate to the UAP?

   1. a client whose IV infiltrated and needs replacing

   2. a client on BiPAP who needs arterial blood gases (ABGs) drawn

   3. a client with mild dementia who needs assistance with her food tray

   4. a client who needs a wet-to-dry dressing change on an abdominal incision

2. A nurse is preparing a client scheduled for a right mastectomy. Which statement indicates the need for further intervention?

   1. The client refuses to sign the blood consent since she is a Jehovah's Witness.

   2. The client identifies the right breast as the surgical site for a right mastectomy.

   3. The client signs the consent form with an X, which is witnessed by two licensed personnel.

   4. The client expresses doubt over her decision and asks the nurse to explain more about the procedure.

3. An external weather disaster has flooded the emergency department with several new clients. Which client should the nurse see **first**?

   1. the client complaining of chest pain and nausea who is diaphoretic

   2. the client with a simple fracture of the radius from a fall on a staircase

   3. the client complaining of slight redness and itching at the IV site in his hand

   4. the client presenting with a sprained ankle from a tree branch falling on him

4. A nurse is working with an unlicensed assistive personnel (UAP) to perform a bed bath on a client. The nurse notes the smell of alcohol on the UAP's breath. Which is the **priority** nursing action?

   1. Work closely with the UAP during the shift and observe for any signs of impairment.
   2. Complete the bed bath without comment. The unit is already short one staff member.
   3. Offer chewing gum to the UAP. Since she does not give medications, she can do her job as she does not appear impaired.
   4. Call for another nurse to complete the bath and immediately report the UAP to the charge nurse or unit manager.

5. The nurse has received report on the assigned night-shift clients. Which client should the nurse see **first**?

   1. a mildly confused client due for a dressing change on a diabetic ulcer to the heel
   2. an elderly, stable client who just returned from an MRI to rule out a kidney mass
   3. a client whose IV pump has started beeping, indicating that the antibiotic has completed infusing
   4. a client complaining of sudden warmth and pain at an appendectomy incision site 48 hours after surgery

6. The nurse is working triage in the ED when four clients present at the same time. Which client should be seen **first**?

   1. a 45-year-old female on oral contraceptives with unusually heavy menstrual bleeding
   2. a 24-year-old with a dog bite to the leg from the family dog who is current on rabies shots
   3. an irritable 4-month-old with a petechial rash, nuchal rigidity, and temperature of 103.4°F
   4. a 16-year-old football player with a twisted ankle who has no deformity and a pedal pulse

7. The nurse is caring for clients on a medical-surgical floor. Which tasks related to pain management can be delegated to unlicensed assistive personnel (UAP)? **Select all that apply.**

   1. assessing the pain level on a scale of 1 – 10
   2. reminding clients to report pain immediately
   3. reporting facial grimacing in unresponsive clients
   4. asking clients directly, "Are you having any pain right now?"
   5. giving acetaminophen (Tylenol) after the nurse obtains the medication but is interrupted to attend a code blue before she administers it

8. A newly graduated nurse is working in the pediatric unit. Which client assignment is **most** appropriate for this nurse?

   1. a 2-year-old with hemophilia A who has suddenly become less responsive
   2. a 15-year-old with sickle cell disease complaining of lower right quadrant abdominal pain
   3. a 6-year-old who just had a tonsillectomy 2 hours earlier and is frequently swallowing
   4. a 12-year-old with newly diagnosed type 2 diabetes whose parents need teaching on insulin

9. The nurse is preparing to transfer a client from the ICU to the floor. Which of the following ensures continuity of care for the client? **Select all that apply.**

   1. using approved abbreviations in documenting care
   2. providing report on the client using standard hand-off reports
   3. informing the receiving nurse of pending lab results and when they are expected
   4. informing the receiving nurse of any care that needs to be done, such as bathing
   5. telling the receiving nurse that the family is demanding and asks too many questions

10. A client has been admitted to the oncology unit and has a large amount of cash, several credit cards, and several pieces of expensive-looking gold jewelry in her possession. Which action by the nurse is **most** appropriate?

    1. tell the client to hide everything in her purse or a bag and put it in the closet
    2. offer to take her belongings to the charge nurse's office where they can be locked up
    3. suggest that the client put her valuables in a sock and place it in the bottom of the bedside table under some clothing
    4. inform the client of the hospital policy regarding valuables and suggest that she give them to a trusted family member or to security for safekeeping

11. The nurse is caring for a 7-year-old child who presents to the ED with multiple bruises, a fractured ankle, and cigarette burns on the arms. Which action by the nurse is **most** appropriate?

    1. ask the parents if they burned the child with cigarettes
    2. ask the client to tell you what happened to cause the bruising and burns
    3. inform the parents that they cannot leave with the child until they talk to the police
    4. notify the charge nurse immediately so that the suspected child abuse can be reported

SAFE AND EFFECTIVE CARE ENVIRONMENT— SAFETY AND INFECTION CONTROL

12. Which precaution must a nurse take when checking the blood pressure of an HIV-positive client?

    1. wear gloves
    2. wear a gown
    3. use contact precautions
    4. wash hands

13. The pediatric nurse is preparing a child with acute lymphocytic leukemia for discharge. The discharge plan should include all but which of the following statements?

    1. restrict naps to allow more complete rest at night
    2. increase intake of protein, iron, and vitamin C to provide nutrients required for hemoglobin production
    3. keep a food diary to evaluate dietary intake
    4. restrict antacids, tetracyclines, and phosphorous salt

14. The nurse teaches a group of fire fighters about the spread of tuberculosis (TB). Which statement by a fire fighter indicates the teaching has been effective?

    1. "I could get TB if I come in contact with blood from an infected person."
    2. "I can share a cup of coffee with someone who is infected with TB."
    3. "I could get TB if I inhale infected droplets when an infected individual coughs."
    4. "I need to refrain from shaking hands with an infected person."

15. After administering the annual Mantoux tuberculin skin test to employees, the nurse instructs the staff to return within how many hours after administration to have the results determined?

    1. 12 to 24 hours
    2. 24 to 48 hours
    3. 48 to 72 hours
    4. 72 to 84 hours

16. A client is diagnosed with Meniere's disease. Which nursing diagnosis would take **priority** for this client?

    1. risk for injury
    2. disturbed body image
    3. low self-esteem
    4. impaired skin integrity

17. While driving, the client forgets how to get home. Which lobe could be dysfunctional?
    1. temporal
    2. parietal
    3. occipital
    4. frontal

18. At the scene of an accident, which intervention applies to a client with a suspected neck injury?
    1. administer CPR
    2. keep the person warm
    3. do not move the client
    4. ask the client to state her name and birthday

19. Which treatment should be included in the **immediate** management of acute appendicitis?
    1. prevent fluid volume deficit
    2. administer antibiotic therapy
    3. reduce anxiety
    4. relieve pain

20. Medical management of a client with acute diverticulitis should include which treatment?
    1. increased fiber in diet
    2. administration of antibiotics
    3. pain medication administration
    4. liquid diet for 1 – 2 days

21. An enema is prescribed for a client with suspected appendicitis. The nurse should take which action?
    1. tell the client to lie on his left side
    2. explain the procedure to the client
    3. compile necessary equipment
    4. question the physician about the order

22. A 28-year-old client has just given birth. At one minute the baby appears healthy, with the exception of bluish hands. Which of the following would the nurse midwife pronounce?

    1. The Apgar score is 11.
    2. The Apgar score is 9.
    3. The Apgar score is 6.
    4. The Apgar score is 4.

23. The client's first day of her last period was January 24. Which of the following should the nurse tell the client is her expected date of delivery?

    1. September 30
    2. October 31
    3. November 15
    4. December 1

24. The nurse is discussing concerns the parent has with his 3-year-old. The parent identifies limitations in the child's activities. **Select all that should be of concern to the nurse.**

    1. unable to work simple toys
    2. unable to understand simple instructions
    3. unable to say first and last name
    4. unable to name any colors or numbers

25. The nurse is providing education at a senior center. Which of the following measures will the nurse say is **most** effective in attaining normal blood pressure in a client with hypertension?

    1. eating red meat daily
    2. increasing potassium and calcium intake
    3. increasing fluid intake
    4. decreasing sodium intake

26. A 9-month-old child is registered to attend a local childcare clinic. Upon initial intake, the nurse discovers the child has received the first and second dose of the hepatitis B vaccine. What is the **best** course of action for the nurse to recommend to the parents?

    1. no action; a third dose of the vaccine is not recommended
    2. immediately inoculate the child given the high risk of not having a third vaccine
    3. wait until the child is 12 months to give the vaccine
    4. schedule the child for the third vaccine at the earliest convenience

27. The nurse is teaching a smoking cessation program. He will state that which of the following benefits of quitting appear within one year?

   1. risk of coronary heart disease is the same as that of a nonsmoker
   2. carbon monoxide level in blood drops to normal
   3. risk of dying from lung cancer is about half that of a smoker's
   4. risk of having a stroke is reduced to that of a nonsmoker's

28. The nurse is preparing a community educational presentation. The topic is the leading causes of death for people ages 12 – 19. The nurse knows that which of the following should be presented?

   1. unintentional injuries
   2. cancer
   3. homicide
   4. suicide

29. The nurse identifies a client's learning preference as visual. Which of the following would be appropriate when teaching the client about insulin injection?

   1. an audiotape
   2. an orange, an insulin syringe, an alcohol wipe, and a bottle of sterile saline
   3. classroom discussion
   4. an instructional pamphlet

PSYCHOSOCIAL INTEGRITY

30. The nurse is caring for a client with end-stage kidney disease and multiple organ failure. Which action by the nurse indicates an understanding of end-of-life care? **Select all that apply.**

    1. The nurse explains signs and symptoms that indicate death is near.
    2. The nurse explains to the client and family what to expect during the final phase of the illness.
    3. Cultural beliefs are acknowledged, but priority is placed on life-lengthening treatment options.
    4. The nurse avoids talking to the client about impending death to avoid upsetting him and the family.
    5. The nurse asks the client and family what their goals and wishes are regarding care, pain management, and emergency resuscitation.

31. The nurse is talking in the lounge with other nurses about grief and loss. The nurse understands which to be true regarding grief and loss? **Select all that apply.**

    1. The process of grief is detrimental to physical and emotional health.
    2. Age, gender, and culture are a few factors that influence the grieving process.
    3. The nurse must explore his own feelings about death before he may effectively help others.
    4. The nurse should discourage expression of grief and loss because it may upset other clients nearby.
    5. The nurse can help the family develop ways to relieve loneliness and depression following the death of a loved one.

32. The nurse has assessed the assigned group of clients. Which client would the nurse identify as being at the **greatest** risk for alterations in sensory perception?

    1. a client in a halo vest following an automobile accident
    2. a child with severe autism who is having a tonsillectomy
    3. a teenager who broke her leg during cheerleader practice
    4. a schoolteacher who was hospitalized for shortness of breath

33. The nurse is working in a mental health facility that uses group therapy with the clients. The nurse understands which to be correct regarding group therapy?

    1. The termination stage begins with the initial group meeting.
    2. Members' feelings about their accomplishments are explored in the working stage.
    3. During the working stage, members may be unclear about the purpose of the group.
    4. Group roles and responsibilities are established in the working stage of group therapy.

34. The nurse is caring for a client who is having surgery the next morning. The client says, "I'm really scared about surgery. I've never been put to sleep before and I'm afraid I might not wake up." Which response by the nurse is the **most** therapeutic?

    1. "Why are you worried about such a minor procedure?"

    2. "We can call the doctor and cancel the surgery if you would prefer."

    3. "It's normal to be afraid of something new like surgery. Tell me how you feel."

    4. "Don't worry, you have a really good doctor and he will see to it that nothing goes wrong."

35. The nurse is caring for a client who has just been diagnosed with ovarian cancer. The nurse is using silence as an effective therapeutic response. How is silence an effective therapeutic response?

    1. It is not therapeutic; it implies that the nurse is not listening.

    2. It encourages the client to keep her feelings to herself.

    3. It allows the client time to think and reflect and lead the conversation.

    4. It allows the nurse to think about other tasks she needs to tackle to provide efficient care to all of her clients.

36. The nurse is caring for a client with schizophrenia who is having active hallucinations. The nurse implements which actions to manage the client during the episode? **Select all that apply.**

    1. administers medications as ordered

    2. uses gentle touch to reassure the client

    3. tells the client that others see or hear what he does

    4. distracts the client by placing him in the dayroom with others

    5. asks the client if he hears voices telling him to harm himself or others

    6. goes along with what the client says to decrease the risk of increasing the client's anxiety

37. The nurse is admitting a client with schizophrenia. The client is extremely socially withdrawn, is unable to perform activities of daily living, has an inappropriate affect, and has grimacing mannerisms. The nurse understands that this client is experiencing which type of schizophrenia?

    1. residual schizophrenia

    2. paranoid schizophrenia

    3. catatonic schizophrenia

    4. disorganized schizophrenia

    5. undifferentiated schizophrenia

38. The nurse is precepting a new nurse in the psychiatric unit. The nurse is discussing interventions for schizophrenia. Which statement by the student nurse indicates an understanding of management of schizophrenia? **Select all that apply.**

    1. "I should be warm and friendly to put the client at ease."

    2. "I can reassure the client that he is in a safe environment."

    3. "Puzzles or word games are good activities to engage in."

    4. "I can help the client use art or writing to express his feelings."

    5. "I won't tell the client when I'm leaving him so he won't get upset."

39. The mental health nurse is caring for a client with Cluster B personality disorder. The nurse would expect the client to exhibit which behaviors? **Select all that apply.**

    1. suspicious of others, magical thinking, eccentric behavior, paranoia, relationship deficits

    2. preoccupation with rules and details, hoarding, ritualistic behavior, extremely devoted to work

    3. easily bored, poor and shallow interpersonal relationships, enjoys being the center of attention

    4. impulsivity, unpredictable behavior, extreme mood shifts, easily angered, playing people against each other

    5. suspicious and untrusting of others, argumentative, controlling of others, thoughts of grandiosity

PHYSIOLOGICAL INTEGRITY—
BASIC CARE AND COMFORT

40. The nurse is preparing to receive an 18-month-old client from surgery who had repair of a congenital hip deformity. What type of traction does the nurse anticipate setting up for the client?

_____

41. The nurse is caring for a client whose lab results show triglycerides of 380 and cholesterol level of 240. Which foods would the nurse educate the client about including in his diet when he is discharged? **Select all that apply.**

1. wheat toast with sugar-free jelly
2. grilled salmon seasoned with herbs
3. an egg-white omelet with vegetables
4. natural honey from a local farmer's market
5. plain grilled steak prepared with pepper only

42. The nurse is preparing to discharge a client who was treated for tuberculosis. Which guidelines for home management should the nurse include in his discharge teaching? **Select all that apply.**

1. The client may resume his normal activities.
2. The family should maintain respiratory isolation at home.
3. The medication regimen should be followed diligently as prescribed.
4. The client may return to work when three sputum cultures are negative.
5. The nurse should educate the client about the medication and possible side effects and their management.

43. The nurse is discharging a client who was prescribed prednisone. The nurse tells the client that one of the side effects may be impaired sleep. The client says, "I already have a hard time sleeping. What can I do to help with that?" Which recommendations should the nurse make? **Select all that apply.**

1. avoid alcohol late in the evening
2. keep the bedroom dark and quiet
3. maintain the same consistent sleep schedule
4. eat a large, heavy meal at dinner to help promote sleep
5. read or do another quiet, noncomputer activity before bed
6. do a vigorous exercise routine after work to help him become tired

44. The nurse is caring for a client who has a nasogastric tube for medication administration and tube feedings. How should the nurse care for the tube during her shift? **Select all that apply.**

    1. flush tube every 4 hours with hot water to maintain patency
    2. allow the feeding and tubing to hang until empty, up to 48 hours
    3. maintain the head of bed in a high-Fowler's position during feedings
    4. check residuals and replace them unless the amount is greater than 300 mL
    5. check under the adhesive tape on the nose daily to assess for skin breakdown
    6. assess the bowel sounds before feeding, and feed at half the rate if bowel sounds are absent

45. The nurse is teaching a group of nursing students about proper client positioning. Which statement by a student nurse indicates an understanding of proper positioning?

    1. A client receiving an enema should be placed on the right side in the Sims' position.
    2. A client with a below-the-knee amputation should be positioned with the affected limb elevated at a 45-degree angle.
    3. Clients with pulmonary edema should be positioned upright with the legs dangling over the side of the bed.
    4. Clients with a craniotomy should be positioned with the head of bed at a 20-degree angle with the head in a neutral, midline position.

46. The nurse is caring for a client with deep vein thrombosis (DVT). Which should be included in the plan of care?

    1. bed rest with the affected extremity elevated
    2. bed rest with the bed in reverse Trendelenburg
    3. walking slowly in the hall with assistance to prevent pneumonia
    4. sitting up in the chair for all meals and during visitation time

47. The nurse is assessing a six-month-old infant at the clinic. When the nurse strokes from the heel of the foot upward toward the ball, the infant exhibits no movement. Which action is the **priority** for the nurse?

    1. take the infant's vital signs
    2. order a neurology consult
    3. examine the infant's nose and ears
    4. ask how much formula the infant consumes daily

48. The nurse is caring for a client with COPD who complains of poor quality of sleep. Which question should the nurse ask next?

    1. "Does your partner snore heavily?"
    2. "Do you get exercise during the day?"
    3. "How many pillows do you sleep on?"
    4. "Do you eat large meals right before bed?"

49. The nurse is teaching infant CPR to a group of newly graduated nurses hired to work in the labor and delivery unit. The nurse understands that proper technique with infants includes which action? **Select all that apply.**

    1. The femoral artery is checked for a pulse following each cycle of CPR.
    2. Chest compression depth should be approximately 1.5 inches, or 4 cm.
    3. A single rescuer should use three fingers on the dominant hand to do compressions.
    4. Rest the infant facedown on the forearm with the hand supporting the head and jaw.
    5. If arrest is witnessed the emergency response system should be activated before beginning CPR.

50. The nurse is caring for a comatose client with a Salem sump tube. Which action by the nurse is correct regarding care of this client?

    1. clamp the air vent during tube feedings
    2. place the client on the left side in a high-Fowler's position
    3. assess the position of the Salem sump before each feeding
    4. infuse bolus feedings with a pump or by gently plunging into the stomach

51. The nurse is teaching a client diagnosed with gastroesophageal reflux disease (GERD) about dietary measures to manage symptoms. Which food does the nurse advise the client to avoid?

    1. bananas
    2. tomatoes
    3. white bread
    4. grilled salmon
    5. steel-cut oatmeal

52. The nurse is caring for a client with sternal wires following a coronary artery bypass graft (CABG). The client complains of severe pain when coughing and deep breathing. What nonpharmacological measures can the nurse take to increase client comfort? **Select all that apply.**

    1. apply hot packs to the sternum
    2. give morphine PRN for pain before client coughs
    3. suggest using audio books or relaxing music as a distraction
    4. teach the client how to use a pillow to splint the chest when coughing
    5. encourage the client to engage in prayer, meditation, or other activities
    6. properly position the head of the bed to minimize pressure on the sternum

53. The nurse is caring for a client who is sedated and on the ventilator in ICU. The family expresses concern about controlling the client's pain when he cannot speak. The nurse explains that assessing pain in a nonverbal client involves watching for which of the following signs? **Select all that apply.**

    1. grabbing at the bed rails

    2. biting the ventilator tubing

    3. facial grimacing

    4. stiffness or rigidity of the body

    5. decreased urinary output

    6. increased blood pressure and heart rate as shown on the cardiac monitor

54. The clinic nurse is seeing a pregnant client who is expecting her first child. She complains of morning sickness and nasal stuffiness. The nurse recommends interventions to minimize discomfort from her symptoms. Which should the nurse recommend? **Select all that apply.**

    1. take ginger pills to alleviate nausea

    2. drink a full glass of water at each meal

    3. use a humidifier to help with congestion

    4. eat dry crackers before getting out of bed in the morning

    5. eat three regular meals each day to provide needed nutrients

    6. use an over-the-counter nasal spray such as a saline-based spray

55. The nurse is caring for a client who refuses to get out of bed. He tells the nurse, "I'm too tired to get up. I'm sick. I'm supposed to rest in the hospital." For which complications of immobility does the nurse understand that the client is at risk? **Select all that apply.**

    1. decreased appetite

    2. urinary tract infection

    3. orthostatic hypotension

    4. muscular atrophy and foot drop

    5. boredom, frustration, and anxiety

    6. increased length of hospitalization

56. The nurse is caring for a group of clients in a medical/surgical unit. Which client does the nurse understand to be at **highest** risk for developing decubitus ulcers?

    1. a 27-year-old client who fractured her arm playing volleyball

    2. a 6-year-old client on pelvic skin traction for muscle spasms

    3. a 42-year-old obese client with controlled atrial fibrillation who uses a wheelchair

    4. a 70-year-old client with heart failure who uses a cane for ambulation in the room and hall

PHYSIOLOGICAL INTEGRITY— PHARMACOLOGICAL AND PARENTERAL THERAPIES

57. The nurse is caring for a client receiving total parenteral nutrition (TPN). During the assessment, the nurse notes absence of breath sounds on the right side, where the central catheter is placed. Which of the following does the nurse suspect is responsible for this abnormal assessment finding?

   1. air embolism

   2. fluid overload

   3. pneumothorax

   4. refeeding syndrome

58. The nurse is reviewing a client's morning medication orders. Which of the following orders would prompt the nurse to call the health care provider for order clarification?

   1. famotidine 20 mg PO BID

   2. haloperidol 15 mg IM q4h prn

   3. lithium carbonate 300 mg PO TID

   4. amoxicillin 500 mg PO q12h × 7 days

59. A client with hypertension asks the nurse to explain how amlodipine besylate (Norvasc) lowers her blood pressure. The nurse gives which explanation to the client?

   1. "It prevents calcium from entering the smooth muscle, which relaxes the blood vessels to lower heart rate and blood pressure."

   2. "It is a diuretic that works by removing extra sodium and water from the body through the kidneys, which helps lower blood pressure."

   3. "It causes the body to produce less angiotensin, which allows blood vessels to relax and open up, therefore reducing blood pressure."

   4. "It lowers blood pressure by lowering the heart rate and the workload of the heart, and decreases the amount of blood pumped out of the heart."

60. The nurse is caring for a client who is taking bethanechol chloride (Urecholine) for neurogenic bladder. Which of the following does the nurse understand is correct concerning this medication?

   1. This is the primary treatment for clients with a urinary obstruction.

   2. If the client cannot swallow pills, the medication may be given by the IV or IM route.

   3. Urecholine should be given with food to prevent nausea and vomiting.

   4. Atropine sulfate should be readily available when a client receives this medication.

61. The nurse is caring for a client taking sulfonamides to treat a urinary tract infection. Which of the following should the nurse monitor for in this client? **Select all that apply.**

   1. fever or sore throat
   2. reddish-pink urine
   3. side effects such as dyspnea, chest pains, chills, and cough
   4. urinary output of 1200 mL daily to minimize the risk of renal damage
   5. the need to decrease the dosage if the client takes warfarin sodium (Coumadin) or phenytoin (Dilantin)

62. The nurse is caring for a client diagnosed with tuberculosis. The physician plans to treat the client with a first-line medication. Which medication should the nurse prepare to administer?

   1. rifampin
   2. ciprofloxacin
   3. levofloxacin
   4. streptomycin

63. The nurse is caring for a client who complains of a headache with a pain level of 5 on a scale of 1 to 10. Which PRN pain medication order is **most** appropriate for the nurse to administer?

   1. morphine 2 mg IV q6h PRN
   2. aspirin 325 mg PO q6h PRN
   3. acetaminophen 650 mg PO q6h PRN
   4. nitroglycerin 0.4 mg sublingually every 5 minutes, up to 3 doses over 15 minutes

64. The nurse is preparing to administer 12.4 mL of liquid medication via oral syringe. Which of the following actions by the nurse indicate an understanding of how to give oral medications via syringe?

   1. The nurse uses either an oral or parenteral syringe to administer the medication.
   2. The nurse pours 10 mL of the medication into a 30 mL medicine cup, then adds 2.4 mL with a 3 mL syringe.
   3. The nurse pours 10 mL of the medication into a 30 mL medicine cup, then adds 2.4 mL with a 5 mL syringe.
   4. The nurse pours 10 mL of the medication into a 30 mL medicine cup, then slowly adds the remainder until it is almost halfway between the 10 mL mark and 15 mL mark.

65. The nurse is caring for a client with a staph infection. The client has orders for vancomycin 15 mg/kg per 12 hours. The client weighs 136 pounds. How much of this medication will the client receive every 12 hours?

   _____

66. The nurse is teaching a group of student nurses about drug safety. Keeping in mind Joint Commission guidelines, which of the following does the nurse teach the students? **Select all that apply.**

    1. "Do not abbreviate drug names."
    2. "Use *daily* instead of QD, Q.D., or q.d."
    3. "Rectum can be abbreviated *PR*, *R*, or *Per Rec.*"
    4. "Use *OD* to indicate *right eye* for eye medications."
    5. "Use the letter *u* to indicate units, such as with insulin."

67. The night nurse is preparing to pull night medications for a client. Levofloxacin is scheduled to be given at 0030. The nurse will give this medication at which time?

    1. 1:30 a.m.
    2. 1:30 p.m.
    3. 11:30 p.m.
    4. 12:30 a.m.
    5. 12:30 p.m.

68. The nurse has an order to administer enoxaparin (Lovenox) 40 mg subcutaneously. When the automatic medication dispenser opens, however, the nurse finds enoxaparin 80 mg in the pocket. Which is the correct action by the nurse?

    1. notify the pharmacy to correct the error
    2. skip the morning dose of the medication
    3. call the health care provider for order clarification
    4. waste half of the enoxaparin and give the remaining 40 mg

69. The nurse is caring for a client who has an order for ceftriaxone IV. The client is awake and alert and has been taking PO medications and eating. The IV ceftriaxone is not available in the automatic medication dispenser. What should the nurse do next?

    1. hold the medication since the client is afebrile
    2. call the pharmacy to send up the missing IV medication
    3. obtain the PO ceftriaxone from the medication dispenser and administer it
    4. call the health care provider and see if the client can be switched over to oral ceftriaxone

70. The nurse is preparing to administer furosemide IM to a 6-month-old client with edema. Which location is the **preferred** injection site for this client?

    1. the gluteus medius
    2. the vastus lateralis
    3. the dorsogluteal site
    4. the ventrogluteal muscle

71. The nurse is caring for a client with breast cancer who has an order for doxorubicin IV. The nurse anticipates which common side effect of this medication?

    1. permanent hair loss

    2. halos around objects and blurred vision

    3. red urine for 1 – 2 days after administration

    4. facial flushing and red streaking along the vein

PHYSIOLOGICAL INTEGRITY—
REDUCTION OF RISK POTENTIAL

72. A young child with a rash that's raised and has circumscribed areas filled with fluid comes to the school nurse. What type of rash should the nurse document?

    1. maculopapular rash

    2. heat rash

    3. vesicular rash

    4. pustular rash

73. A 10-year-old is sent home from school with a report of having lice. The nurse should instruct the parent on which intervention?

    1. wash the hair for three continuous days with dandruff shampoo

    2. isolate all clothing of the child for one week

    3. treat with an approved pediculicide agent according to directions

    4. shave the child's head, then cleanse with herbal shampoo

74. A nurse in intensive coronary care is caring for a client with an endotracheal tube who underwent coronary bypass surgery. The client awakens and attempts to communicate. Which nursing interventions should the nurse perform? **Select all that apply.**

    1. offer a communication board

    2. ask simple yes/no questions

    3. ask open-ended questions

    4. offer an electrolarynx

75. A nurse is teaching a client with left-sided hemiparesis to walk with a cane. The nurse should include which points about safe cane use when teaching the client? **Select all that apply.**

    1. hold the cane in the right hand

    2. hold the cane in the left hand

    3. move the cane and step forward with the right leg

    4. move the cane and step forward with the left leg

76. The nurse is assessing a client with Addison's disease. The nurse expects to note which of the following?

    1. craving of salty foods

    2. weight gain

    3. craving of sweet foods

    4. hyperactivity

77. An elderly man is admitted to the ED during the night shift. He reports slipping and hitting his forehead on the bathtub several hours earlier. The nurse is assessing the client's frontal lobe function. Which of the following questions/statements should the nurse ask the client?

    1. "Tell me when you feel me touch your arm."
    2. "Tell me when you stop hearing the tuning fork sound."
    3. "Do you have problems with balance?"
    4. "How much is two plus four plus seven?"

78. A client is admitted to the ED after complaining of acute chest pain radiating down the left arm. The client is diaphoretic and anxious, and has difficulty breathing. Which laboratory studies would the nurse anticipate?

    1. blood urea nitrogen (BUN)
    2. white blood cell count
    3. LDH
    4. myoglobin

79. A nurse is monitoring a client's intracranial pressure (ICP) after a motor vehicle accident. Upon checking the ICP, the nurse knows to contact the physician. What reading would warrant this action?

    1. 8 mm Hg
    2. 14 mm Hg
    3. 18 mm Hg
    4. 22 mm Hg

80. A nurse is caring for a client, diagnosed with Parkinson's disease, who scored as a high-risk fall candidate on the St. Thomas Risk Assessment Tool in Falling Elderly Inpatients. Which nursing interventions should the nurse implement? **Select all that apply.**

    1. provide the client with a call-light device
    2. keep the bed in the lowest position
    3. use a beveled floor mat at bedside
    4. implement a bed alarm

81. While preparing a client for a colonoscopy, the nurse would be correct to implement which interventions? **Select all that apply.**

    1. instruction on high fiber diet the day before the procedure
    2. instruction that a sedative will be administered before the procedure
    3. instruction not to eat or drink 6 – 12 hours before the procedure
    4. instruction not to eat or drink 18 hours before the procedure

82. A nurse is preparing discharge instructions for a client with a below-the-knee amputation. Which instruction would be a **priority**?

    1. sterile wound management

    2. elevation of residual limb

    3. performing prescribed exercises

    4. reporting occurrence of phantom limb pain immediately

83. A nurse is following the progress of a client being treated for hypothyroidism. Which findings indicate the client is experiencing side effects of the thyroid replacement therapy? **Select all that apply.**

    1. excessive sweating

    2. constipation

    3. inability to tolerate cold

    4. leg cramps

84. A client is having a tonic-clonic seizure. Which of the following should the nurse do **first**?

    1. call for assistance

    2. restrain the client

    3. turn the client on her side

    4. provide a safe environment

85. The nurse is preparing to discharge a client with an ileal conduit done for treatment of bladder cancer. Which statement by the client indicates the need for further instruction?

    1. "I look forward to returning to my local health club to swim."

    2. "The local ostomy support group meets on Wednesday morning at 10 a.m."

    3. "My stoma should be cleaned daily with soap and water."

    4. "During the day I will wear a leg bag to collect my urine."

86. The nurse is caring for a client with a history of cirrhosis of the liver. Lab values reveal rising ammonia levels. Which of the following actions should the nurse anticipate performing? **Select all that apply.**

    1. replace electric razor with a straight razor

    2. encourage frequent periods of rest

    3. instruct on a potassium-restricted diet

    4. monitor the client's mental status

PHYSIOLOGICAL INTEGRITY— PHYSIOLOGICAL ADAPTATION

87. The nurse is assessing a client with Graves' disease. Which assessment finding would the nurse expect in this client?

  1. bradycardia

  2. constipation

  3. exophthalmos

  4. recent weight gain

88. The nurse is caring for a client who is HIV-positive. The nurse understands which of the following to be true regarding HIV and AIDS?

  1. Viral load testing monitors disease progression and evaluates effectiveness of treatment.

  2. The Western blot test is positive if antibodies to at least three major HIV antigens are present.

  3. Patients with AIDS present with a white blood cell (WBC) count between 5,000 and 10,000 cells/mm^3.

  4. An enzyme-linked immunosorbent assay (ELISA) test can detect the presence of antibodies within 2 weeks of exposure.

89. The nurse is performing hemodialysis on a client, with the understanding that air embolus is a complication of this treatment. Which assessment findings by the nurse indicate an air embolus?

  1. cold intolerance

  2. chest pain and anxiety

  3. decreased respirations

  4. hypertension and widening pulse pressure

90. The nurse is teaching a client about peritoneal dialysis. Which complication of this treatment would the nurse instruct the client to report?

  1. bone pain

  2. confusion

  3. muscle cramps

  4. cloudy outflow

91. The nurse is caring for a 9-year-old boy who presented to the ED after a penetrating injury from a BB gun. The client is diagnosed with a hyphema. The nurse proceeds to place the client in which position?

  1. flat in bed

  2. semi-Fowler's

  3. Trendelenburg's

  4. lateral on the unaffected side

92. The nurse is caring for a client at risk for postpartum hemorrhage. Which **early** sign of hemorrhage should the nurse monitor for this client?

1. coma
2. hypotension
3. restlessness
4. cool, clammy skin

93. The nurse is caring for a client who presents to the ED with the following arterial blood gas (ABG) results:

pH 7.32
PaCO2 47 mm Hg
HCO3 24 mEq/L
PaO2 91 mm Hg

Which clinical manifestation would the nurse anticipate, based on these findings?

1. confusion
2. nausea and vomiting
3. deep, rapid respirations
4. hypoventilation with hypoxia

94. The nurse is caring for a client with abdominal aortic aneurysm. Which observation by the nurse indicates the need for **immediate** intervention?

1. complaints of yellow-tinted vision
2. sudden onset of frothy, pink sputum
3. urinary output of 75 mL/hr. per urinary catheter
4. complaints of sudden and severe back pain and shortness of breath

95. The nurse is caring for a client who has been diagnosed with pulseless electrical activity (PEA). Following effective CPR and administration of epinephrine, which is the next **priority** nursing action?

1. check for a pulse
2. insert a urinary catheter
3. prepare to shock the client
4. administer a bolus of sodium bicarbonate

96. The nurse is caring for a client with cardiogenic shock. The nurse expects which signs present with this client? **Select all that apply.**

1. hypertension; slow, labored breathing
2. decreased urine output; warm, pink skin
3. increased urine output; cool, clammy skin
4. hypotension; weak pulse; cool, clammy skin

97. The nurse is caring for a client with a sacral wound. The wound is full thickness, measures 4 cm × 6 cm with irregular borders, and is covered by a layer of black collagen. Which is this wound stage?

    1. Stage I

    2. Stage II

    3. Stage III

    4. unstageable

98. The nurse is caring for a client with a Braden score of 13. How does the nurse interpret this client's risk of skin breakdown?

    1. high risk

    2. mild risk

    3. severe risk

    4. moderate risk

99. The nurse is performing the Glasgow coma scale on a client. The assessment is as follows: eye opening, to pain; motor response, localizes pain; verbal response, inappropriate words. The nurse interprets which score is correct for this client?

    1. 9

    2. 10

    3. 11

    4. 12

100. The nurse is reviewing morning labs for a client. Which lab value requires **immediate** intervention by the nurse?

    1. calcium 9.8 mg/dL

    2. sodium 137 mEq/L

    3. chloride 104 mEq/L

    4. potassium 3.1 mEq/L

1. Number 3 is correct.

Rationale: Assessing the IV site and inserting an IV is beyond the scope of practice for a UAP and should be performed only by the licensed nurse. Drawing ABGs should be performed by the licensed nurse or respiratory therapist per facility policy. Assisting a client with a meal tray is within the scope of practice for a UAP. Dressing changes should be performed by the licensed nurse. UAPs may not provide direct nursing care or perform nursing interventions requiring specialized nursing knowledge, judgment, or skill.

2. Number 4 is correct.

Rationale: Expressing doubt and asking further questions of the nurse indicates that the client may not be fully informed and should confer further with the health care provider. The nurse may clarify facts, but it is the health care provider's responsibility to give detailed information about the surgical procedure. The nurse is responsible for ensuring that the client has been adequately informed. A client may refuse to sign a blood consent due to religious beliefs prior to surgery. The client has correctly identified the surgical site, which is to be expected. The client who cannot write may sign with an X as long as it is witnessed by two people.

3. Number 1 is correct.

Rationale: Triage works on the principle that clients with the highest acuity have priority over clients with injuries or conditions that are not considered life-threatening. Chest pain, nausea, and diaphoresis indicate a possible myocardial infarction, which can be life-threatening and requires immediate intervention. Fractures and sprains are nonurgent and can wait for treatment. Redness and itching at an IV site indicates a need to assess the site and remove and replace the IV, but is not immediately life-threatening.

4. Number 4 is correct.

Rationale: The professional nurse works under the framework of six ethical principles. Nonmaleficence emphasizes protecting the client from harm. Client safety is always a priority. Another nurse may step in and complete the bath, ensuring that the client is not left alone with impaired personnel. Options 1, 2, and 3 allow the impaired UAP to remain on duty, possibly causing harm to the client. The nurse also has an ethical and legal duty to report situations that may cause client danger. Failure to do so may result in disciplinary action by the board of nursing for the nurse involved, regardless of whether harm comes to the client.

5. Number 4 is correct.

Rationale: Classic signs of localized infection include sudden warmth, redness, pain at the site, and swelling caused by the inflammatory process. This client should be assessed first due to the risk of infection following surgical procedures. The health care provider should be notified immediately so that lab work can be ordered and an appropriate course of treatment started. The client needing a dressing change is not as urgent as a client with infection. A stable client returning from MRI is not the priority. The client with an IV pump beeping can be seen once the health care provider has been notified. The risk of infection and subsequent complications take priority over a beeping IV pump.

6. Number 3 is correct.

Rationale: Petechial rash, nuchal rigidity, and fever are signs of meningitis, which is a medical emergency, especially in an infant. The client with heavy menstrual bleeding is not as urgent as the infant. Dog bites from a known pet current on rabies shots are less urgent than bites from a dog with an unknown rabies status. A twisted ankle with a pedal pulse and no deformity is not life-threatening and can be seen after more urgent clients.

7. Numbers 2, 3, and 4 are correct.

Rationale: Asking clients if they currently have any pain and reminding clients to report pain are within the scope of practice for the UAP. The UAP may also report facial grimacing to the nurse, who can then assess the pain. Assessing pain using the pain scale should be done by the nurse, as assessment is a nursing action. No medications, even over-the-counter ones, may be given by anyone other than the licensed nurse. If the nurse is interrupted for an emergency, another nurse may administer the medication after assessing the client's pain and checking the chart for any allergies, if facility protocols permit this. The nurse is ultimately responsible for the task that has been delegated.

8. Number 2 is correct.

Rationale: Clients with sickle cell disease commonly present with pain during a crisis. The newly graduated nurse is qualified to assess the client's pain and administer ordered pain medications. A client with a clotting disorder and a decreased level of consciousness is an emergency situation due to possible intracerebral bleeding and is not appropriate for an inexperienced nurse. Swallowing after a tonsillectomy indicates possible bleeding and should be assessed by the more experienced nurse. Client teaching is an important and more advanced skill that takes time to develop. Insulin is a high-alert drug, and incorrect information from the new nurse may cause harm to the client.

9. Numbers 1, 2, 3, and 4 are correct.

Rationale: Ensuring continuity of care is especially important when the client is being transferred to another area of the hospital. Options 1, 2, 3, and 4 are guidelines that ensure continuity of care. Addressing pending lab results, listing client requests that the nurse was unable to do, and informing the receiving nurse of upcoming medications or glucose checks that will need to be done shortly after the client arrives make it easier for the receiving nurse to be sure that upcoming tests or medications are not missed. Complaining about the family is unprofessional and takes the focus away from client needs. A smooth transition is essential to ensure that no orders are overlooked. The nurse should be prepared to answer questions from the receiving nurse if needed for clarification after the client is transferred.

10. Number 4 is correct.

Rationale: Most hospitals provide security to lock up client's valuables, along with a receipt or form for identification for claiming the items. All items placed in security must be documented on the admission form and signed. The facility is not responsible for valuables left in the room by clients, and the nurse should be sure that the client is aware of this policy and understands it. Options 1 and 3 still leave the valuables subject to theft. Locking them up in the charge nurse's office is not an appropriate option, as this places the charge nurse in a position of responsibility. Many hospital admissions are unplanned, and the best advice the nurse can give a new client is to send home anything of value.

11. Number 4 is correct.

Rationale: Any suspected cases of abuse and neglect must, by law, be reported to the authorities. The ED will have policies and procedures to guide staff on appropriate responses to suspected child abuse cases. Option 1 assumes that the parents are responsible for the burns and may provoke a violent response. While it is appropriate to ask the client what happened, the nurse should be aware that many abused children are coached to say that they fell off a swing or had another type of accident when asked about their injuries by authority figures. Option 3 is both presumptive and accusatory. Additionally, it may also provoke a violent response. The nurse must objectively assess the client and chart the findings, including descriptions of injuries. Child abuse cases require collaboration among nurses, physicians, social workers, police, and family services. The nurse should remain alert to verbal or nonverbal cues that the situation may intensify, and follow facility guidelines.

12. Number 4 is correct.

Rationale: Washing hands is sufficient since taking a client's blood pressure does not involve contact with blood or secretions. The other listed precautions would be appropriate if blood or secretions is involved.

13. Number 1 is correct.

Rationale: Arranging rest periods throughout the day helps promote the client's ability to participate in an array of desired activities. Increasing intake of protein, iron, and vitamin C aids in hemoglobin production. Keeping a food diary helps document actual nutritional intake. Restricting antacids, tetracyclines, and phosphorous salts will avert absorption of iron.

14. Number 3 is correct.

Rationale: TB bacteria is spread through the air from one person to another. When a person breathes in TB bacteria, the bacteria can settle in the lungs and begin to grow. TB is not transmitted through blood, sharing a cup of coffee, or shaking hands with an infected person.

15. Number 3 is correct.

Rationale: The Center for Disease Control recommends the skin test be read 48 – 72 hours after administration. A test is considered positive if an induration of 5 – 15 millimeters is observed at the injection site. Results read after 72 hours are not accurate and another skin test needs to be conducted.

16. Number 1 is correct.

Rationale: Meniere's disease occurs when the pressure of the fluid in part of the inner ear gets too high. As a result, the client is at risk for injury related to altered mobility because of gait disturbance and vertigo. While hearing loss may occur, this does not result in disturbed body image, low self-esteem, or impaired skin integrity.

17. Number 4 is correct.

Rationale: The frontal lobe regulates intellectual functions, such as complex problem solving. The temporal lobe regulates memory, speech, and comprehension. The parietal lobe regulates reading ability, writing ability, and spatial relationships. The occipital lobe is responsible for vision function.

18. Number 3 is correct.

Rationale: Do not move a client whose neck is in an awkward position or who is unconscious. Instead, keep the client immobilized and get help immediately. In this situation, CPR is not needed for the client. Keeping the client warm is necessary but not a priority. Asking the client to state her name and birthday may be appropriate if a brain injury is suspected, not a neck injury.

19. Number 4 is correct.

Rationale: Relieving pain is the most immediate need for management. Preventing fluid volume deficit by infusion of IV fluids should occur once the client has experienced initial control of pain. Administration of antibiotic therapy will be important during the recovery phase. Reducing anxiety is important and will be partially addressed with the reduction of pain.

20. Number 2 is correct.

Rationale: Acute diverticulitis results from inflammation of the diverticula, typically from an infection. As such, the priority treatment is administration of antibiotics to address the root cause of the condition. Gradually increasing fiber in the diet will occur during the recovery stage of the disease. Pain medication for residual pain would be a second management approach after initiation of antibiotic protocol. To promote rest of the intestinal tract, a liquid diet is advisable for an undeterminable time.

21. Number 4 is correct.

Rationale: An enema is contraindicated for a client with suspected appendicitis as increased intestinal motility may aggravate the suspected appendicitis. When enema administration is appropriate, the other answers are correct.

22. Number 2 is correct.

Rationale: Apgar scoring consists of 5 areas (muscle tone, heart rate, reflex response, color, breathing) with a possible score of 0, 1, or 2 for each area. An Apgar of 9 is correct: four of the five categories for this example rate a score of 2 (subtotal of 8) with 1 point for good color with bluish hands (or feet). The maximum score achievable is 10. A score of 4 or 6 will require support, typically in breathing.

23. Number 2 is correct.

Rationale: Due date is determined by adding 9 months and 7 days to the first day of the client's last menstrual cycle, making October 31 the correct date. September 30 is one month too early. November 15 and December 1 would make the baby overdue.

24. Numbers 1 and 2 are correct.

Rationale: By the age of 3 a child should be able to work simple toys and understand simple instructions. In contrast, the ability to say the first and last name and to name colors or numbers are milestones that occur at 4 years old.

25. Number 4 is correct.

Rationale: Decreasing sodium intake is an effective way to reduce blood pressure in a client with hypertension. Eating red meat daily, increasing potassium and calcium intake, and increasing fluid intake are not measures that affect blood pressure readings.

26. Number 4 is correct.

Rationale: The nurse should recommend the child receive the third vaccine at the earliest convenience as it should be routinely administered anytime from 6 to 19 months of age. Thereafter, the third dose may be safely administered through the age of 18 years old. A third dose of the hepatitis B vaccine is advisable. The child is not in immediate danger by not having had the third vaccine.

27. Number 2 is correct.

Rationale: Within 12 months after quitting, the carbon monoxide level in a smoker's blood drops to normal. At 15 years after quitting, the risk of coronary heart disease is the same as that of a nonsmoker. At 10 years after quitting, the risk of dying from lung cancer is about half that of a smoker's. At 5 to 15 years after quitting, the risk of having a stroke is reduced to that of a nonsmoker's.

28. Number 1 is correct.

Rationale: According to the Centers for Disease Control and Prevention, accidents (unintentional injuries) account for nearly one half of all teenage deaths. The other four leading causes of death among teenagers are homicide, suicide, cancer, and heart disease.

29. Number 4 is correct.

Rationale: The instructional pamphlet is visual, allowing the client to see words and pictures, which is appropriate given the client's preference. The audiotape and classroom discussion are auditory, allowing the client to hear words. The orange/syringe/alcohol wipe/bottle are tactile, allowing the client to touch.

30. Numbers 1, 2, and 5 are correct.

Rationale: In providing end-of-life care, the nurse explains to the client and family the signs and symptoms that death is approaching. Explaining what to expect during the final phase of the illness may help alleviate fear and anxiety as the family observes their loved one transitioning through the stages of death. Addressing client and family wishes regarding care, pain management, and emergency resuscitation respects their wishes and ensures that their choices are carried out as much as possible. Cultural beliefs are acknowledged, and life-lengthening treatment options may give way to maintaining comfort. The nurse should not avoid the difficult topic about end-of-life care, but ensure that open discussion is a central part of the client's care.

31. Numbers 2, 3, and 5 are correct.

Rationale: Age, gender, and culture are a few factors that influence the grieving process. The nurse must explore his own feelings about death before he may effectively help others. Nurses can help families find ways to cope with the loneliness and depression that follow the death of a loved one. The process of grief is normal following a loss, and expression of grief is essential for physical and emotional well-being. The expression of grief should never be discouraged; family members should have a quiet room in which they may express their feelings in private.

32. Number 2 is correct.

Rationale: A child with severe autism who is having a tonsillectomy is at greatest risk for alterations in sensory perception. Clients with severe autism experience altered thought processes. Adding an unfamiliar environment (the hospital) with pain from a surgical procedure compounds the risk of altered sensory perception. The client in the halo vest may have pain and restricted mobility, but he does not have as great a risk for altered perception as the child with severe autism. A teenager who broke her leg during cheerleader practice is more likely to have a large social group and be less isolated. A schoolteacher is more likely to work in a stimulating environment and have many social contacts. Risk factors for altered perception include emotional disorders, a non-stimulating environment, acute illness, limited mobility, pain, decreased cognitive ability, and impaired hearing or vision.

33. Number 1 is correct.

Rationale: The termination stage begins with the initial group meeting. Members' feeling about their accomplishments are explored during the termination stage. Members may be unclear about the group's purpose during the initial stage. Group roles and responsibilities are established in the initial stage of group therapy.

34. Number 3 is correct.

Rationale: Telling the client that it is normal to be afraid and asking how he feels is the most therapeutic option. Asking the client why he is worried about such a minor procedure puts the client on the defensive and trivializes the procedure. What the nurse may see as a minor procedure may feel like major surgery to the client. Offering to call the doctor and cancel the surgery may not be an option, depending on the procedure the client is having. It also does not allow for exploration of the client's feelings and may increase the client's fear if the nurse is quick to offer canceling the procedure. Telling the client not to worry and that the doctor will be sure that nothing goes wrong offers false reassurance and dismisses the client's feelings.

35. Number 3 is correct.

Rationale: Silence allows the client time to think and reflect and lead the conversation in the desired direction. Silence does not imply that the nurse is not listening, nor does it encourage the client to keep her feelings to herself. Silence is part of listening; the nurse should be focused on the client and not thinking ahead to what else she needs to do.

36. Numbers 1 and 5 are correct.

Rationale: During an active hallucination, safety is the first priority. The nurse should administer medications as ordered to manage the hallucinations. Asking the client if he hears voices telling him to harm himself or others is important for both client and nurse safety, as well as others in the area. A client having hallucinations should not be touched. The nurse should not tell the client that others are experiencing the same thing as this only reinforces the hallucination and false beliefs. The client should be moved to an area with decreased stimuli, not taken to the dayroom with others. The nurse should gently attempt to reorient the client to reality. Going along with what the client says he is experiencing reinforces false beliefs and interferes with reorienting the client to reality.

37. Number 4 is correct.

Rationale: Characteristics of disorganized schizophrenia include extreme social withdrawal, inability to perform activities of daily living, inappropriate affect, and grimacing mannerisms. Residual schizophrenia is characterized by being diagnosed with schizophrenia in the past, extreme social isolation, and impaired role functioning. Several years may pass between episodes. Paranoid schizophrenia includes hostility, delusions, violence, persecutory themes, and suspiciousness. Clients with catatonic schizophrenia experience waxy flexibility, psychomotor disturbances, stupor, and excessive purposeless motor activity. They may also be automatically obedient to directions and exhibit stereotypical or repetitive behaviors. Undifferentiated schizophrenia does not meet the definition of paranoid, disorganized, or catatonic schizophrenia. It is characterized by disorganized speech, delusions and hallucinations, flat affect, social withdrawal, and catatonic or disorganized behavior.

38. Numbers 2, 3, and 4 are correct.

Rationale: Interventions for schizophrenia include reassuring the client that the environment is safe and engaging in simple, concrete activities such as puzzles or word games. Art, writing, and music can help the client safely express his feelings. A neutral approach is less threatening than an overly warm and friendly approach. The nurse should inform the client when she is leaving to orient the client to reality and reassure him.

39. Numbers 3 and 4 are correct.

Rationale: Clients who are easily bored, have poor and shallow interpersonal relationships, and enjoy being the center of attention have histrionic personality disorder, which is one of the four types of Cluster B personality disorders. Clients who are impulsive, exhibit unpredictable behavior, experience extreme mood shifts, are easily angered, and play people against each other exhibit borderline personality disorder, which is a Cluster B personality disorder. Other Cluster B personality disorders include narcissistic and antisocial personality disorders. Preoccupation with rules and details, hoarding, ritualistic behavior, and extreme devotion to work are characteristics of obsessive-compulsive personality disorder, which is one of the Cluster C personality disorders. Other Cluster C personality disorders include dependent and avoidant personality disorders. Clients who are suspicious of others and engage in magical thinking, eccentric behavior, paranoia, and relationship deficits exhibit schizoid personality disorder, which is a Cluster A personality disorder. Clients who are suspicious and untrusting of others, are argumentative, are controlling of others, and have thoughts of grandiosity have paranoid personality disorder, which is a Cluster A disorder. The other Cluster A disorder is schizotypal personality disorder.

40. Correct response: Bryant's traction

Rationale: Bryant's traction is used following corrective surgery to repair congenital hip deformities. It involves wrapping the child's legs with moleskin tape and an adhesive elastic bandage which is attached to a series of ropes and weights. The tension helps keep the end of the femur in the hip socket during the healing process.

41. Numbers 2 and 3 are correct.

Rationale: Salmon is a cold-water fish that is rich in omega-3 fatty acids, a good fat that can help lower triglycerides. Grilling eliminates the need for oils or butter, which are high in saturated fat. Herbs offer a very low-calorie way to add flavor to grilled fish. An egg-white omelet eliminates the yolks, which contain the bulk of fat, and vegetables add flavor and nutrients. Animal-based foods are naturally higher in fat; therefore, vegetables such as spinach or red peppers are a better choice than cheese. Wheat toast is not a good choice since it is high in carbohydrates; too many carbohydrates convert into sugar which raises triglycerides. Although the jelly is sugar free, the high amount of carbohydrates in the whole wheat bread make it a poor choice. Natural honey is still very high in sugar, which should be avoided when trying to lower triglyceride levels. Plain grilled steak is not a good choice as it is an animal-based product that is high in fat. A four-ounce serving of sirloin contains about 16 grams of fat, 6 grams of which is saturated. The average person, especially a male, tends to eat far larger servings, which exponentially increases the amount of fat. Skinless poultry is a lower fat choice.

42. Numbers 3, 4, and 5 are correct.

Rationale: The medication regimen for tuberculosis may last up to 12 months, depending on the medications. Strict adherence is important to prevent a relapse. The client may return to most jobs after three sputum cultures are negative. Teaching the client about possible side effects and management of medication helps ensure compliance with treatment. The client should return to his previous activity level gradually, following the health care provider's recommendations. There is no need for the family to maintain respiratory isolation at home since they have already been exposed.

43. Numbers 1, 2, 3, and 5 are correct.

Rationale: The nurse will educate the client on good sleep hygiene. Keeping the bedroom dark and quiet helps promote sleep. Rooms that are too light due to outside lights should be fitted with dark shades or curtains. Going to bed and getting up at the same time helps the body maintain a circadian rhythm. Sleeping in late on weekends can disrupt weekday sleep. Reading and other quiet activities help the client relax and prepare for sleep. Computers and TVs emit blue light, which stimulates the brain to stay alert. Despite common belief, alcohol does not help with sleep. It may make it easier to fall asleep initially, but later disrupts REM sleep, making it easier to wake. A heavy meal before bed stimulates the metabolism and can cause discomfort, leading to difficulty sleeping. Vigorous activity close to bedtime will stimulate the body, making sleep harder.

44. Numbers 3 and 5 are correct.

Rationale: In order to prevent aspiration, the head of the bed should be in a high-Fowler's position whenever feedings are infusing. The tape on the nose should be removed daily and the skin assessed for breakdown; the tape should then be replaced, using care not to move the tube. The tube should be flushed every 4 hours using tepid water, not hot. Using hot water can cause discomfort and possibly burn the client. Tubing and feedings must be changed every 24 hours, even if there is still feeding left in order to prevent bacterial growth. Residuals should be replaced unless the amount is greater than 250 mL. In that case, discard the extra and consider slowing the feeding rate using the health care provider's guidelines. If no bowel sounds are present, hold the feeding and contact the health care provider.

45. Number 3 is correct.

Rationale: Clients with pulmonary edema should be positioned upright with the legs dangling over the side of the bed to decrease venous return. Clients receiving an enema should be positioned on the left side in the Sims' position to allow the gravity flow of the solution to follow the direction of the colon. Client with lower limb amputations should have the affected limb supported but not elevated in order to prevent flexion contractures. Clients with a craniotomy should be positioned with the head of bed at a 30- to 45-degree angle to promote venous drainage from the head.

46. Number 1 is correct.

Rationale: Clients with DVT should be on bed rest to prevent movement of the DVT and pressure changes that occur with walking and other weight-bearing activities. The affected extremity should be elevated. Placing the bed in reverse Trendelenburg will increase pressure on the affected extremity. Walking is contraindicated for clients with DVT; while preventing hospital-acquired pneumonia is important, client safety takes priority over pneumonia prevention at this time. The client may still use an incentive spirometer and practice coughing and deep breathing to clear the lungs without ambulating. Sitting up in a chair is also contraindicated until the DVT has resolved and the health care provider has prescribed activity for the client.

47. Number 2 is correct.

Rationale: The infant is failing to exhibit the Plantar reflex, or Babinski's sign. This is a normal reflex present until 1 year of age. Lack of the reflex indicates the need for further neurological assessment by the health care provider. Taking the infant's vital signs is a necessary part of every visit but is not the priority here. Examining the nose and ears is not indicated at this time and is not as urgent as determining if the infant has neurological deficits. Determining how well the infant feeds is important to track, but is not the primary concern for this client.

48. Number 3 is correct.

Rationale: Asking the client how many pillows she sleeps on evaluates the client for orthopnea, which is shortness of breath caused by lying down. The more pillows the client requires, the worse the orthopnea. This provides important information to the health care provider. Snoring partners, the amount of daily exercise the client gets, and eating heavy meals before bed also affect sleep; however, in the client with COPD, determining the extent of orthopnea will best help prescribe treatments.

49. Numbers 2 and 5 are correct.

Rationale: CPR on infants less than 1 year of age includes a chest compression depth of approximately 1.5 inches, or 4 cm. A witnessed arrest calls for activating the emergency response system before initiating CPR. An automated external defibrillator should be retrieved before starting CPR. The pulse checkpoint on an infant is the brachial artery. A single rescuer should use two fingers for compression, regardless of which hand is dominant. Resting the infant facedown on the forearm is proper positioning for performing the Heimlich maneuver. CPR is performed with the infant lying face up and flat on a firm surface.

50. Number 3 is correct.

Rationale: The Salem sump's position should be checked before each feeding by aspirating gastric content and measuring pH (should be 3.5 or less). Administering feedings through an improperly positioned tube may cause aspiration. The air vent should not be clamped and should be kept above stomach level. The comatose client should be placed on the right side in the high-Fowler's position. Bolus feedings should be infused via a pump or allowed to flow by gravity. Feedings should never be forcibly plunged into the client.

51. Number 2 is correct.

Rationale: The nurse should instruct the client to eat a low-fat, high-fiber diet, avoiding acidic foods. Tomatoes are highly acidic and consumption of tomatoes or tomato-based sauces can worsen the symptoms of GERD. Bananas are low in fat and acid and contain fiber. White bread does not contain acid and has fiber. Grilled salmon is a low-fat choice that avoids fried foods, which are high in fat and irritating to clients with GERD. Steel-cut oatmeal is a low-fat, high-fiber option.

52. Numbers 3, 4, 5, and 6 are correct.

Rationale: Listening to audio books or music can take the client's focus off the pain. Distraction is a useful tool to shift focus away from pain and also includes music therapy and art therapy when appropriate for the client. Splinting the sternum when coughing is one of the most important things post-CABG clients can do to increase their comfort. If the client engages in prayer, meditation, or other rituals at home, he should be encouraged to continue those practices in the hospital. This is respectful to the client and his beliefs and/or culture and allows him to have some measure of control on maintaining normal routines. The bed should be positioned so as to not increase pressure on the sternum. Hot or cold packs should not be used on the sternum, as this area is a fresh post-op site and should be kept clean. Also, the packs may place pressure on the sternum and cause more discomfort. Warm, not hot, heat packs may be used on the back to relieve aches from bed positioning if approved by the health care provider. Morphine is a pharmacological method of pain relief.

53. Numbers 1, 2, 3, 4, and 6 are correct.

    Rationale: Grabbing at the bed rails and general restlessness may indicate pain. Biting the ventilator tubing and breathing over the vent due to increased respiratory rate are other indicators of pain. Facial grimacing and frowning is another pain indicator. Guarding an area of the body during the "sedation vacation" or stiffness or rigidity can indicate a pain response. Blood pressure and heart rate generally increase when experiencing pain. Decreased urinary output is not an indicator of pain. Based on the client's injury, disease process, or surgical procedures, the nurse should be able to anticipate what type and intensity of pain the client may experience. When multiple indicators suggest pain, the nurse should administer pain medications as ordered. It is important to remember that just because a client is sedated does not mean he is not experiencing pain.

54. Numbers 3 and 4 are correct.

    Rationale: A humidifier can help with congestion and stuffiness. Eating dry crackers before getting out of bed in the morning helps with morning sickness. Ginger pills should not be taken unless prescribed by the health care provider, as they can cause miscarriage in higher doses. Liquids should be consumed between meals rather than at meals. Several small meals during the day are better than three regular meals. Over-the-counter nasal sprays should not be used without the health care provider's recommendation.

55. Numbers 2, 3, 4, 5, and 6 are correct.

    Rationale: Prolonged immobilization can lead to urinary stasis, which can cause a urinary tract infection. Decreased cardiac circulation leads to orthostatic hypotension, which can cause dizziness upon standing. Lack of physical exercise can cause the muscles to atrophy, especially over a long period of time. Foot drop is another side effect of prolonged lack of exercise. Lack of mental stimulation causes boredom, frustration, and anxiety in some clients. In addition, respiratory effects of immobility can cause pneumonia. Complications of immobility can lead to longer hospital stays, particularly in clients who have multiple complications or comorbidities.

56. Number 2 is correct.

    Rationale: The client in pelvic traction is on bed rest wearing a traction belt around the pelvis. This client is the most immobile of the clients listed. The client who fractured her arm playing volleyball is able to get up and easily change positions, even with an arm brace. The client who uses a wheelchair is able to be out of the bed. The client who uses a cane for ambulation is walking in the room and hall and is active. The client's condition, medical diagnosis, and treatment plan—not age—determine how great the risk is for developing decubitus ulcers. The greater the immobility, the greater the risk.

57. Number 3 is correct.

    Rationale: A pneumothorax is one of the complications of TPN. It is caused by improper central catheter placement or by a catheter that has migrated. Absence of breath sounds on the affected side, chest or shoulder pain, tachycardia, cyanosis, and sudden shortness of breath are indications of pneumothorax. The nurse should notify the health care provider and prepare the client for a portable chest X-ray. An air embolism is another complication of TPN. Signs and symptoms of air embolism include respiratory distress; a weak, rapid pulse; chest pain; dyspnea; hypotension; and a loud churning sound auscultated over the pericardium. Fluid overload would not present as absence of breath sounds; instead, expected findings include hypertension, bounding pulses, increased respiratory rate, distended veins in the hands and neck, and moist crackles. Signs of refeeding syndrome include arrhythmias, vomiting, shortness of breath, weakness, ataxia, and seizures. It occurs in severely malnourished clients who are undergoing nutritional replacement therapy.

58. Number 2 is correct.

    Rationale: The typical dosage for haloperidol is 2 – 5 mg IM. This dose is three times the normal dose and should be questioned by the nurse. Options 1, 3, and 4 reflect average dosing ranges for those medications.

59. Number 1 is correct.

Rationale: Norvasc is a calcium channel blocker. Calcium causes the heart to beat stronger and harder, so by blocking it, the blood pressure is lowered. Option 2 describes the action of diuretics, such as furosemide. Option 3 describes ACE (angiotensin-converting enzyme) inhibitors, such as lisinopril. Option 4 describes the action of beta-blockers, such as metoprolol tartrate.

60. Number 4 is correct.

Rationale: Atropine sulfate is the antidote for Urecholine, which can cause transient complete heart block. Urecholine is contraindicated in clients with urinary obstructions or strictures. It should never be given by IV or IM routes. It should be given on an empty stomach to decrease the risk of nausea and vomiting.

61. Numbers 1, 4, and 5 are correct.

Rationale: The nurse should monitor for fever or sore throat, as sulfonamides can cause leukopenia, hemolytic anemia, thrombocytopenia, and agranulocytosis. If the client develops a fever or sore throat, the health care provider should be notified. The client should drink 8 – 10 glasses of water daily to maintain daily urinary output of 1200 mL to minimize the risk of renal damage. If the client takes warfarin sodium, phenytoin, or oral hypoglycemics, it may be necessary to reduce the dosage of the medication: sulfonamides potentiate the effects of those drugs. Sulfonamides can cause the urine to turn dark brown or red when taken with some combination sulfonamide medications. Dyspnea, chest pains, chills, and cough are side effects of urinary tract antiseptics such as Macrodantin and Macrobid.

62. Number 1 is correct.

Rationale: Rifampin is one of the first-line agents for tuberculosis. Ciprofloxacin, levofloxacin, and streptomycin are second-line medications for tuberculosis.

63. Number 3 is correct.

Rationale: Acetaminophen is commonly given to relieve mild headache pain, and this is a typical dose. Morphine is an opioid and would not be the first choice, due to the risk of dependency and/or abuse. It may also make the client drowsy, which increases the risk of falls. Aspirin increases the risk of bleeding, especially at doses greater than 81 mg, so this would not be a first choice. Nitroglycerin is given for angina pain, not headaches.

64. Number 2 is correct.

Rationale: Administering 12.4 mL of liquid medication requires using a 3 mL syringe to most accurately draw up the 2.4 mL to add to the 10 mL in the medicine cup. A 5 mL syringe is less accurate and increases the risk of an incorrect dosage. Only oral syringes should be used to administer oral medications. In option 4, the nurse is essentially estimating the amount to add to the cup, increasing the risk of an incorrect dosage.

65. Answer: The client will receive 930 mg of vancomycin every 12 hours.

Solution:

$\frac{136\text{ lbs}}{2.2\text{ kg}}$	Convert pounds to kilograms.
= 61.8 kg = 62 kg.	Round up to find patient's weight in kilograms.
15 mg × 62 kg	Multiply milligrams of vancomycin by client's weight in kilograms.
= 930 mg	Solve for dose per 12 hours.

66. Numbers 1 and 2 are correct.

Rationale: Joint Commission guidelines dictate which abbreviations can or cannot be used. Drug names should be spelled out fully. For example, *MS* can be *magnesium sulfate* or *morphine sulfate*; therefore, drug abbreviations should be avoided. The word *daily* should no longer be abbreviated, but spelled out in full. The rectal route should not be abbreviated, but should be spelled out as *per rectum*. The designation of right eye or left eye should be spelled out and not abbreviated. The word *units* should not be abbreviated, since it can be confused with a zero, the number 4, or the term *cc*.

67.   Number 4 is correct.

Rationale: Medication times are given in military times, based on a 24-hour clock. Midnight is 2400 hours, at which time the clock resets to 0000. Medications due at 0030 are then due at 12:30 a.m. Using a 24-hour clock instead of a 12-hour clock eliminates the need to designate a.m. or p.m. for medication times.

68.   Number 1 is correct.

Rationale: The nurse should notify the pharmacy to correct the error. A pharmacy tech should come and place the proper dose of the medication in the dispenser pocket. Not reporting the error to the pharmacy may lead to a client receiving double the ordered dose if the nurse administering it is not paying close attention. Skipping the medication increases the risk of clots. There is no need for an order clarification from the health care provider. Wasting half of the medication does not solve the problem; it leaves others vulnerable to a dosing error and still allows room for error if the amount wasted is not precise. The nurse should never try to adapt an incorrect dosing pack by wasting it.

69.   Number 4 is correct.

Rationale: If the client is eating and tolerating meals, the nurse should ask the health care provider if the client can take the medication in PO form. The oral form is more convenient for the client and lessens the need to repeatedly access the IV, which increases the risk of infection. If the health care provider declines to change the form of the medication, the nurse would then contact the pharmacy for the missing medication. The nurse should not hold medication without notifying the health care provider, nor should the nurse administer medication in a form different from what was ordered.

70.   Number 2 is correct.

Rationale: The vastus lateralis is the preferred injection site for babies under 7 months of age. It may be used from birth to adulthood. The gluteus medius and the ventrogluteal site should be used only in infants older than 7 months. The dorsogluteal site should not be used for injections due to the risk of damaging the sciatic nerve and puncturing blood vessels.

71.   Number 3 is correct.

Rationale: Doxorubicin causes red urine for 1 – 2 days after administration. Hair loss is temporary; regrowth begins 2 – 3 months after treatment is completed. Visual changes are not a side effect of this medication. Facial flushing and red streaking along the vein only occur when infused too rapidly; therefore, this should not be an expected side effect.

72.   Number 3 is correct.

Rationale: Vesicular rashes contain small raised, sacs filled with clear liquid. A maculopapular rash is characterized by a flat, red area on the skin covered with small confluent bumps. A heat rash appears as tiny red pimples, bumps, or spots usually on the back of the neck or lower back. Pustular rash presents with pustules smaller than 5 – 10 mm filled with pus.

73.   Number 3 is correct.

Rationale: Treating hair lice most commonly requires application of an over-the-counter pediculicide (medication that kills lice). Leave on the hair according to label instructions. If the child has long hair, a second bottle may be necessary. Washing the hair with dandruff shampoo is ineffective. For clothing and items that cannot be washed in hot water/hot heat drying, sealing them in a plastic bag for two weeks is recommended. Shaving the child's head and cleansing with herbal shampoo is ineffective.

74. Numbers 1 and 2 are correct.

Rationale: Communication boards are highly effective in allowing clients to express their needs. Similarly, yes/no questions allow ease in communicating needs with minimal frustration. Open-ended questions require oral communication the client with an endotracheal tube cannot perform. An electrolarynx, a battery-powered handheld device that transmits sound when pressed against the oropharyngeal cavity, is used for clients with a tracheostomy.

75. Numbers 1 and 4 are correct.

Rationale: The client should hold the cane in the hand opposite the weaker leg, the right hand. The client should move the cane and step forward with his weaker leg, left, at the same time.

76. Number 1 is correct.

Rationale: The impaired ability of the adrenal gland to produce the hormone aldosterone (a mineralocorticoid), which helps the kidney retain sodium, results in a craving for salty foods. Weight loss is associated with the disease. Loss of appetite, rather than craving for sweet foods, is consistent with Addison's disease. Fatigue and muscle weakness are typically seen with Addison's disease.

77. Number 4 is correct.

Rationale: Asking the client to add a simple series of numbers tests problem solving, a function of the frontal lobe. Tactile sensation is a parietal lobe function. Hearing function is a temporal lobe function. Balance is a function of the cerebrum.

78. Number 4 is correct.

Rationale: Myoglobin, a small hemeprotein, becomes abnormal within 1 – 2 hours of myocardial infarction (MI). BUN and white blood cell levels do not provide relevant information when an MI is suspected. LDH, lactate dehydrogenase, will begin to rise 2 – 5 days after an MI.

79. Number 4 is correct.

Rationale: In a healthy adult the ICP is 5 – 15 mm Hg. Any pressure greater than 20 mm Hg after a head injury is abnormal.

80. Numbers 2, 3, and 4 are correct.

Rationale: Keeping the bed in the lowest position reduces the impact if the client falls from the bed. Special flooring provides a cushioned surface that reduces impact. A bed alarm will notify staff if the client moves from the bed. Providing a call-light device to a client with Parkinson's is ineffective as the client's ability to use the device is impaired because of fine motor movement limitation.

81. Numbers 2 and 3 are correct.

Rationale: Before the procedure a sedative will be administered. The typical pre-procedure diet is low fiber or clear liquids only for one to three days prior to the procedure. Clients should not eat or drink 6 – 12 hours pre-procedure.

82. Number 3 is correct.

Rationale: The nurse should advise the client to exercise as instructed to prevent contracture formation. Aseptic dressing wound management is acceptable. Elevation of the residual limb should be avoided to prevent contracture formation. As phantom limb pain is common, reporting on an imminent basis is unnecessary.

83. Numbers 1 and 4 are correct.

Rationale: Excessive sweating and leg cramps are side effects of thyroid replacement therapy. Diarrhea rather than constipation is a side effect of thyroid replacement therapy. Inability to tolerate heat rather than cold is a side effect as well.

84. Number 4 is correct.

Rationale: As safety is the top priority during seizure activity, the nurse should remove any objects in the immediate area that may cause the client harm. Calling for assistance is not the first course of action. Restraining a client during a seizure is contraindicated. Turning the client on her side is important yet it is a secondary action.

85. Number 1 is correct.

Rationale: During the initial postoperative period after an ileal conduit, the client should not swim due to the risk of infection. Attendance at an ostomy support group will help the client deal with altered body image. Cleaning the stoma with soap and water will help reduce chance of infection. Wearing a leg bag during the day to collect urine allows the client to return to a normal lifestyle. At night, a larger urine collection bag will be needed.

86. Numbers 2 and 4 are correct.

Rationale: Due to diffuse destruction of hepatic cells with cirrhosis of the liver, the client will experience fatigue and need frequent rest periods throughout the day. An inability of the liver to filter toxins can lead to hepatic encephalopathy making assessment of the client's mental status imperative. Due to impaired clotting function, clients need safety measures implemented such as replacing a straight shaving razor with an electric one. Sodium rather than potassium should be restricted with cirrhosis of the liver.

87. Number 3 is correct.

Rationale: Exophthalmos, or a "startled" look, is caused by edema in the extraocular muscles. Clients may report difficulty in focusing, dry eyes, or photophobia. Graves' disease causes tachycardia, not bradycardia. The client may report an increase in bowel movements. Unplanned weight loss is also common.

88. Number 1 is correct.

Rationale: Viral load testing measures the level of HIV RNA or other viral proteins and monitors disease progression and evaluates effectiveness of treatment. The Western blot test is positive if antibodies to at least two major HIV antigens are present. Clients with AIDS are frequently leukopenic, with a WBC less than 3,500 cells/mm^3. The ELISA test cannot detect antibodies before 3 weeks to 3 months. The client can test negative although HIV infection is present until sufficient antibodies are made.

89. Number 2 is correct.

Rationale: Signs of air embolus include chest pain, anxiety, changes in sensorium, and decreased oxygen saturation. Cold intolerance is not an indication of air embolus. Tachypnea, dyspnea, and hypotension are other findings.

90. Number 4 is correct.

Rationale: Cloudy outflow is a sign of peritonitis, which is life-threatening if left untreated. Other signs include distention, pain, fever, and tenderness. The classic sign is a rigid, boardlike abdomen. Bone pain is a sign of dialysis encephalopathy. Confusion and muscle cramps occur with disequilibrium syndrome.

91. Number 2 is correct.

Rationale: The client should be in a semi-Fowler's position to keep the hyphema away from the cornea's optical center. Positioning the client flat in bed or in Trendelenburg's increases pressure on the site. The lateral position should be avoided until after the hyphema resolves.

92. Number 3 is correct.

Rationale: Restlessness is one of the first signs of shock. Coma is a late sign of shock. Hypotension occurs later in shock. Skin may appear pale early in shock, but coolness manifests later if shock is not corrected.

The presenting signs vary slightly depending on which type of shock the client is experiencing. Middle and late signs may overlap, or progress differently in the client depending on previous health history. With hemorrhagic shock, acute bleeding is obvious and the client can quickly enter the late stages of shock if blood loss is fast enough or high volume loss persists.

93. Number 4 is correct.

   Rationale: These ABGs indicate acute respiratory acidosis. Common signs of respiratory acidosis include hypoventilation with hypoxia, disorientation, and dizziness. Untreated respiratory acidosis can progress to ventricular fibrillation, low blood pressure, seizures, and coma. The other options are signs of metabolic acidosis. If metabolic acidosis is severe, it can cause nausea and vomiting.

94. Number 4 is correct.

   Rationale: Sudden back pain and shortness of breath indicate rupture of the aneurysm, which is an emergency. The nurse should notify the health care provider, monitor neurological and vital signs, and remain with the client. Yellow-tinted vision is a finding of digitalis toxicity. Frothy, pink sputum is a sign of pulmonary edema. Urinary output of 75 mL/hr. is a normal urinary output.

95. Number 1 is correct.

   Rationale: Following CPR, the most important priority is to check the client for a pulse. Often the cardiac monitor may display normal sinus rhythm when there is no pulse present. A urinary catheter would not be the first priority. PEA is never shocked. Once airway is established, the client should be monitored for a pulse, regardless whether the monitor displays an organized rhythm or not.

96. Number 4 is correct.

   Rationale: Classic signs of cardiogenic shock include a rapid pulse that weakens; cool, clammy skin; and decreased urine output. Hypotension is another classic sign.

97. Number 4 is correct.

   Rationale: A full-thickness wound covered with black collagen, known as eschar, is unstageable. Wounds covered in eschar or slough cannot be staged because the full depth of the wound is not visible.

98. Number 4 is correct.

   Rationale: This client is at moderate risk for skin breakdown. The Braden scale is a tool used to assess client's risk of skin breakdown. A score of 15 – 16 indicates mild risk, 12 – 14 indicates moderate risk, and a score of less than 11 indicates severe risk.

99. Number 2 is correct.

   Rationale: The Glasgow coma scale ranges from 3 to 15 and is a measure of neurological function. Based on the findings for this client, the score is 10.

100. Number 4 is correct.

   Rationale: Normal potassium ranges from 3.5 to 5 mEq/L. Hypokalemia can manifest with weak peripheral pulses, orthostatic hypotension, diminished breath sounds, lethargy, confusion, and coma. EKG changes include ST depression and T wave changes. Severe hypokalemia (less than 2.5 mEq/L) can cause death without emergent treatment. The health care provider should be notified for orders. The other laboratory findings are within normal limits.

ONE: Practice Test One

READ THE QUESTION, AND THEN CHOOSE THE MOST CORRECT ANSWER.

1. The nurse is caring for a group of clients in an alcohol rehabilitation facility. A local news station is doing a story on addiction, and a representative comes to the facility, asking to interview a client. A client agrees to appear in the story, and the crew films an interview in the dayroom, showing a glimpse of other clients. Which violation has the nurse committed?

    1. allowing clients in a substance abuse facility to be interviewed by the media

    2. violating the HIPAA *need to know* rule

    3. releasing information about a minor without parental consent

    4. There is no violation.

2. The nurse is talking with a client who has been diagnosed with thyroid cancer. The client is asking about different treatment options. Which response by the nurse is **most** appropriate?

    1. "There are several local support groups you can join after you have completed chemo."

    2. "Don't worry about it. Your doctor will explain the best course of treatment for you."

    3. "What information has your health care provider shared about the different treatment options?"

    4. "I wouldn't take chemo if I were you. I've seen so many clients say that they wish they hadn't done it."

3. The nurse is working in the ED when a client in labor comes in and says that she does not have health insurance, but wants to know if a doctor will see her. The nurse understands that the client's right to emergency services, regardless of ability to pay, is provided by which piece of legislation?

    1. HIPAA

    2. the Continuity of Care Act

    3. the Patient's Bill of Rights

    4. the Code of Ethics for Nurses

4. An RN is working with an LPN to care for a group of clients. Which client would the RN **most** likely assign to the LPN?

   1. a client receiving blood following back surgery
   2. a client who has just returned from having a left heart catheterization
   3. a client with an arterial line who is on a nitroprusside drip to control blood pressure
   4. a client with an abdominal wound requiring dressing changes every 4 hours and PRN

5. The nurse is caring for an elderly client following a total knee replacement. The client is disoriented to time and place, and has pulled out multiple IVs. The health care provider writes an order for soft wrist restraints. Which of the following are appropriate nursing actions for this client? **Select all that apply.**

   1. secure restraints with a double knot
   2. offer toileting and nutrition every 2 hours
   3. ask for a new restraint order every 48 hours
   4. check restraints for proper placement and check the skin every 2 hours
   5. document the type of restraint, need for continued use, and trial release results

6. The nurse is in the medication room drawing up insulin for a client when a code blue is called. In his haste to respond to the call, the nurse places the syringe of insulin on the counter and responds to the code. Afterward, the nurse returns to the medication room and retrieves the syringe of insulin. Which action by the nurse is correct?

   1. return the insulin to the insulin vial and draw up a new syringe
   2. administer the insulin after labeling the syringe with the date, dose, and client name
   3. dispose of the syringe in the sharps container, and draw up a new dose in a new syringe
   4. administer the insulin that was drawn up, since the syringe is still in the medication room

7. The nurse is preparing to administer the first dose of IV antibiotic to the client. Halfway through the infusion, the nurse realizes that the antibiotic dosage is not the same as ordered by the health care provider. Which action should the nurse take **first**?

   1. stop the infusion
   2. fill out an incident form
   3. notify the health care provider
   4. only give part of the antibiotic to obtain the correct dose

8. The nurse is entering several orders that the health care provider has just ordered for a new admission. One of the medication orders is illegible. Which action by the nurse is correct?

   1. ask another nurse to transcribe the order
   2. call the prescribing physician for clarification
   3. scan the order to the pharmacy and let the pharmacy staff decipher it
   4. figure it out based on the client's diagnosis and home medications

9. A client who just delivered is concerned about her neonate's Apgar scores of 7 at 1 minute and 8 at 5 minutes. She has been told a score lower than 9 is associated with learning disabilities. Which response is **best**?

   1. "Your infant is fine. Don't worry."
   2. "Apgar scores indicate a need for extra medical care at birth. Your baby's score of 7 is fine."
   3. "There are many good special education programs available I can recommend."
   4. "I'll ask the physician to speak with you."

10. An elderly client's wife tells a nurse she is concerned because her husband insists on talking about past events. The nurse assesses the client and finds him alert, oriented, and responsive to questions. Which statement should the nurse make to the client's wife?

    1. "Your husband is choosing to live in a happier time in his life."
    2. "Redirect your husband to speak about current events when he begins regressing into the past."
    3. "If he were my husband, I would call our minister to speak to him."
    4. "Your husband is reflecting on his life. This is normal at his age."

11. A client who is postmenopausal asks the nurse how to prevent osteoporosis. Which statement should the nurse make to the client?

    1. "Eat 2 ounces of cheese each day and walk a mile a day."
    2. "There are no known ways to prevent osteoporosis."
    3. "Do weight-bearing exercises regularly and take hormones as ordered by your physician."
    4. "Take potassium supplements daily."

12. The nurse is caring for a client who recently experienced a massive stroke. Which of the following statements by the spouse indicates a need for further teaching by the nurse?

    1. "My spouse may not return to normal for some time."
    2. "I plan on returning to work full time as soon as my spouse returns home."
    3. "Home health care will help us once my spouse is discharged."
    4. "You will provide me with support during this difficult time."

13. The nurse is on a memory care unit. A client insists on leaving to go home. Which of the following should the nurse do?

    1. review the reality orientation board in the client's room
    2. take the client to the activity room to interact with others
    3. contact the client's primary health care provider for a medication order
    4. provide the client with a glass of milk and a sandwich

14. A client who is Muslim is refusing to eat food served to him by a nursing assistant. The nurse should do which of the following? **Select all that apply.**

    1. arrange a mealtime that will avoid prayer times

    2. remove farm-raised catfish from the food tray

    3. arrange with the family for halal food to be brought from home

    4. deliver food by a nursing assistant of the same sex

15. The nurse is taking care of a 12-year-old male who sustained 30% full-thickness burns on his chest and arms 20 hours ago. To maintain optimal fluid and electrolyte balance, the nurse expects to administer which of the following?

    1. lactated Ringer's

    2. D10W

    3. plasma

    4. normal saline

16. The nurse working in an outpatient pain clinic has the opportunity to teach a client with chronic back pain about nonpharmacological pain management. Which of the following would be **most** appropriate for the nurse to include when teaching? **Select all that apply.**

    1. music

    2. therapeutic massage

    3. stretching exercises

    4. relaxation

17. The nurse working in an outpatient clinic has the opportunity to teach a client recently diagnosed with irritable bowel syndrome (IBS). Which of the following topics would be **most** appropriate for the nurse to include? **Select all that apply.**

    1. daily iced tea intake

    2. stress reduction techniques

    3. limit fluids

    4. daily probiotic

18. The nurse is caring for an elderly female client in an extended-care facility who has dry age-related macular degeneration (AMD). Which nursing intervention would be the **most** appropriate?

    1. provide written materials to explain medications

    2. stand in front of the client when addressing her

    3. limit room lighting to create a relaxed environment

    4. encourage use of radio and CDs

19. The nurse working in an outpatient clinic is preparing to teach insulin injection to an elderly male client who is hard of hearing yet refuses to wear prescribed hearing aids. Which of the following communication strategies would be **most** appropriate for the nurse to use?

   1. speak in a high-pitched voice
   2. use sign language
   3. ensure the room is well lit
   4. refrain from touching the client

20. A student nurse is preparing to administer the client's first dose of tetracycline while the charge nurse observes. What statement by the student nurse prompts the charge nurse to provide further teaching? **Select all that apply.**

   1. "Tetracycline may be given with grapefruit juice."
   2. "After taking tetracycline, the client should wait two hours before eating."
   3. "It should be given with caution in clients with liver or renal dysfunction."
   4. "The client may have an antacid along with the tetracycline if it causes GI upset."
   5. "It should be taken on an empty stomach at least one hour before meals with a glass of milk."

21. The nurse is caring for a group of clients in an infectious disease unit. The nurse understands that which of the conditions listed are required to be reported by the CDC? **Select all that apply.**

   1. tetanus
   2. scarlet fever
   3. chlamydia
   4. Lyme disease
   5. group B streptococcal infection

22. The nurse administers ciproflaxin to a client and then realizes that the client is allergic to the medication. What nursing action is the **priority** for this client?

   1. induce vomiting
   2. obtain the client's vital signs
   3. complete an incident report
   4. notify the health care provider

23. The nurse is monitoring a client taking chlordiazepoxide hydrochloride (Librium). Which adverse effect would be of **greatest** concern?

   1. hiccups
   2. lethargy
   3. drowsiness
   4. respiratory depression

24. The client has a nitroprusside drip infusing at 0.3 mcg/kg/min. The concentration is 50 mg nitroprusside in 250 mL D5W. The client weighs 70 kg. What will the IV infusion rate be?

_____

25. The nurse has an order to give 1,000 mL of 0.9% NS with 20 meQ of potassium chloride over 8 hours. The IV set has a drop factor of 15. How many gtts/min should the client receive?

_____

26. The nurse has an order to give 500 mL of 0.45% NS over 12 hours. The IV set has a drop factor of 10. How many gtts/min should the client receive? **Fill in the blank.**

_____

27. The nurse is monitoring the labs of a client admitted with viral hepatitis. Which of the following lab findings would the nurse expect for this client? **Select all that apply.**
    1. decreased ALT levels
    2. increased AST levels
    3. elevated ammonia levels
    4. low serum albumin levels
    5. shortened prothrombin time

28. The nurse is talking to a client and his family about hepatitis. Which of the following statements by a family member indicate understanding of the nurse's teaching? **Select all that apply.**
    1. "Hepatitis D only occurs with hepatitis B."
    2. "Hepatitis A can occur at any time of the year."
    3. "Hepatitis D is transmitted through contaminated drinking water."
    4. "Hepatitis A can be spread by uncooked shellfish and contaminated water or milk."
    5. "Hepatitis B is spread by contact with blood or body fluids, sexual contact, or sharing dirty needles."

29. The nurse is caring for a client who just had a supratentorial craniotomy to remove a tumor. The nurse will implement which of the following in the client's plan of care? **Select all that apply.**
    1. check the dressing every 8 hours for excessive drainage
    2. assess the pupils for signs of increased intracranial pressure
    3. position the client flat with the head rotated away from the surgical site
    4. monitor the client's respiratory status, including rate and pattern of breathing
    5. notify the health care provider if the dressing is saturated or the client has more than 50 mL of drainage in 8 hours

30. A nursing student is assigned to a client with an endotracheal tube on a ventilator. Upon entering the client's room the primary care nurse is alerted by observing which of the following?

    1. The head of the bed is elevated 45 degrees.
    2. The cuff on the endotracheal tube is inflated.
    3. Normal saline is present at the bedside table.
    4. The client is wearing an intermittent compression device on each leg.

31. The nurse is assessing a client at home who is receiving outpatient hemodialysis 12 hours a week. The nurse knows the client needs further instruction about proper diet when he states which of the following?

    1. "I drink prune juice when I'm constipated."
    2. "I drink ginger ale with lunch."
    3. "I drink 1 cup of milk with my dinner."
    4. "My bread choice is white rather than whole grain."

32. A 22-year-old female primigravida who is at 36 weeks' gestation is seen in the ED with a low platelet count, ALT of 68 U/L, AST of 55 U/L, and a continuous, severe headache that has lasted three days. The nurse prepares for what to occur?

    1. amniocentesis
    2. ultrasound of the baby
    3. delivery of the baby
    4. C-section

33. The nurse is teaching a female client who is experiencing urge incontinence how to manage her condition at home. Which statement by the client indicates a need for further explanation by the nurse?

    1. "I will be cured in four weeks if I follow the bladder retraining instructions."
    2. "I will perform the pelvic muscle exercises daily."
    3. "I will wait five minutes once I get the urge to urinate to go to the bathroom."
    4. "I will empty my bladder when I first get up in the morning.

34. A nurse has received report on the day's clients. In planning morning rounds, which client is the **priority** to see?

    1. a new admission with a UTI and fever
    2. a client who is NPO for surgery later in the morning
    3. a client complaining of nausea after eating breakfast
    4. a client recently complaining of shortness of breath

35. A nurse has been floated to the ICU from the step-down unit. Which client assignment would be **best** for this nurse?

    1. a client awaiting a bed on the medical floor
    2. a client receiving continuous renal replacement therapy (CRRT)
    3. a client on an insulin drip with a large abdominal wound attached to a wound vacuum
    4. a client who has just returned from surgery to replace pacemaker wires and is being externally paced

36. A client has signed the consent form for a right radical mastectomy. Shortly before the client is to be taken to surgery, she tells the nurse, "I'm not really sure that this is what I want to do. Everything was so sudden." Which response by the nurse is **most** appropriate?

    1. "You will be glad you did it once it's over."
    2. "What are your thoughts right now on this procedure?"
    3. "I will notify the surgeon and let her know you have concerns about having the surgery."
    4. "The OR has been prepared for you, and the doctor will be mad if you mess up the surgery schedule."

37. The nurse is working with an unlicensed assistive personnel (UAP). In planning the morning's care, which tasks can the nurse delegate to the UAP? **Select all that apply.**

    1. feeding a client who has lost the use of his hands
    2. starting an IV in a confused client who pulled her IV out
    3. assisting a stable and alert client up to the bedside commode
    4. checking an apical pulse in a client prior to administering digoxin
    5. ambulating a client in the hall for the first time since surgery to repair a fractured T5 vertebra

38. A client is on contact and airborne precautions. In which order should the nurse don personal protective equipment (PPE) before entering the room?

    1. perform hand hygiene, don the gown, don the mask, don eye protection, apply gloves
    2. don the gown, perform hand hygiene, don the mask, apply gloves, don eye protection
    3. don the mask, don eye protection, perform hand hygiene, don the gown, apply gloves
    4. don eye protection, don the mask, perform hand hygiene, apply gloves, don the gown
    5. perform hand hygiene, apply gloves, don the gown, don the mask, don eye protection

39. The nurse is caring for a client on airborne precautions. Which of the following would the nurse expect to see in the client's medical record?

    1. measles
    2. influenza
    3. Lyme disease
    4. herpes simplex

40. Four 6-month-old children arrive at the clinic for diphtheria-pertussis-tetanus immunization. Which child can safely receive the immunization at this time?

    1. the child with a runny nose
    2. the child who experienced a seizure after the last immunization
    3. the child who experienced a life-threatening allergic reaction after the last immunization
    4. the child with a temperature of 102°F

41. The nurse is preparing to pull a thin, frail client up in the bed. No one responds to the nurse's call for lifting assistance. Which is the **best** action by the nurse?

    1. call again and apologize to the client for the wait
    2. stand behind the bed at the client's head, and pull her up gently from her armpits
    3. since the client is small, pull her up in the bed by pulling on the draw sheet, alternating sides
    4. if the client is able to roll and bend her knees, lower the head of the bed and place it in Trendelenburg's position while helping the client bend her knees and push up

42. A client asks what diabetes mellitus does to the body over time. Which condition should the nurse include in teaching as a common chronic complication of diabetes mellitus?

    1. hyperglycemia
    2. diabetic ketoacidosis
    3. hyperglycemia
    4. retinopathy

43. An 88-year-old client fractured a hip after a fall in her home. Because of her peripheral vascular disease and asthma, surgery is not an option. The client tells the nurse she does not know how she is going to get better. Which response by the nurse is **best**?

    1. "You'll do just fine."
    2. "You can't live alone anymore."
    3. "What are you most worried about?"
    4. "You should get a second opinion."

44. A client has recently lost her best friend to cancer. The client tells the nurse, "I'm very sad about the loss of my friend." Which of the following responses by the nurse is the **most** appropriate?

    1. "I lost my best friend two years ago, but I feel better now."
    2. "It's important for you to keep busy."
    3. "Why do you feel this way?"
    4. "It's normal to feel loss. Tell me about your friend."

45. The nurse is caring for a client in the intensive care unit. The nurse recognizes that to prevent sensory alteration in a client, the nurse needs to do which of the following interventions? **Select all that apply.**

   1. orient the client to person, place, and time during every contact

   2. limit visitors to one 15-minute visit per 8-hour shift

   3. explain all nursing care

   4. keep the lighting level consistent throughout the day

46. The nurse is taking a history from a client in an outpatient clinic. The client has been taking duloxetine (Cymbalta) for fibromyalgia. Which of the following over-the-counter medications would cause the nurse some concern if the client says she is taking it?

   1. aspirin

   2. garlic supplements

   3. vitamin B6

   4. cough medicine with dextromethorphan

47. The nurse is caring for a client with Crohn's disease. How should the nurse educate the client regarding nutrition and hydration?

   1. Drink coffee each morning, as this can help stimulate the appetite.

   2. Avoid enteral supplements, as they may decrease the appetite for solid foods.

   3. Select high-calorie, low-fiber, high-protein, and high-vitamin foods for each meal.

   4. Drink clear liquids as soon as they are tolerated, and then progress the diet rapidly in order to obtain needed nutrients.

48. The nurse is caring for a 7-year-old child with constipation. The child's mother asks the nurse what she can do to help prevent another episode. What information would the nurse include in her response?

   1. "Give enemas until the child runs clear."

   2. "Give laxatives daily on a regular basis."

   3. "Provide lots of milk and sugary foods to promote defecation."

   4. "Have the child sit on the toilet for 5 to 10 minutes about 20 to 30 minutes after meals to encourage defecation."

49. The nurse is caring for a first-time mother who is asking how to help her baby sleep through the night as the baby gets older. Which recommendation should the nurse tell the mother?

   1. "Rock her to sleep every night until she is in a deep sleep."

   2. "Give diphenhydramine 12.5 mg orally to put the baby to sleep."

   3. "If she starts waking up a lot in the middle of the night, put her in the bed with you."

   4. "Give the last feeding as late as possible, and put her in the bed awake without a bottle."

50. The nurse is caring for a client diagnosed with a cerebral aneurysm. Which precautions would the nurse put in place for this client? **Select all that apply.**

   1. keep the room dark and avoid direct, bright lights
   2. allow frequent visitors to provide social interaction to the client
   3. administer deep vein thrombosis (DVT) prophylaxis as ordered
   4. encourage the client to breathe deep and cough to clear secretions
   5. keep the client on bed rest in a side-lying or semi-Fowler's position

51. The nurse is caring for a client who is at risk for altered fluid balance. Which signs and symptoms of dehydration would the nurse expect to find in this client? **Select all that apply.**

   1. bounding pulses
   2. increased hematocrit
   3. orthostatic hypotension
   4. diminished bowel sounds
   5. decreased urine specific gravity

52. The nurse is caring for a client who has stage 3 lung cancer and is in renal failure. The client indicates that he does not wish to have life-sustaining treatment and wants to die a natural death. What document does the nurse anticipate this client completing? **Fill in the blank.**

   _____

53. The nurse is caring for a client post-op day 1 for a bowel resection. The client is receiving pain medication via a patient-controlled analgesic pump (PCA) but states that her pain is severe and the pain pump is not providing adequate relief. Which is the **priority** nursing action for this client?

   1. assess vital signs and pain for location, quality, and intensity
   2. reposition the client with the head of bed elevated 30 degrees
   3. offer nonpharmacologic pain relief measures since the medication dose cannot be increased
   4. press the PCA button to deliver a bolus and ask family members to press the button for the client if she is asleep

54. The nurse is caring for a client receiving IV heparin therapy for a pulmonary embolism. Which lab values would the nurse expect to order on this client?

   1. hematocrit
   2. HDL and LDL
   3. PT, PTT, INR
   4. troponin level

55. The nurse on a physical rehabilitation unit is assigned a 63-year-old male client post-amputation of his left lower limb above the knee two weeks prior. The client has a history of peripheral vascular disease due to diabetes mellitus. Which statement by the client indicates a need for further teaching?

    1. "I had my leg removed because of diabetes."
    2. "My exercises are going well."
    3. "My left leg hurts after I wrap my stump."
    4. "I use canes to walk to the bathroom."

56. The nurse is caring for a client admitted to ICU following a heart attack. The nurse notes on the chart that the client has named his spouse to make decisions regarding his care if he is unable to speak for himself. What is the name of the document the client has signed? **Fill in the blank.**

    _____

57. The nurse is reviewing labs on a client receiving IV heparin and notes an INR of 4.6. Which order by the health care provider does the nurse anticipate?

    1. an order for vitamin K IM
    2. an order for protamine sulfate
    3. an order to redraw labs in 6 hours
    4. an order to increase the infusion rate

58. The nurse is providing client education on self-administration of insulin. Which action by the client indicates the need for further education?

    1. The client gently rubs the insertion site after removing the needle.
    2. The client verifies the type of insulin and checks the expiration date.
    3. The client cleans and grasps the skin, inserting the needle at a 90-degree angle.
    4. The client cleans the rubber stopper on the bottle with an alcohol swab before drawing a dose.

59. The nurse is caring for a client who fractured her leg in a motor vehicle accident. A cast is applied. The nurse will assess which of the following? **Select all that apply.**

    1. pulses
    2. capillary refill
    3. skin temperature
    4. squeeze the cast every hour to check for firmness
    5. assess for pain, numbness, tingling, or inability to move the toes

60. The nurse is providing post-op education to a client who had a splenectomy. Which statement by the client indicates that the nurse's teaching was successful?

1. "I can resume yoga classes in two weeks."
2. "I need to eat a diet low in fiber to rest my digestive tract."
3. "I will need to be careful when I go to the NFL game next month."
4. "I need to talk to my doctor about getting influenza, pneumococcal, and meningococcal vaccines."

61. The nurse is caring for a client with dementia who has pulled out three peripheral IVs. Which intervention by the nurse is the **best** way to manage this client?

1. place the client in restraints or mitts
2. tell the family that they need to stay with the client
3. replace the IV and wrap it in gauze to hide it from view
4. tell the client that if she pulls another IV out, she will have to have a PICC line placed

62. The nurse is preparing a 73-year-old client for cataract surgery on the left eye. Which statement by the client indicates a need for further teaching?

1. "I will wear glasses when going outside."
2. "I will avoid bending below the waist."
3. "I will stop taking Coumadin after surgery."
4. "I will still be able to work out on weight training."

63. A client admitted for treatment of a deep venous thrombosis of the calf complains of dyspnea and chest pain. What is the **best** response by the nurse?

1. administer oxygen at 2L/min as ordered prn
2. place client in a semi-Fowler's position
3. prepare client for diagnostic tests
4. obtain vital signs

64. The nurse in an ambulatory care clinic is admitting a 27-year-old client with severe systemic lupus erythematosus (SLE). In assessing the client's health history, the nurse knows to question which of the following statements?

1. "I avoid being outside on sunny days."
2. "The medications I take make me bloated."
3. "My work schedule is down to four hours a day."
4. "I get an eye exam annually."

65. The nurse is working in a small hospital that still uses paper charting for client assessments. While writing the nurse's note, the nurse makes an error. Which method does the nurse utilize to make the correction?

    1. use Wite-Out® to cover the error, and proceed after it dries

    2. throw away the nurse's note and start over with a fresh note

    3. mark through the error in red ink and place her initials afterward

    4. mark a single line through the error in black ink and place her initials afterward

66. The unit manager believes that each member of the care team should have input regarding unit goals and problem solving techniques. The manager is concerned for each individual member and serves primarily as a resource person for the unit. The unit nurse understands that this style of leadership is which of the following?

    1. autocratic

    2. situational

    3. democratic

    4. laissez-faire

67. A nurse working in ICU has a client on a propofol (Diprivan) drip while on the mechanical ventilator. The nurse needs another bottle, which must be picked up in person in the hospital pharmacy. Which is the correct action by the nurse concerning this medication?

    1. ask the unit secretary to go to the pharmacy and pick it up

    2. send the unlicensed assistive personnel (UAP) to pick it up since the nurse is busy

    3. ask the client's health care provider to bring it when he or she rounds on the client

    4. ask another nurse to watch the clients while the nurse goes to the pharmacy to get the medication

68. A 68-year-old woman newly diagnosed with diabetes is preparing for discharge. Which of the following activities **best** describes the nurse's role as an advocate?

    1. teach the client how to test her glucose level

    2. provide a short-term supply of insulin syringes

    3. refer the patient to home health care follow-up

    4. reinforce the follow-up visit to her primary care provider in two weeks

69. The nurse answers a call to the unit, which turns out to be a bomb threat. Which actions by the nurse are correct? **Select all that apply.**

    1. dismiss the call as a prank

    2. follow facility protocol to ensure client and staff safety

    3. try to find out where the bomb is and when it will go off

    4. alert the charge nurse, security, and the police department

    5. start evacuating clients, starting with those who are most mobile first

70. The nurse enters the client's room and smells cigarette smoke. When confronted, the client says, "I only smoked one cigarette because I was having a bad craving." Which action by the nurse is **most** appropriate?

   1. escort the client outside to smoke
   2. call the health care provider to obtain an order for a nicotine patch
   3. remind the client that oxygen is in use and smoking is banned in the facility
   4. tell the client that if he continues to smoke in the room, he will be discharged from the hospital

71. The nurse is caring for a client with a history of schizophrenia, alcohol abuse, bipolar disorder, and noncompliance with treatment and medications. The client has also been arrested in the past for violent behavior. Which action by the nurse is the **most** important when caring for a potentially violent client?

   1. treat the client with courtesy and respect
   2. always maintain an open pathway to the door
   3. be sure the client swallows his pills and does not "cheek" them
   4. ask permission from the client before drawing blood or performing other invasive procedures

72. A client arrives at the emergency department in her third trimester of pregnancy with painless vaginal bleeding. Which condition is suspected?

   1. placental abruption
   2. urinary tract infection
   3. placenta previa
   4. uterine polyps

73. The nurse gives a 35-year-old primigravida client a RhoGAM injection in her 27th week of pregnancy. Which of the following client situations requires the nurse to take this action?

   1. Rh-negative mother and Rh-positive father
   2. Rh-negative mother and Rh-negative father
   3. Rh-positive mother and Rh-negative father
   4. Rh-positive mother and Rh-positive father

74. A community center is having a health fair. Which of the following main food courses should the nurse recommend as most healthful for a 20-year-old adult whose total cholesterol level is 300 mg/dL?

   1. fettuccine alfredo
   2. fried chicken
   3. grilled cheese sandwich with bacon
   4. natural peanut butter and banana sandwich on whole wheat bread

75. The family of a hospice client wishes to visit at midnight. Which of the following actions by the nurse would be the **most** appropriate?

   1. tell the family that visiting hours are over
   2. ask the client if he wishes to see his family
   3. allow two family members to visit at a time
   4. provide entrance for the entire family to visit

76. The nurse on the inpatient memory care unit is caring for a client with Alzheimer's who exhibits wandering behavior. The 24-hour observer calls the nurse to report that the client left the unit. It would be **most** appropriate for the nurse to take which of the following actions?

   1. notify the family
   2. notify security along with a description of the client
   3. ask the observer in what direction the client headed
   4. ask other staff on the unit to assist in finding the client

77. A client is admitted to an inpatient psychiatric unit after being found unresponsive as a result of prescribed opioid drugs. Upon awakening she attempts to get out of bed and is unsteady. The nurse is concerned that the client will fall. The doctor ordered a vest restraint to be applied as necessary to maintain client safety. The client refuses the restraints. The nurse should take which of the following actions?

   1. move the client closer to the nursing station to allow close monitoring
   2. apply the restraint in compliance with hospital policy
   3. consult with a more experienced nurse on a course of action
   4. check on the client every 30 minutes to ensure her safety

78. A client who is three days postpartum and is bottle-feeding her infant calls the nurse at the gynecology clinic with complaints of breast engorgement. What instruction should the nurse provide?

   1. reduce fluid intake to 1,500 ml/day
   2. take a warm shower twice a day
   3. apply a tight binder around her breasts
   4. come in to see the physician immediately as this is abnormal

79. A nurse is giving instructions to parents of a child who had a tonsillectomy. Which instruction is the **most** important?

   1. drink orange juice to relieve discomfort
   2. drink extra milk to relieve discomfort
   3. avoid drinking from a straw
   4. rinse twice a day with antiseptic mouthwash

80. A client with a colostomy is experiencing mild diarrhea. Which instruction should the nurse give the client?

   1. drink two 8-oz glasses of water

   2. eat two bananas

   3. eat five prunes

   4. eat a salad with vinaigrette dressing

81. A 92-year-old male client with Alzheimer's frequently experiences urinary incontinence. Which intervention should the nurse do **first**?

   1. apply a condom catheter

   2. insert an indwelling catheter

   3. apply a diaper

   4. offer the urinal every 2 hours

82. Along with traditional therapy, a client asks the nurse about alternative therapies for chronic pain. Which could the nurse provide to the client?

   1. yoga

   2. acupuncture

   3. music therapy

   4. hypnosis

83. The nurse is caring for a client newly diagnosed with diabetes type 2. The health care provider plans to start the client on a rapid-acting insulin. Which insulin does the nurse anticipate noting on the order?

   1. Lantus

   2. Levemir

   3. Humalog

   4. Humulin 70/30

84. The nurse is caring for a client receiving TPN. The nurse understands that TPN management includes which of the following? **Select all that apply.**

   1. monitor daily weights and intake and output

   2. monitor serum electrolytes and glucose levels daily

   3. change IV tubing every 48 hours or per facility protocol

   4. change the IV site dressing every 24 hours or per facility protocol

   5. if TPN is unavailable, OK to give D10W or D20W until TPN becomes available

85. A student nurse is precepting on the unit and caring for a client with a Dobbhoff nasoenteric tube. Which statement by the student nurse indicates the need for further teaching on caring for a client with this tube? **Select all that apply.**

   1. "I should wait for X-ray confirmation before using the tube."
   2. "I can confirm placement by auscultating over the epigastric area."
   3. "I can mix liquid medications in with the tube feeding for administration."
   4. "I will flush the tube with 20 to 30 mL of water every 4 hours during continuous tube feeding."
   5. "I will observe the client for diarrhea, abdominal distention, nausea and vomiting, and tube dislodgement."

86. A client recently diagnosed with atrial fibrillation is being discharged home on digoxin (Lanoxin). The nurse is providing education to the client and family. Which client statement indicates the need for further teaching?

   1. "I should take my medicine at the same time each day."
   2. "If I miss a dose, I can take it as soon as I remember it."
   3. "I need to call my doctor if my heart rate goes below 60 or above 110."
   4. "Changes in my vision could be toxicity and should be reported immediately."

87. The nurse is caring for a client who just arrived in the PACU following a colonoscopy with polyp removal. The client's level of sedation is assessed using the Ramsay Sedation Scale (RSS). The client responds quickly, but only to commands. What Ramsay score would the nurse chart for this client?

   1. RSS 1
   2. RSS 2
   3. RSS 3
   4. RSS 4
   5. RSS 5
   6. RSS 6

88. The nurse is caring for a client who has a lithium level of 2.2 mEq/L. Based on this lab value, what would the nurse anticipate to do in order to care for this client? **Select all that apply**.

   1. prepare to administer IV fluids
   2. notify the health care provider
   3. order a mechanical soft diet for the client
   4. administer the next dose of lithium when it is due
   5. observe the client for confusion and slurred speech

89. The nurse is caring for a client receiving hemodialysis. During hemodialysis, the client becomes anxious, experiencing tachypnea and hypotension. The nurse suspects which complication of hemodialysis?

    1. air embolism
    2. clotting of the graft site
    3. dialysis encephalopathy
    4. disequilibrium syndrome

90. The nurse is assisting the health care provider to perform a renal biopsy. Which position should the nurse place the client in?

    1. in the semi-Fowler's position
    2. on the same side of the kidney to be biopsied
    3. on the side opposite of the kidney to be biopsied
    4. prone with a pillow under the shoulders and abdomen

91. The nurse is seeing a client in the clinic who has shingles (herpes zoster). The client is concerned about spreading the disease to others. How should the nurse respond?

    1. It is only possible to have one episode of the disease.
    2. Persons with leukemia are at higher risk.
    3. Persons of all ages should receive the zoster vaccine (Zostavax).
    4. Persons between 30 and 40 years old are at high risk.

92. The nurse is caring for a client after he experienced a seizure (postictal). Which intervention would the nurse expect **not** to perform?

    1. return client to pre-seizure activity
    2. administer medications as appropriate
    3. reorient as necessary
    4. assess neurologic and vital signs

93. The nurse is teaching feeding protocol to the spouse of a client who experienced a severe stroke. Which statement by the spouse indicates a need for further explanation by the nurse?

    1. "I will not let him use a straw."
    2. "I will turn on the television during meals."
    3. "Instead of whole pills, I will crush the pill and place it in custard."
    4. "He will sit up for a half hour after eating."

94. The nurse is preparing to transfer a client from the ED to the orthopedic unit. She knows that adhering to the hospital policy for client handoffs **best** ensures which of the following?

    1. privacy
    2. Patient's Bill of Rights
    3. continuity of care
    4. case management

95. On the diagram, identify the location of the following pedal pulses.

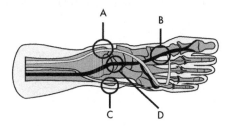

    1. posterior tibial
    2. peroneal
    3. dorsalis pedis
    4. anterior tibial

96. An RN is in charge of a team on a medical/surgical unit that includes an LPN. The RN understands that which of the following is an activity that falls within the scope of practice of an LPN?

    1. contact the physician for prescription orders
    2. formulate a nursing diagnosis
    3. administer oral medications to a client
    4. collaborate with physical therapy to develop a discharge plan

97. A client is being treated for irritable bowel syndrome (IBS). The nurse knows that the involvement of nursing, pharmacy, gastroenterology, and nutritional services is an example of which of the following approaches?

    1. continuity of care
    2. multidisciplinary
    3. managed care
    4. case management

98. The nurse on a pediatric unit has just admitted a 3-year-old diagnosed with measles. Which precautions should the nurse initiate? **Select all that apply.**

    1. droplet precautions
    2. hazmat precautions
    3. contact precautions
    4. airborne precautions
    5. universal precautions

99. The nurse is preparing to hang a unit of blood on a client. The blood has been checked off with two RNs and the pre-infusion vitals recorded. The nurse is at the bedside monitoring the infusion. Shortly after beginning the infusion, the pump alarm sounds. The IV has infiltrated. No blood has yet reached the client. The client is a hard stick, and the nurse realizes that a line cannot be placed within the time frame to begin the infusion. Which action by the nurse is correct?

    1. return the blood and the tubing to the blood bank for storage until an IV can be placed
    2. place the blood bag and tubing in the medication refrigerator until an IV can be restarted
    3. cancel the order for blood and notify the health care provider that the client has no access
    4. wait until 30 minutes has passed while IV placement is attempted, and then waste the blood and chart it as expired
    5. return the blood to the blood bank and notify the next shift when they arrive that they need to start an IV and administer the blood

100. A nurse is working in the cardiac unit when a Code Pink (infant abduction) is called. Which action by the nurse is the **best** response to the code?

    1. nothing; she does not work in the pediatric area
    2. search in empty rooms or unlocked closets for the infant
    3. avoid taking the elevator down to the lab until the all clear is called
    4. stay alert for someone who matches the description of the person of interest
    5. tell the visitors that they must leave since a code was called for an infant abduction

101. The nurse is caring for an elderly client with dementia. The family wishes to take the client home instead of placing her in an assisted living facility. Which information should the nurse include in his discharge teaching? **Select all that apply.**

   1. the names of community resources that can help families who provide care at home

   2. that the health care provider will not be happy that the client is going to live at home

   3. the advantages of having the client cared for in an assisted living facility instead of at home

   4. the contact information for the social worker in case the family has questions or needs after returning home

   5. home safety information, such as removing trip hazards and having adequate lighting at night for the client

102. The nurse is educating a couple about permanent methods of birth control. Vasectomy for the male is discussed. The nurse explains that which organ is cut or sealed off to prevent sperm from entering semen?

   _____

103. A client scheduled for a cardiac catheterization tells the nurse, "My mother died during this same procedure 10 years ago. I'm afraid the same thing will happen to me." Which of the following responses by the nurse is the **most** appropriate?

   1. "It's normal to be scared. You are safe here. Let's discuss the procedure."

   2. "I'll ask the cardiologist to come and speak with you about your concerns."

   3. "We have the best outcomes of any facility in the area for this procedure."

   4. "Don't worry. The procedure has improved a lot in the last 10 years."

104. The nurse is interviewing a client with clinical depression. Which of the following risk factors would the nurse expect to find in the client's history? **Select all that apply.**

   1. normal childhood

   2. family history of depression

   3. recent major life change

   4. Lipitor used to treat high blood pressure

105. A young male client who has recently become a quadriplegic makes a sexually inappropriate comment to the nurse. Which of the following statements by the nurse would be **most** appropriate?

   1. "It is inappropriate to speak me or any nurse that way."

   2. "While you're attractive, I'm married."

   3. "Don't you have a fiancé?"

   4. "I'm old enough to be your parent."

106. The nurse is infusing total parenteral nutrition (TPN) through a peripherally inserted central catheter. The client's TPN was turned off for 1 hour for an MRI. Which action by the nurse is **most** appropriate for this client?

    1. notify the health care provider for further orders

    2. discard the volume of the TPN that should have been administered and make a note in the chart

    3. double the flow rate on the infusion for 1 hour to keep the TPN on schedule, and then resume the normal flow rate

    4. increase the flow rate on the infusion for two hours to keep the TPN on schedule, and then resume the normal flow rate

107. The nurse is precepting a student nurse on the medical-surgical unit. The student nurse is preparing to administer insulin. Which action by the student nurse calls for immediate intervention?

    1. The student nurse verifies the insulin dose with another nurse.

    2. The student nurse draws up regular insulin to be given intravenously.

    3. The student nurse draws up intermediate-acting (NPH) insulin, and then regular insulin.

    4. The student nurse draws up regular insulin, and then intermediate-acting (NPH) insulin.

108. The nurse is providing discharge teaching to a client newly diagnosed with heart failure. Which statement by the client indicates an understanding of the side effects of furosemide (Lasix)?

    1. "I should eat bananas, dried dates, or peaches every day."

    2. "I should check my heart rate before taking this medicine."

    3. "I will avoid foods containing tyramine while on this medicine."

    4. "I will not take the medicine when I have to go on a long car trip."

109. The nurse is preparing to deliver an infusion of vancomycin through a client's peripherally inserted central catheter (PICC). Shortly after the infusion begins the IV pumps beeps, indicating a blockage. How should the nurse proceed? **Select all that apply.**

    1. start a peripheral IV in the opposite limb

    2. notify the PICC nurse if unable to clear the blockage

    3. use a 5 mL syringe to flush the PICC with sterile saline

    4. ask the client to raise and lower the arm or cough

    5. attempt to flush the line by aggressively pushing heparin to clear the blockage

    6. use a 10 mL syringe to gently flush the PICC with sterile saline or tPA as ordered

110. The nurse is caring for a client taking vancomycin. The nurse anticipates drawing a peak and trough on this client. Which statement regarding peak and trough levels is correct?

   1. The peak is drawn 1 hour after the infusion, and the trough is drawn right before the next scheduled dose.

   2. The peak is drawn 2 hours after the infusion, and the trough is drawn 1 hour before the next scheduled dose.

   3. The peak should be drawn immediately after infusion, and the trough is drawn right before the next scheduled dose.

   4. The peak should be drawn 30 minutes before the next scheduled dose, and the trough drawn immediately after the infusion.

111. The nurse is caring for a client receiving IV vancomycin. The trough level is 14 mcg/mL. The next dose is now due. What is the correct response by the nurse?

   1. give the next dose as ordered

   2. wait 2 hours and redraw the trough

   3. wait 30 minutes and redraw the trough

   4. hold the dose and notify the health care provider

112. The nurse is preparing to discharge a client diagnosed with gout. Which statement by the client indicates understanding of dietary restrictions while managing gout?

   1. "I should avoid beer, anchovies, and liver."

   2. "I should avoid bananas, grapefruit, and oranges."

   3. "I should avoid dairy products such as milk and ice cream."

   4. "I should avoid red wine, dark chocolate, and aged cheeses."

113. The nurse is assessing a client who has a sacral pressure ulcer. The wound has partial thickness, loss of dermis and a red-pink wound bed. No slough is present. How would the nurse chart this wound?

   1. Stage I

   2. Stage II

   3. Stage III

   4. Stage IV

   5. unstageable

114. A child who ingested 18 500-mg acetaminophen tablets 30 minutes ago is seen in the ED. Which of these orders should the nurse do **first**?

   1. activated charcoal per pharmacy

   2. start an IV with D5W to keep the vein open

   3. gastric lavage PRN

   4. acetylcysteine (Mucomyst) for age per pharmacy

115. The nurse is caring for a client with a stage II sacral ulcer. Which nursing intervention would be most effective in promoting healing?

    1. a heat lamp positioned 12 inches from the skin for 10 minutes twice a day
    2. antibiotic therapy as ordered
    3. increasing the client's nutritional intake of protein and calories
    4. wet to dry dressings once every shift

116. The nurse is preparing the client for surgery. The pre-op medication includes atropine sulfate 0.4 mg, meperidine (Demerol HCl) 50 mg, and promethazine hydrochloride (Phenergan) 25 mg IM. Which action should the nurse do **first**?

    1. make sure the surgical permit is signed
    2. ask the client to go to the bathroom
    3. explain the purpose of the medication to the client
    4. ask family members to exit the room

117. A nurse on the medical floor notices an increase in urinary tract infections (UTIs) among clients with indwelling urinary catheters. He records the findings and works with the unit manager and another nurse to develop a UTI risk assessment tool. Which is the correct description of the nurse's actions?

    1. advocacy
    2. client rights
    3. consultation
    4. quality improvement

118. The nurse is admitting a client directly from a health provider's office. The client has a rash and has been diagnosed with measles. Which room assignment by the nurse indicates an understanding of the disease process of measles?

    1. a private negative-pressure room
    2. a semiprivate room with a client who has a broken femur
    3. a semiprivate room with a client diagnosed with type 1 diabetes
    4. a private room at the end of the hall away from the nurses' station

119. The charge nurse in a cardiac ICU is precepting a student nurse. Which action by the student nurse requires **immediate** intervention by the charge nurse?

    1. The student nurse stops the tube feeding to measure residual.
    2. The student nurse lifts the urinary catheter bag up and over the client while turning her.
    3. The student nurse scans the client armband and the medication barcode when administering medication.
    4. The student nurse observes two other nurses verifying and administering blood to the client while the student nurse records the vital signs just prior to administration.

120. The nurse is caring for a group of clients who are experiencing pain. Which client is the **priority** for the nurse to see first?

   1. a client with dull abdominal pain and constipation

   2. a client complaining of pain 6/10 due to sickle cell crisis

   3. a client with severe chest pain experiencing an acute myocardial infarction (MI)

   4. a client who had a laparoscopic appendectomy yesterday with mild incision pain

121. The nurse is caring for a client diagnosed with C. diff. The client has soiled the bed and the nurse is preparing to change it. Which action by the nurse is correct in regard to handling soiled linens that have been exposed to C. diff?

   1. throw the linens in the trash can in the soiled utility room

   2. leave the dirty linens in a bag in the client's room until he is discharged

   3. place the items in a red biohazard bag and place them in the soiled utility room

   4. place the soiled linen in a regular dirty linen bag and place in the soiled utility room

122. A nurse is planning care for a client with human immunodeficiency virus. The nurse knows to wear gloves under the following circumstance(s). **Select all that apply.**

   1. when there is an open wound

   2. during all client contact

   3. when starting an IV

   4. when drawing blood for a specimen

123. The nurse is caring for a client admitted with chest pain and atrial fibrillation. The nurse accidentally gives the client the wrong dose of digoxin. The client is monitored throughout the shift and no ill effects are noted. Which actions by the nurse are correct? **Select all that apply.**

   1. fill out an incident report and make a note of it in the nurse's notes

   2. print out rhythm strips every 2 hours and place on the client's chart

   3. fill out an incident report and notify the health care provider for further orders

   4. notify the health care provider at the end of the shift, since no ill effects were observed

   5. notify the pharmacy that they loaded the wrong dose in the automatic medication dispensing system

124. Two nurses are preparing to pull a client up in the bed. Which actions by the nurses are correct in regard to safe client handling? **Select all that apply.**

   1. place the bed in the lowest position possible

   2. ask the client to cross her arms over her chest if she is able

   3. use a patient lifting device, such as a Hoyer lift, if needed

   4. extend the elbows out away from the body while pulling client up

   5. place the head of the bed flat or slightly Trendelenburg if the client can tolerate it

125. The nurse is preparing her client for an MRI to evaluate intracranial hemorrhage. Which finding in the client history would prompt the nurse to notify the health care provider?

    1. vertigo

    2. atrial fibrillation

    3. allergy to contrast dye

    4. past military duty in Iraq

126. The nurse finds a client crying after she was told hemodialysis is needed due to the development of acute renal failure. Which intervention is **best**?

    1. refer the client to the chaplain

    2. quietly sit with the client

    3. arrange for a hemodialysis client to speak with her

    4. leave the client alone

127. While terminating the therapeutic nurse-client relationship, which action should be avoided?

    1. raise a new issue with the client

    2. review accomplishments of the relationship

    3. refer the client to a community support group

    4. allow the client to express his feelings about ending the relationship

128. A 53-year-old client had a colostomy 2 days ago due to colon cancer and is having trouble adjusting to it. Following this procedure, which condition is **most** common?

    1. disturbed body image

    2. panic attacks

    3. impaired mobility

    4. acute pain

129. The oncology nurse is caring for a 24-year-old male client with testicular cancer. Cisplatin IV has been ordered. Which lab value would the nurse notify the health care provider about before administering this medication?

    1. iron 129 mcg/dL

    2. ammonia level 52 mcg/dL

    3. creatinine clearance 23 mL/minute

    4. brain natriuretic peptides (BNP) 36 pg/mL

130. The nurse is caring for a client in the clinic who takes captopril and ramipril for hypertension. The health care provider renews the client's prescriptions and leaves the room. Which comment by the client would prompt the nurse to notify the health care provider **immediately**?

   1.   "I am able to start walking longer at the gym without getting tired."
   2.   "Occasionally I am slightly dizzy when standing, so I get up slowly."
   3.   "I don't get short of breath anymore now that my blood pressure is controlled."
   4.   "I am going to my gynecologist tomorrow for my 12-week pregnancy checkup."

131. The nurse is preparing to administer streptomycin 0.25 g. The directions say to reconstitute with 9 mL of sterile water for a concentration of 400 mg/2 mL. How many mLs will the nurse give? **Fill in the blank.**

   _____

132. A client has orders for ampicillin 350 mg IM daily. The directions state to reconstitute with 3.5 mL of sterile water for a concentration of 500 mg/mL. How much will the nurse give?

   _____

133. The nurse is caring for a client with a wound that presents with full-thickness tissue loss and eschar covering the wound bed. The nurse would record this wound as which stage?

   1.   Stage I
   2.   Stage II
   3.   Stage III
   4.   Stage IV
   5.   unstageable

134. The nurse is monitoring the labs of a client admitted with viral hepatitis. Which of the following lab findings would the nurse expect for this client? **Select all that apply.**

   1.   decreased ALT levels
   2.   increased AST levels
   3.   elevated ammonia levels
   4.   low serum albumin levels
   5.   shortened prothrombin time

135. The clinic record for a client reads: *gravida 3, para 2*. The admitting nurse is most correct to confirm which prenatal history?

    1. The client has been pregnant three times and had two stillbirths.

    2. The client has been pregnant three times and had two children born after 20 weeks' gestation.

    3. The client has been pregnant three times and had two miscarriages.

    4. The client has been pregnant three times and had two children born after 24 weeks' gestation.

136. A nurse is floated to oncology from the postsurgical floor. The assigned client is almost finished with an infusion of doxorubicin for breast cancer. The floated nurse is not chemotherapy certified. Which nursing action is the **priority** in this situation?

    1. assess the client's pain

    2. ask another nurse about side effects of the drug

    3. assess the IV site, including the date on the tubing and IV site

    4. inform the charge nurse that she is not chemotherapy certified and ask for another assignment

137. The nurse is teaching a newly diagnosed client about Crohn's disease but discovers that the client has several barriers to learning. The nurse understands that socioeconomic barriers to learning include which factors? **Select all that apply.**

    1. cognitive delays

    2. low level of literacy

    3. adequate health insurance

    4. lack of access to health resources

    5. lack of interest in learning about disease

138. A client has orders for a heparin drip with 20,000 units in a 250 mL bag. The heparin must be delivered at 750 units per hour. What rate will the nurse set for the IV?

_____

139. A school nurse is approached by a student who says that her friend has been cutting herself on the arms. The student asks the nurse not to tell anyone. Which response by the nurse is correct?

    1. "I have to notify her parents, because this affects her personal safety."

    2. "I won't tell anyone, but let me know if she starts talking about suicide."

    3. "I will call the hospital and let them send a psychiatrist to do an evaluation on your friend."

    4. "I will make it a point to run into her in the hall and notice the cuts on her arms so I can ask about them."

140. Place in order the steps a nurse should take when removing a gown from a client in isolation. All steps are to be used.

   1. peel gown from shoulder toward hand on each arm

   2. hold removed gown away from body

   3. unfasten neck and then waist ties

   4. roll gown into a bundle and discard into an appropriate receptacle

141. A client is scheduled for a CT with and without contrast to rule out diverticulitis. Which medication on the client's medication list would be of concern to the nurse?

   1. paroxetine (Paxil)

   2. gabapentin (Neurontin)

   3. metformin (Glucophage)

   4. methocarbamol (Robaxin)

142. The nurse is caring for a client taking levothyroxine (Synthroid) for hypothyroidism. Which finding indicates a side effect of this medication?

   1. weight loss

   2. weight gain

   3. light sensitivity

   4. excessive sleepiness

143. Mix and Match: Match the therapeutic position with a reason for assuming the position.

Position	Reason
1. Fowler's	prevent pulmonary aspiration
2. lithotomy	nasogastric tube in place
3. prone	administering an enema
4. reverse Trendelenburg's	gynecological procedures
5. Sim's	post neck surgery

144. A client admitted with hepatic encephalopathy continues to attempt ambulation without assistance despite repeated instruction. Which intervention should the nurse take to promote safety?

   1. administer Xanax 6 mg PO

   2. apply a vest restraint device

   3. request a family member stay with the client around the clock

   4. move the client closer to the nurses' station

145. A 23-year-old woman who is 16 weeks pregnant is seen by the nurse for a routine maternal-child clinic appointment. The client has had erratically controlled type 1 diabetes since 12 years old. The client asks the nurse if she is at risk during her pregnancy. The nurse instructs the client she should do which of the following actions to limit complications for both her and her baby? **Select all that apply.**

    1. eat healthy foods
    2. refrain from exercise
    3. take medications as directed
    4. monitor her blood sugar before every meal

146. The nurse is teaching a client with limited mobility about preventing blood clots. Which statement by the nurse is correct?

    1. "Do not cross your legs when sitting."
    2. "Avoid riding in a car for more than two hours."
    3. "Put a pillow under your knees when lying in bed."
    4. "You should ask your doctor to give you a blood thinner."

147. A client is scheduled for a hypophysectomy following the discovery of a pituitary gland tumor. The nurse is teaching the client about the procedure. Which statement by the client indicates effective learning? **Select all that apply.**

    1. "I should brush my teeth with a soft toothbrush."
    2. "I can remove the pad under my nose the next morning."
    3. "I will avoid bending my head down or bending forward."
    4. "I will not blow my nose until cleared by my health care provider."
    5. "I will need to breathe through my mouth due to the nasal packing."

148. The nurse has orders for dopamine at 20 mcg/kg/min. The bag has 500 mg of dopamine in 500 mL. The client weighs 60 kg. What rate will the nurse set?

    _____

149. The oncoming nurse receives report on a group of clients. Which client should have **priority** during the nurse's rounds?

    1. a client who just returned from surgery for an open appendectomy
    2. a client with a blood pressure of 184/86 who has not received the morning dose of lisinopril
    3. a client who is on a 100% non-rebreather mask with an oxygen saturation level of 96%
    4. a client with COPD who is on 2L of oxygen via nasal cannula with an oxygen saturation level of 90%

150. The client has an order for Claforan 665 mg. The directions say to reconstitute with 10 mL of bacteriostatic water to yield a concentration of 95 mg/mL. How many milliliters of solution should the nurse administer to give the dose of 665 mg?

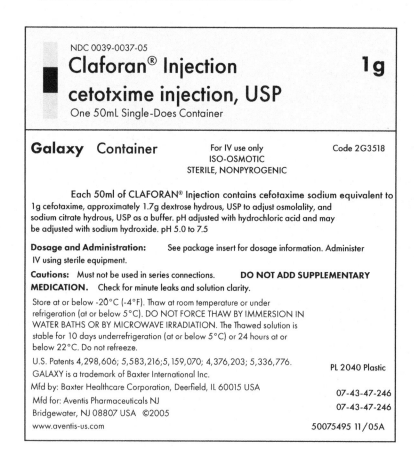

NDC 0039-0037-05

Claforan® Injection

cetotxime injection, USP

One 50mL Single-Does Container

1g

Galaxy Container

For IV use only
ISO-OSMOTIC
STERILE, NONPYROGENIC

Code 2G3518

Each 50ml of CLAFORAN® Injection contains cefotaxime sodium equivalent to 1g cefotaxime, approximately 1.7g dextrose hydrous, USP to adjust osmolality, and sodium citrate hydrous, USP as a buffer. pH adjusted with hydrochloric acid and may be adjusted with sodium hydroxide. pH 5.0 to 7.5

Dosage and Administration: See package insert for dosage information. Administer IV using sterile equipment.

Cautions: Must not be used in series connections.   **DO NOT ADD SUPPLEMENTARY MEDICATION.**   Check for minute leaks and solution clarity.

Store at or below -20°C (-4°F). Thaw at room temperature or under refrigeration (at or below 5°C). DO NOT FORCE THAW BY IMMERSION IN WATER BATHS OR BY MICROWAVE IRRADIATION. The Thawed solution is stable for 10 days underrefrigeration (at or below 5°C) or 24 hours at or below 22°C. Do not refreeze.

U.S. Patents 4,298,606; 5,583,216;5,159,070; 4,376,203; 5,336,776. GALAXY is a trademark of Baxter International Inc.

Mfd by: Baxter Healthcare Corporation, Deerfield, IL 60015 USA

Mfd for: Aventis Pharmaceuticals NJ
Bridgewater, NJ 08807 USA ©2005

www.aventis-us.com

PL 2040 Plastic

07-43-47-246
07-43-47-246

50075495 11/05A

PRACTICE TEST ONE ANSWER KEY

1.   Number 1 is correct.

Rationale: HIPAA rules do not allow clients in a substance abuse facility to be interviewed, even if the client agrees to do so. Not only was the client shown on TV, but other clients were also shown in the dayroom, which violates their right to privacy. The *need to know* rule applies when releasing client information to those providing direct care to the client, but not to others who are not involved in the client's care. There is no indication in this scenario that the client is a minor.

2.   Number 3 is correct.

Rationale: Before launching a discussion, the nurse must be aware of the client's knowledge and understanding of the different treatments. Understanding the client's background will guide the nurse in what information to reinforce to the client, or highlight areas the client may want to explore further with the health care provider. Telling the client about local support groups is helpful, but the nurse's response implies that the client will choose chemo. Telling the client not to worry because the doctor will select the best course of treatment is belittling and also implies that the decision will be made for her, not with her. Telling the client not to take chemo is offering the nurse's opinion, giving advice, and shuts down the opportunity for further discussion.

3.   Number 3 is correct.

Rationale: The Patient's Bill of Rights was adopted by the President's Advisory Commission on Consumer Protection and Quality in the Health Care Industry. This bill states that all clients are entitled to be screened and receive stabilizing treatment from emergency services, regardless of the ability to pay. HIPAA prohibits the release of private health information. There is no Continuity of Care Act. The Code of Ethics for Nurses provides guidance on professional practice based on ethical principles.

4.   Number 4 is correct.

Rationale: The LPN can perform wound dressing changes without oversight from an RN. An LPN cannot hang blood, so the client receiving blood would not be the best assignment. Clients who have had a heart catheterization require frequent site assessments of the puncture site, which is beyond the scope of practice for an LPN. The client on the nitroprusside drip may require titration, which is also beyond the scope of practice for an LPN. Caring for an arterial line requires site assessment, troubleshooting, and calibrating the transducer, which is an advanced RN skill.

5.   Numbers 2, 4, and 5 are correct.

Rationale: Clients in restraints must be offered toileting and nutrition every 2 hours. Restraints should be checked every 2 hours for proper placement, and the skin assessed. Documentation of restraints includes type of restraint, the need for continued use, and the results of a trial release. Many facilities require that a trial release be performed on clients with restraints at least once per shift. Restraints should be tied with a quick-release knot in case of emergency. Restraint orders must be renewed every 24 hours, and they may not be written on a PRN basis. Follow facility guidelines when caring for restrained clients.

6.   Number 3 is correct.

Rationale: Since the medication was left out, there is no way to be sure that it was not tampered with or contaminated; therefore, the nurse should dispose of the syringe in the sharps container and draw up a new dose of insulin. Returning the insulin to the vial increases the risk of cross-contamination, since the contents of the syringe may be contaminated. Administering the insulin after labeling it still leaves the client vulnerable, since the medication was left unattended. Option 4 is risky because the insulin in the syringe may have been contaminated or replaced by something else. Nurses should never give medications that were drawn up and then out of their sight for any period of time. If a medication error or adverse reaction occurs, the nurse is responsible due to negligence.

7. Number 1 is correct.

Rationale: The first step after discovering any medication error is to stop the infusion. The nurse should also notify the health care provider for further orders and complete an incident report. The nurse should observe the client for any signs of allergic reaction or overdose and be prepared to report to the health care provider exactly how much of the medication infused. If the wrong dose of a medication is hung, the nurse should never try to give the ordered amount by adjusting the amount to infuse. This can cause an error and may lead to serious side effects if the client is overdosed.

8. Number 2 is correct.

Rationale: The nurse should always call for clarification. Asking another nurse to transcribe the order may still result in a medication error. While most medication orders are scanned to the pharmacy in facilities using computerized medication systems, the nurse should still know which medications the client is receiving. The pharmacy may also misread the order, so the nurse should return to the source for clarification. The nurse should not attempt to guess at the medication based on the client's diagnosis or home medications, because this may also be incorrect. The nurse has a duty to clarify any unclear orders with the health care provider who wrote the orders.

9. Number 2 is correct.

Rationale: Developed in 1952 by anesthesiologist Virginia Apgar, the test rates five areas on a scale of 0 – 2, for a possible score of 10. The scores of 7 and 8 are considered acceptable. Response 2 provides an explanation to the client about the test while confirming the acceptability of her neonate's score. It is inappropriate to tell the client not to worry. Information on a special education program is unwarranted in this situation. NCLEX-RN wants to know the action of the nurse in this situation, not the physician.

10. Number 4 is correct.

Rationale: Reminiscing is a common occurrence by the elderly. The nurse should confirm this behavior with the client's wife. Redirecting the husband to speak on current events interferes with the normal pattern of reminiscing. Stating what you would do is contraindicated when interacting with the client's wife. Additionally, this statement assumes the client's wife is involved in organized religion.

11. Number 3 is correct.

Rationale: Hormone replacement therapy and weight-bearing exercises (such as walking) are recommended to prevent osteoporosis. A therapeutic dose of calcium to influence bone density for women 51 and older is 1,200 mg/day. Two ounces of hard cheese contains 500 mg of calcium, which is suboptimal. Potassium supplements are not effective in preventing osteoporosis.

12. Number 2 is correct.

Rationale: The spouse will likely need to limit her work hours at least initially to remain available to the client upon discharge. The goal of hospitalization is to return the client to maximum independence, although he may not return to normal for some time, if at all. Home health care will assist the client at home upon discharge. Nursing care involves the family as well as the client. Providing support to the client and family are within the scope of nursing practice.

13. Number 1 is correct.

Rationale: Reorienting the client to her surroundings by reviewing the reality orientation board in the room is advisable. Taking the client to a noisy room with strangers is not advisable. Obtaining an order for medication may be necessary should other activities be ineffective, but it is not the best initial intervention. Providing food and fluids would be helpful if the client is thirsty or hungry, but it is not the best initial intervention.

14. Numbers 1, 3, and 4 are correct.

    Rationale: From an Islamic perspective, prayer time is sacred and other activities should be avoided. Food brought by family members from home is beneficial as it is prepared using Islamic traditions. Modesty and privacy are honored in the Muslim tradition where care by a staff member of the same sex is preferable. Fish killed by removal from water are considered halal (lawful) and may be eaten.

15. Number 1 is correct.

    Rationale: Lactated Ringer's is typically administered in the first 24 hours because its composition is similar to the extracellular fluid that has shifted from damage to the skin. D10W is less ideal than Lactated Ringer's at this time post-burn as it lacks sodium, chloride, lactate, potassium, and calcium. Plasma would be administered in the next 24 hours. Normal saline will not meet the fluid and electrolyte requirements for the client at this stage in his recovery.

16. Numbers 1, 2, and 4 are correct.

    Rationale: Music, stretching exercises, and relaxation are proven nonpharmacological pain management techniques that the nurse is able to teach the client. Therapeutic massage for the purpose of pain management is performed by a licensed massage therapist.

17. Numbers 2 and 4 are correct.

    Rationale: Anxiety increases sympathetic stimulation to the bowels, thereby increasing symptoms. Reducing anxiety will lessen the incidence of IBS episodes. The precise mechanism on how probiotics aid in IBS symptoms is not known, but it is thought to alter the bacteria found in the intestines. Ingestion of cold liquids will increase intestinal mobility that is contraindicated in IBS. Further, caffeine is considered a trigger food for symptoms of IBS. Fluid intake should be increased to compensate for fluid loss associated with frequent bowel elimination.

18. Number 4 is correct.

    Rationale: Auditory diversional activities, such as radios and CDs, should be encouraged. Regular-size printed material will not be readable. Instead, provide the client with large-size printed instructions. Stand to the side of the client when addressing her as central vision is impaired with AMD. Adequate lighting, such as natural or halogen, is preferred to improve vision for patients with limited acuity.

19. Number 3 is correct.

    Rationale: Proper lighting allows the client to see your face, improving communication. In many types of hearing loss, the ability to hear higher-pitched tones is lost. Unless you know the client knows sign language, this communication form will frustrate the client. Gentle touching allows the client to know where you are located.

20. Numbers 4 and 5 are correct.

    Rationale: Antacids interfere with absorption of tetracycline, along with food, milk, and milk products. Aluminum, calcium, and magnesium decrease absorption of the drug. It may be taken on an empty stomach with another liquid besides milk. Grapefruit juice does not interfere with tetracycline, which should be given on an empty stomach at least one hour before meals or two hours afterward. Tetracycline should be given with caution in clients with renal or liver dysfunction, and blood panels should be monitored.

21. Numbers 1, 3, and 4 are correct.

    Rationale: Tetanus, chlamydia, and Lyme disease are designated as reportable diseases by the CDC. Reportable diseases are considered to be a national concern due to their seriousness, the risk of death, or the ease with which they spread. Untreated tetanus can lead to laryngospasm, pneumonia, pulmonary embolism, and difficulty breathing. Chlamydia can cause permanent damage to a woman's reproductive system and may cause a potentially fatal ectopic pregnancy. Lyme disease can spread to any organ in the body and may cause permanent damage to the brain, heart, and neurological system. Scarlet fever and group B streptococcal infection are not reportable under current CDC guidelines.

22. Number 4 is correct.

    Rationale: The first action is to notify the health care provider for further orders. The nurse should never induce vomiting, as this may cause more harm to the client. Obtaining vital signs is important but can be done after the health care provider is notified. An incident report should be completed following the facility guidelines once the situation is under control and the client has been stabilized.

23. Number 4 is correct.

    Rationale: Respiratory depression can become life-threatening if not treated early. Hiccups are not life-threatening. Lethargy and drowsiness are common side effects with anxiolytic and benzodiazepine medications.

24. The infusion rate is 7mL/hr.

    Solution:

$\dfrac{\text{ordered amount of drug} \times \text{weight in kg} \times 60 \text{ (min per hr)}}{\text{drug concentration}}$ = mL/hr	Solve using the formula.
$\dfrac{50 \text{ mg nitroprusside}}{250 \text{ mL D5W}}$ = 0.2 mg/mL	Find dose per milliliters
0.2×1000 = 200 mcg/mL	Convert milligrams to micrograms.
$\dfrac{0.3 \text{ (ordered amount)} \times 70 \text{ kg} \times 60 \text{ min}}{200 \text{ mcg/mL}}$	Input into formula and solve.
$\dfrac{1260}{200}$ = 6.3 mL/hr	
= 7 mL/hr	Round up to find the IV infusion rate.

25. The client should receive 32 gtts/min.

    Solution:

$\dfrac{\text{volume (mL)} \times \text{drop factor (gtts)}}{\text{time (min)}}$ = flow rate in gtts/min	Solve using the formula.
$8 \times 60 = 480$ min	Convert hours to minutes.
$\dfrac{1{,}000 \text{ mL} \times 15 \text{ gtts}}{480 \text{ min}}$	Input into formula and solve.
$\dfrac{15{,}000}{480}$ = 31.25	
= 32 gtts/min	Round up to find gtts/min.

26. The client should receive 7 gtts/min.

Solution:

$\dfrac{\text{volume (mL)} \times \text{drop factor (gtts)}}{\text{time (min)}}$ $= \text{flow rate in gtts/min}$	Solve using the formula.
$12 \times 60 = 720$ min	Convert hours to minutes.
$\dfrac{500 \text{ mL} \times 10 \text{ gtts}}{720 \text{ min}}$	Input into formula and solve.
$\dfrac{5,000}{720} = 6.94$	
= 7 gtts/min	Round up to find gtts/min.

27. Numbers 1, 2, 3, and 4 are correct.

Rationale: With viral hepatitis, lab findings include increased AST and ammonia levels. Serum albumin and ALT levels decrease. Prothrombin time is prolonged in viral hepatitis.

28. Numbers 1, 2, 4, and 5 are correct.

Rationale: Hepatitis D coexists with hepatitis B and intensifies the acute symptoms. Hepatitis A can occur at any time of the year and is spread via uncooked shellfish, contaminated water or milk, and contaminated fruits and vegetables. Hepatitis B is spread by contact with blood or body fluids, sexual contact, sharing dirty needles, and contact with infected semen or saliva. Hepatitis A is seasonal and tends to occur mainly during the fall and early winter. Hepatitis D is spread by contact with blood and blood products.

29. Numbers 2, 4, and 5 are correct.

Rationale: Following a craniotomy, the nurse should monitor the pupils for signs of increased intracranial pressure. Report dilated or pinpoint pupils or pupils that are slow to react or nonreactive to light to the health care provider. Respiratory status is monitored closely, as even minor hypoxia can increase cerebral ischemia. Notify the surgeon immediately if the dressing is saturated or if the client has more than 50 mL drainage in 8 hours, as this can cause hypovolemic shock. Immediately post-op the nurse should check the dressing every 1 or 2 hours. The drainage area can be marked once a shift to obtain a baseline. Clients with supratentorial craniotomies should be positioned with the head elevated 30 degrees in a neutral, midline position. Avoid extreme hip or neck flexion, which can cause increased intracranial pressure.

30. Number 3 is correct.

Rationale: The presence of normal saline is of concern as it should not be used in the endotracheal tube to promote secretion removal. The head of the bed should be elevated 30 – 45 degrees at all times to prevent ventilator-associated pneumonia. The cuff on the endotracheal tube should be sufficiently inflated to ensure the patient receives proper ventilator parameters. Wearing an intermittent compression device on both legs provides deep vein thrombosis prophylaxis, an appropriate measure.

31. Number 1 is correct.

Rationale: Potassium will accumulate in the blood with renal disease. As a potassium-rich food, prune juice should be avoided. Phosphorous can accumulate with renal disease. Because soft drinks contain phosphorous, only clear ones, such as ginger ale, are allowed. Dairy foods contain phosphorous, so milk intake is limited to 1 cup/day. White bread has less phosphorous than whole-grain bread and is preferred over whole-grain bread.

32. Number 3 is correct.

Rationale: The client is experiencing preeclampsia. The only cure for preeclampsia is to deliver the baby. The mother, rather than the baby, is in danger, making an amniocentesis or an ultrasound unnecessary. A C-section is not medically necessary in this situation. Given the pregnancy is 36 weeks' gestation, the lung function of the baby is sufficiently developed for delivery.

33. Number 1 is correct.

Rationale: The standard time for a bladder-retraining program to be successful is 6 to 12 weeks. The other statements are consistent with bladder retraining instructions.

34. Number 4 is correct.

Rationale: Shortness of breath is a medical emergency and can be life-threatening, so this client should be seen first. A client with a UTI and fever may be uncomfortable, but is not in any immediate danger. The client who is NPO awaiting surgery is stable and can wait to be seen. The client with nausea can be seen after attending to the client who is short of breath.

35. Number 1 is correct.

Rationale: The client awaiting a bed on the medical floor is the most stable client for this nurse, who may not be familiar with the more complicated ICU clients. Clients receiving CRRT are usually a one-on-one assignment due to the extreme complexity of managing bedside dialysis. The client on the insulin drip may require titration, which the nurse may not be familiar with. A client who is being externally paced requires special training to care for the pacer wires, and it is likely that the floated nurse will not have the experience to care for this client.

36. Number 3 is correct.

Rationale: The nurse should notify the surgeon and ask her to come talk to the client and address her concerns, even if it means the client withdraws consent and decides not to have surgery. The client may withdraw consent at any time. Telling the client she will be glad she had the surgery fails to acknowledge the client's feelings and assumes that she will proceed with surgery. Asking the client what her thoughts are will only delay the discussion with the surgeon; the client has already expressed sufficient doubt about the procedure. Telling the client that the doctor will be mad because the OR has been prepared may make the client feel guilty and possibly coerce her into having surgery she does not want. If the surgery is performed anyway, the client has a case for a lawsuit.

37. Numbers 1 and 3 are correct.

Rationale: Feeding clients and assisting stable clients up to the bedside commode are within the scope of practice for a UAP. Starting IVs is beyond the scope of practice for a UAP. The nurse must be the one to check an apical pulse before giving digoxin, as this cannot be delegated to a UAP. The nurse is using the apical pulse to determine whether or not to give a medication. Ambulating a client for the first time since surgery to the T5 should be done by the nurse to determine how well the client can balance and manage walking. Once the nurse determines that the client can safely ambulate following the surgery, a UAP may ambulate the client in the future.

38. Number 1 is correct.

Rationale: Hand hygiene is the first step in performing client care. Hand hygiene is done first to minimize contamination risk. The gown is donned and securely tied in the back. The mask is applied to fully cover the nose and mouth, forming a secure seal. Eye goggles or a face shield are donned once the mask is in place. Gloves are applied, making sure they cover the wrist of the gown.

39. Number 1 is correct.

Rationale: Measles requires airborne precautions. Droplet precautions apply to influenza. There are no special precautions for Lyme disease other than universal precautions (hand washing, avoid touching areas with a rash unless gloves are used). Lyme disease is caused by a tick bite and cannot be transmitted from one person to another. Contact precautions would be used for herpes simplex.

40. Number 1 is correct.

Rationale: A child with minor illness, such as a runny nose, may be vaccinated. The child who experienced a seizure after the last immunization should not get another dose of pertussis vaccine but may get the diphtheria and tetanus vaccine. A child who experienced a life-threatening allergic reaction after the last immunization should not get another dose. The child who has a high temperature should wait until he recovers before getting the immunization.

41. Number 1 is correct.

Rationale: The nurse should never attempt to pull a client up in bed without assistance, no matter how small the client is. The nurse risks injuring her back by doing so. The nurse should call again and wait a few moments for help. Pulling the client up by the armpits increases the risk of skin shear or a skin tear to the client. Trying to pull the client up by pulling on one side of the draw sheet at a time is ineffective and may result in skin shear on the client. If other help is not available, a lifting assistive device should be used for the client. With a client who can self-position, option 4 may be used if no other help is available and if the client can tolerate the position with the head down; however, another person or a lifting device should be used whenever possible to avoid injury to the nurse and client.

42. Number 4 is correct.

Rationale: Retinopathy, an eye complication due to breakdown of blood vessels in the back of the eye, is a chronic complication of diabetes mellitus. Hyperglycemia, diabetic ketoacidosis, and hyperglycemia are short-term complications of diabetes mellitus.

43. Number 3 is correct.

Rationale: Asking an open-ended question allows the client to verbalize her feelings and discuss health care options. Telling the client she is fine allows no opportunity to discuss her feelings. Telling the client she cannot live alone or that she should get a second opinion closes communication channels.

44. Number 4 is correct.

Rationale: Confirming how the client feels confirms the client's experience. Allowing verbalization of the loss is consistent with therapeutic communication. The first response places the need of the nurse above the client's. The second response fails to listen to the client. The third response implies disapproval of what the client is saying.

45. Numbers 1 and 3 are correct.

Rationale: Manage the therapeutic environment to provide an appropriate level of stimuli to the client. Orienting the client and explaining interventions actively engages the client in normal cognitive activities. Limiting visitors to one 15-minute visit per 8-hour shift will produce a nonstimulating environment. The level of lighting should be varied throughout the day to provide the client with a sense of normalcy.

46. Number 4 is correct.

Rationale: Cymbalta increases the body's serotonin level. A rare but life-threatening condition called serotonin syndrome may occur when someone takes two or more medications that increase the body's serotonin levels. Cough medicines that contain dextromethorphan may interact with Cymbalta and cause serotonin syndrome. The other over-the-counter medications have no known interaction with Cymbalta.

47. Number 3 is correct.

Rationale: Clients with Crohn's must have adequate nutrition to promote wound and fistula healing and prevent loss of lean muscle mass. High-calorie, low-fiber, high-protein, and high-vitamin foods should be available at every meal to maximize nutritional benefits. Coffee should be avoided, since clients with Crohn's should avoid caffeine. Enteral supplements may be given through a gastrostomy tube to supplement solid foods eaten by the client and should not cause a decrease in appetite. The diet should progress slowly, not rapidly.

48.   Number 4 is correct.

Rationale: Having the child sit on the toilet for 5 to 10 minutes about 20 to 30 minutes after meals can encourage defecation. Enemas should only be given if instructed to do so by the health care provider. The nurse cannot prescribe enemas, as this constitutes practicing medicine without a license. The nurse should also not instruct the parent to give laxatives on a daily, regular schedule. Enemas and laxatives can exacerbate certain gastrointestinal conditions. Milk and sugar intake should be decreased, not increased.

49.   Number 4 is correct.

Rationale: Feeding the infant as late as possible and putting her in bed awake without a bottle helps the infant learn to recognize cues for bedtime, and learn to fall asleep on her own. Rocking the infant will not allow her to learn to self-soothe. The infant should never be given diphenhydramine simply to make her sleep for the parents' convenience. The nurse should not act in the role of a prescriber by advising the mother to give medication to make her sleep. Infants should never share the bed with parents for safety reasons.

50.   Numbers 1, 3, and 5 are correct.

Rationale: Clients with a cerebral aneurysm need a quiet, non-stimulating environment. This client is at risk for DVT, so the appropriate DVT prophylaxis should be administered as prescribed. The client should be on bed rest in a side-lying or semi-Fowler's position. Visitors should be limited to avoid overstimulation. The client should not be encouraged to cough or perform other activities that mimic the Valsalva maneuver. Stool softeners should be given to avoid straining with bowel movements.

51.   Numbers 2, 3, and 4 are correct.

Rationale: Clients with dehydration experience increased hematocrit, orthostatic (postural) hypotension, and diminished bowel sounds. Thready pulses are a sign of dehydration. Bounding pulses would be found in clients with fluid volume excess. Urine specific gravity increases in clients with dehydration.

52.   (Correct response: DNR form)

Rationale: A DNR, or do not resuscitate order, allows the client to make his wishes known regarding care and treatments desired should he be unable to speak for himself. A DNR covers specific life-prolonging treatments such as tube feedings, artificial hydration, and code status. A DNR is a legally binding document; if a client requests to be a no-code and a code is run on him and he survives, the family or client may bring legal action against the health care provider and the facility. DNR status should be determined as soon as possible following client admission.

53.   Number 1 is correct.

Rationale: The first priority is to evaluate pain, including vital signs. Clients on a PCA must have vital signs monitored regularly due to the risk of respiratory depression from oversedation. The nurse can contact the health care provider with this information for further orders. Repositioning the client may increase comfort but is not the first priority for this client with severe pain. Nonpharmacologic measures are not likely to offer much relief to this client, and the nurse should not assume that dosages cannot be adjusted. In teaching the client and family proper use of the PCA, emphasis should be placed on the client being the only one to administer pain medication in order to avoid oversedation. If the client is unable to use the PCA, other means of pain relief should be considered.

54.   Number 3 is correct.

Rationale: PT, PTT, and INR are blood tests that monitor effectiveness of anticoagulant therapy. Hematocrit measures packed red blood cells and is not a specific study of anticoagulant effectiveness.

HDL and LDL are components of cholesterol measurement. Troponin levels measure myocardial muscle injury.

55. Number 3 is correct.

Rationale: Pain in the residual limb indicates the wrapping is too tight and should be reapplied. Peripheral vascular disease due to diabetes mellitus is a common reason for surgical removal of a lower limb. Range-of-motion exercises are standard after an amputation. Use of adaptive devices such as canes to ambulate is standard post-amputation.

56. (Correct response: Health care Power of Attorney)

Rationale: A Health care Power of Attorney is the document that names a specific person to be in charge of making health care decisions for the client if he is unable to communicate. This differs from a living will, which states which treatments the client wants to have or does not want to have.

57. Number 2 is correct.

Rationale: An INR of 4.6 indicates that the client is at risk for bleeding. Protamine sulfate is the antidote for heparin. Vitamin K is the antidote for warfarin. Redrawing labs in 6 hours is only ordered when INR is therapeutic and no changes to therapy must be made. Increasing the infusion rate greatly increases the risk of bleeding in this client.

58. Number 1 is correct.

Rationale: Rubbing the injection site is not advised as it can affect absorption. The client should check the vial of insulin for the correct type and expiration date. Insulin is a high-risk medication, and some clients may be on more than one type. Grasping the skin and inserting the needle at a 90-degree angle is correct injection technique. Prior to drawing up the dose, the rubber stopper should be cleaned with alcohol.

59. Numbers 1, 2, 3, and 5 are correct.

Rationale: Pulses and capillary refill are assessed and compared to the unaffected limb. Pulses should be equal in both feet, with brisk capillary refill. The skin should be warm. The nurse should assess the client's pain and ask her to report numbness, tingling, or inability to move the toes. Decreased pulses or capillary refill, cool skin, and changes in sensation and movement indicate a possible complication. The client is at risk of necrosis if unusual findings are not reported immediately. The nurse should not squeeze the cast for any reason. The cast can take 24 – 48 hours to completely harden, and squeezing it can create pressure points inside that can damage the skin.

60. Number 4 is correct.

Rationale: Clients without a spleen are at increased risk of infection. The spleen manufactures many antibodies, so clients should consult their health care provider about receiving vaccinations two weeks following surgery. Regular activity cannot be resumed for a period of 4 – 8 weeks after surgery. Two weeks is too soon to return to yoga. There is no need to eat a low-fiber diet to rest the digestive tract following a splenectomy. Large crowds should be avoided due to the risk of infection, so the client should not attend a sporting event within a month of surgery.

61. Number 3 is correct.

Rationale: Many clients with dementia pull out an IV because they see it and know that they don't normally have one. Placing the IV in an inconspicuous place, such as where it can be covered by the gown or wrapped up in gauze, prevents the client from pulling it out, because he cannot see it. Restraints should not be the first-line intervention for this client, as this may increase confusion and agitation. If the family can stay with the client, they can help watch, but many clients do not have family close by that can stay with them around the clock. Threatening the client with a more invasive procedure should never be used as a means of obtaining cooperation.

62. Number 4 is correct.

Rationale: Lifting heavy objects is contraindicated after cataract surgery as this will increase intraocular pressure on the newly operated eye. Wearing glasses outside is recommended after surgery to protect from infectious agents. Bending below the waist increases intraocular pressure on the newly operated eye and is contraindicated. Anticoagulants should be stopped as this predisposes the patient to hemorrhage.

63. Number 2 is correct.

Rationale: The client is experiencing symptoms of a pulmonary embolism. The best action by the nurse is to place the client in a semi-Fowler's position to enable a clear airway. Obtaining vital signs would be action number 2, to compare to established baseline data. Administering oxygen as ordered would be the third response to provide adequate oxygenation of the client. Last, prepare the client for diagnostic tests such as blood gases, ventilation-perfusion lung scan, and pulmonary angiography.

64. Number 4 is correct.

Rationale: SLE is a chronic autoimmune disorder treated with a variety of medications. One such drug is an antimalarial drug that produces retinal toxicity. Eye exams every six months, rather than annually, are advised to monitor ocular changes. Avoidance of sunlight prevents the skin rash that occurs with SLE. Also, sensitivity to light is seen in persons with lupus. High-dose prednisone, commonly prescribed with severe SLE, will result in water retention and the appearance of being bloated. Due to fatigue, the work schedule is limited for persons with lupus.

65. Number 4 is correct.

Rationale: The nurse should mark a single line through the error in black ink and initial afterward. This alerts whoever reads the note that the nurse wrote information in error and has signed her initials acknowledging the correction. Some facilities may require the nurse to use *m.e.* with her initials to indicate *medical error* or a similar designation. Use the facility guidelines regarding corrections on paper charts. Wite-Out® is never used in the hospital setting. The note should not be thrown away, especially if it has charting by other nurses. Drawing a line through the error saves time in replicating a new form from scratch. Red ink should not be used to draw the line, as all paper charting should be in black, unless otherwise required by the facility.

66. Number 3 is correct.

Rationale: In the democratic form of management, the manager is concerned for each individual member and serves primarily as a resource person for the unit. The manager encourages all members of the care team to participate in setting unit goals and developing problem-solving techniques. In autocratic management, the leader is strongly focused and maintains full control over all decisions. Individuals are told what to do and are not asked for input or problem-solving strategies. The situational leader responds to current circumstances and uses a mix of the above styles as he or she sees fit. The laissez-faire form of management is very laid back; the manager has a passive approach and the group makes decisions with little direction from the manager.

67. Number 4 is correct.

Rationale: Propofol is an anesthetic agent and therefore a controlled substance. Most hospitals require licensed nurses to pick up controlled substances. Asking the unit secretary or the UAP to pick up propofol is outside their scope of practice. The health care provider is not responsible for picking up medications from the hospital pharmacy. The nurse should ask another nurse to look after her clients while she runs the errand to the pharmacy. Before leaving the unit, the nurse should give report to the nurse who will watch the clients, as this is important for client safety.

68. Number 1 is correct.

Rationale: The focus of the nurse's role as an advocate is to teach the client the necessary skills to manage her diabetes, making number 1 correct. The other actions, while important, do not directly provide the client with the necessary skills to manage her disease.

69. Numbers 2, 3, and 4 are correct.

Rationale: Facility guidelines should always be followed in this situation in order to protect clients and staff. Mock drills can be beneficial training tools so that each staff member understands his or her role in crisis management. If possible, the nurse can try to obtain details about the bomb, which can help security and police locate the bomb and determine the level of risk. The nurse should immediately notify authorities so that the facility's emergency plan can be activated. Bomb threats or other threats should always be taken seriously in order to protect lives. The nurse should not evacuate or move clients until directed to do so by security or police; they can determine the safest area if evacuation is necessary.

70. Number 3 is correct.

Rationale: Remind the client that oxygen is highly flammable and that smoking is banned throughout the facility. If the client continues to smoke in the room, notify security so that they can intervene. There have been documented cases of explosions in facilities caused by smoking around oxygen, so this situation should be taken seriously and not dismissed. Escorting the client outside to smoke places the client at risk for falling, especially if he has an IV pole. It also encourages behavior that is not healthy and takes a staff member off the unit without good cause. To help prevent cravings, clients who smoke should be offered a nicotine patch upon admission when the smoking history is documented. The nurse should check and see if the health care provider ordered one as a PRN medication. If not, the nurse can ask the client if he would like a patch. Threatening the client with discharge if he is not compliant with the smoking ban does not address the situation in a safe manner and can escalate the situation.

71. Number 2 is correct.

Rationale: When caring for mentally unstable or possibly violent clients, staff safety is the primary concern. The nurse should avoid getting blocked into a corner between the client and the door. If possible, the client should be in a room near the nurses' station, and the nurse should notify someone else before he enters the room. Taking another nurse or client care technician when entering the room is another way to maintain safety. All clients should be treated with courtesy and respect, especially someone who may be prone to paranoia. It may be necessary to observe the client closely for "cheeking" pills instead of swallowing them. Some medications may be ordered in IV form in order to ensure that the client receives the medication if he has surreptitiously avoided swallowing pills in the past. Always ask permission before touching or approaching the client to avoid startling him. If the client refuses medications or blood draws, do not argue. Chart the refusal in the medical record and notify the health care provider.

72. Number 3 is correct.

Rationale: Placenta previa presents with painless vaginal bleeding. Placental abruption is the separation of the placenta from the uterine wall before delivery and is associated with serious vaginal bleeding. A urinary tract infection is associated with painful urination or discomfort in the bladder area. Uterine polyps present as irregular and/or heavy bleeding associated with a menstrual period or postmenopause.

73. Number 1 is correct.

Rationale: Problems occur during pregnancy when the mother is Rh-negative and is exposed to Rh-positive fetal blood (via a Rh-positive father). Administration of RhoGAM to the Rh-negative woman with a Rh-positive father is done twice, once between 26 and 28 weeks of pregnancy and again within 72 hours of birth.

74. Number 4 is correct.

Rationale: A cholesterol level less than 200 mg/dL is desirable for an adult without heart disease. At the stated level, this client needs to consume a low-cholesterol diet. Natural peanut butter contains no cholesterol, making this sandwich the best choice. The remaining options are high in fat that will elevate the cholesterol level.

75. Number 2 is correct.

Rationale: The nurse should give the client a sense of control by asking if he wishes to see his family. Clients in hospice typically have open visiting hours. Hospice environments encourage family visits, and neither limit the number of visitors (in this case, to two) nor disallow large groups of visitors.

76. Number 3 is correct.

Rationale: To locate the client, the nurse must first determine the direction the client went. The observer is most likely to know which path the client took. Notifying family members can wait until the client is located. Security may not be readily available. Staff will first need to know the direction the client took in order to assist in recovery.

77. Number 2 is correct.

Rationale: Applying the restraint is in compliance with hospital policy and, as ordered, provides for client safety. Moving the client closer to the nursing station is inadequate to provide a safe environment. The NCLEX-RN exam wants to see what the test taker would do rather than passing the responsibility to someone else. Monitoring the client consistent with hospital policy would be in addition to appropriate use of a restraining device.

78. Number 3 is correct.

Rationale: A tight binder is recommended for the client bottle-feeding her baby to reduce engorgement. Limiting fluid intake will not impact breast engorgement. A warm shower will stimulate milk production. As engorgement is normal several days postdelivery, seeing the physician is not necessary.

79. Number 3 is correct.

Rationale: Drinking from a straw is very problematic post-tonsillectomy for two reasons: First, the sucking motion may disrupt the clot at the operative site. Second, insertion of the straw into the mouth may disrupt the clot at the operative site. Orange juice and antiseptic mouthwash will irritate the tissue at the operative site. Milk promotes mucus production, which increases the need to swallow, potentially irritating the operative site. Still, drinking from a straw presents the most potential harm.

80. Number 2 is correct.

Rationale: Bananas help to bind the stool thereby reducing diarrhea. Drinking additional fluids should be encouraged but will not reduce the diarrhea. Prunes promote peristalsis thereby increasing diarrhea. A salad has fiber that will increase diarrhea.

81. Number 1 is correct.

Rationale: Using a condom catheter to drain urine in the least intrusive manner is the best intervention for maintaining skin integrity and preventing infection. An indwelling catheter puts the client at risk of an infection. A diaper would allow the urine to be kept in contact with the skin thereby affecting skin integrity. Offering the urinal every 2 hours is unlikely to be effective in controlling urine output.

82. Number 3 is correct.

Rationale: Music therapy is effective as an alternative therapy for chronic pain and may be done by the nurse. Yoga, acupuncture, and hypnosis may be effective alternative therapies but are not within the domain of nursing.

83. Number 3 is correct.

Rationale: Humalog, NovoLog, and Apidra are all rapid-acting insulins. Lantus and Levemir are long-acting insulins. Humulin 70/30 is an intermediate-acting insulin.

84.   Numbers 1, 2, and 5 are correct.

Rationale: TPN tubing should be changed every 24 hours or per facility protocol. IV site dressing changes should be performed every 48 to 72 hours or per facility protocol.

85.   Numbers 2 and 3 are correct.

Rationale: The most accurate method to confirm placement is by X-ray. Auscultation may not be reliable, especially with small-bore tubes. Medications should never be mixed with the tube feeding. The student nurse should hold the feeding and flush with 20 to 30 mL of water before giving any medications. She should follow medication administration with another flush and then resume feeding. Options 1, 4, and 5 are correct tube management techniques.

86.   Number 2 is correct.

Rationale: Digoxin must be taken exactly as prescribed without skipping or doubling up on doses. It should be taken at the same time each day. Options 3 and 4 indicate potential problems that need to be addressed by the health care professional.

87.   Number 3 is correct.

Rationale: The client who responds quickly, but only to commands has a Ramsay score of 3. The client with an RSS of 1 is restless, anxious, or agitated. Clients with an RSS of 2 are alert, oriented, and cooperative. Clients with an RSS of 4 respond briskly to stimulus. A client with a sluggish response to stimulus is scored as a 5. A client with an RSS of 6 is deeply sedated and does not respond to stimulus.

88.   Numbers 1, 2, and 5 are correct.

Rationale: Lithium has a narrow therapeutic range of 0.6 to 1.2 mEq/L. A level of 2.2 mEq/L indicates moderate toxicity. The nurse should notify the health care provider immediately, as severe toxicity can cause tonic-clonic seizures, coma, or death. Treatment typically involves administering IV fluids to dilute the concentration of the medication, holding the medication, and possible hemodialysis in severe cases. The client may exhibit signs of toxicity such as confusion, slurred speech, and severe diarrhea. A mechanical soft diet will not treat the toxicity. The nurse would hold the next dose and prepare to draw lab work, including lithium and electrolyte levels, BUN and creatinine, and a CBC.

89.   Number 1 is correct.

Rationale: This client is exhibiting signs of an air embolism, which is a complication of hemodialysis. The nurse should stop the dialysis immediately and turn the client on the left side in the Trendelenburg's position. The health care provider should be notified immediately. The nurse should administer oxygen and assess vital signs and pulse oximetry. Positioning the client in this manner helps to trap the air in the right side of the heart so it cannot travel to the lungs. Clotting at the graft site would be present when there is no thrill to palpate or a bruit to auscultate. A clotted graft site would not produce this client's signs. Dialysis encephalopathy is caused by aluminum toxicity from dialysate water that contains aluminum. Signs include mental cloudiness, speech disturbances, bone pain, and seizures. Disequilibrium syndrome is characterized by nausea and vomiting, headache, hypertension, muscle cramps, and confusion.

90.   Number 4 is correct.

Rationale: Clients having a renal mass removed should be placed in a prone position with a pillow under the shoulders and abdomen. Options 1, 2, and 3 are incorrect positions for this procedure.

91.   Number 2 is correct.

Rationale: Persons with suppressed or compromised immune systems, such as occurs with leukemia, are at higher risk to acquire shingles. Although rare, a second and even third episode of shingles can occur. A zoster vaccine is recommended for persons 60 years and older, the timeline for highest risk of acquiring herpes zoster.

92.   Number 1 is correct.

Rationale: The client should be allowed to gradually assume normal activities at his own pace to prevent aggression or combativeness. Medications may be administered to reduce anxiety post-seizure. The client may become disoriented, confused, or anxious as a result of the seizure, making reorientation necessary. Assessment of neurologic and vital signs should occur until the client is stable to ensure complete recovery.

93.   Number 2 is correct.

Rationale: The client will need to focus his attention on proper swallowing technique during meals, making television undesirable. Talking while eating should also be avoided. Unless recommended by a speech pathologist, use of a straw can increase aspiration by administering a bolus of liquid. As approved by the pharmacist, whole pills may be crushed and placed in a soft food item such as custard to allow complete administration. To prevent the chance of aspiration, the client should remain sitting upright after consuming a meal.

94.   Number 3 is correct.

Rationale: Continuity of care is effective in allowing each care provider to communicate complete and accurate information as the patient progresses through the health care system. Privacy, the Patient's Bill of Rights, and case management do not address the issue of handoffs between caregivers.

95.   1. posterior tibial (A)

    2. peroneal (C)

    3. dorsalis pedis (B)

    4. anterior tibial (D)

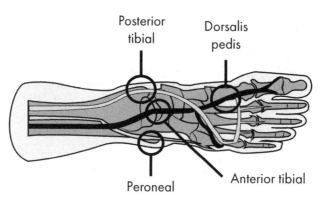

96.   Number 3 is correct.

Rationale: Administering oral medications is an appropriate activity for the LPN. The other activities fall within only the registered nurse's scope of practice.

97.   Number 2 is correct.

Rationale: Providing a comprehensive and individualized approach requires involvement of members from a variety of disciplines. The other approaches are not related to a multidisciplinary approach.

98.   Numbers 4 and 5 are correct.

Rationale: Airborne precautions are used with measles, since measles is highly contagious. The virus can remain in the air for up to 2 hours if an infected person sneezes or coughs. The client should be placed in a negative pressure room to minimize the risk of spreading the infection. All clients are placed on universal precautions. Droplet precautions are used with infections that do not usually travel farther than 3 feet from the client. Examples of illnesses requiring droplet precautions include influenza, pneumonia, and bacterial meningitis. Droplet precautions are not adequate for the measles. There is no such thing as hazmat precautions. Contact precautions are used with infections that are transmitted by direct contact, such as C. diff and MRSA.

99.   Number 1 is correct.

Rationale: Before blood is picked up, the nurse should check the IV for good blood return and verify that it is working. This saves time and is more efficient than picking up the blood first. Blood must be administered within 30 minutes of the time it leaves the blood bank. This does not leave a lot of time to restart an IV if needed. If the nurse determines that the blood cannot be started within the guidelines, the blood should be returned to the blood bank before it is spiked for administration. Once blood is spiked, there is potential for contamination. The blood should never be placed in the medication refrigerator on the unit; it must be returned to the blood bank. The nurse should not cancel the order and notify the provider that there is no access. All reasonable attempts must be made to restart the IV. If the client appears to need a PICC or other central line due to being a difficult stick, the nurse can notify the health care provider, but should not cancel an order for blood. The blood has been ordered for a reason. Blood should never be wasted. Once it is apparent that time is an issue, the blood should be returned to the blood bank before the last minute. Delaying administration and telling the next shift to start an IV is inappropriate. Blood is too important to delay to another shift, and the nurse has the duty to complete orders given on her shift. The client needing blood should never be without an IV for a long period of time, in case other fluids or emergency resuscitation is needed.

100.   Number 4 is correct.

Rationale: If a Code Pink is called, the staff should remain alert for anyone matching the description of the person of interest, even if they do not work in the pediatric area. The staff should observe anyone who is wearing a bulky coat or has a large package in their arms. While searching empty rooms and unlocked closets may be of some help, it is far more helpful to look for a person matching the description of the abductor. Elevators will not work when a Code Pink or other emergency abduction code has been called, so the nurse should take the stairs if she needs to go to the lab. It is best for visitors to remain in place and not be wandering around the facility while a search is on for the abductor.

101.   Numbers 1, 4, and 5 are correct.

Rationale: The nurse should provide information regarding client safety, as well as community resources available to the family. Providing a list of community resources will likely contain many agencies that the family is not aware of that can help them. A social worker's contact information is good to provide in case the family needs further assistance or decides to utilize home health to help the client with ADLs. Home safety is key, and the family may not be aware of all the potential hazards that the client may encounter. The nurse should address handrails in bathrooms, adequate lighting at night, avoiding the rugs since they are a fall hazard, and securing medications and chemicals. A home assessment may be conducted by a home health nurse if home health is ordered. The nurse should not tell the family that the health care provider will be unhappy or upset at their decision. The family has the ultimate right to do what they feel is best for the client, and only they understand how their financial and living situation affects how they will care for the client. Likewise, being too aggressive in pointing out the advantages of assisted living belittles the family's choice and implies that they are incapable of making a good decision for the client.

102.   (Correct answer: vas deferens)

Rationale: Vasectomy involves cutting or otherwise sealing the vas deferens to prevent sperm from entering the semen. It is considered a permanent form of birth control and is the only permanent option for men.

103.   Number 1 is correct.

Rationale: Demonstrating empathy for the client is an essential component for a therapeutic relationship, as is allowing an opportunity to verbalize feelings. Contacting the cardiologist passes responsibility for therapeutic communication on to someone else. Stating a record of good outcomes is not a component of therapeutic communication. Dismissing the client's concerns is inconsistent with establishing a therapeutic relationship.

104. Numbers 2, 3 and 4 are correct.

Rationale: Known risk factors associated with clinical depression include family history of depression and a recent major life change. Certain medications are known to cause depression in some patients including prednisone, calcium channel blockers, birth control pills, and statins. High levels of anxiety—demonstrated as irritability—are commonly seen in childhood.

105. Number 1 is correct.

Rationale: Setting appropriate boundaries is necessary to establish a therapeutic relationship. Confirming an attraction is contraindicated. Questioning the client's relationship status avoids the fundamental issue of establishing limits. Identifying an age difference between the client and the nurse fails to set limits.

106. Number 1 is correct.

Rationale: The health care provider should be notified so that the client's ability to tolerate an increased flow rate can be determined. If orders are given to increase the flow rate, the nurse should monitor for signs of fluid overload such as increased respirations and heart rate, and lung congestion. The TPN should not be discarded. Increasing TPN rates may result in electrolyte imbalance or osmotic diuresis, which can lead to severe dehydration and hypovolemic shock. It is outside the scope of practice for a nurse to adjust IV flow rates without a prescriber's order.

107. Number 3 is correct.

Rationale: If both regular and intermediate-acting (NPH) insulins are ordered for a client, the regular insulin should be drawn up first to prevent contamination with the intermediate-acting (NPH) insulin. Insulin is a high-alert drug that requires two nurses to verify the dosage. Regular insulin is the only type that may be given intravenously.

108. Number 1 is correct.

Rationale: Furosemide causes loss of potassium. Daily consumption of high-potassium foods helps prevent potassium depletion. The heart rate should be checked before taking digoxin. Foods containing tyramine should be avoided when taking MAOIs for depression. This medicine should be taken even if traveling; some patients are reluctant to take medications that cause more frequent urination while traveling. Convenience is not a reason to withhold the medication unless directed to do so by the health care provider.

109. Numbers 2, 4, and 6 are correct.

Rationale: After attempting to clear the PICC following facility protocol, the nurse should notify the PICC nurse if he is unsuccessful. The catheter may be positional, which can be corrected by having the client raise and lower the arm or cough. A 10 mL syringe should be used to flush PICCs, as smaller syringes can increase pressure within the catheter and cause it to rupture or damage the blood vessels. Starting a peripheral IV in the opposite limb would not be a first-line intervention. Depending on the IV medications the client is receiving and length of expected therapy, the health care provider will determine if the PICC can be removed and a peripheral IV placed. This should only be done with a prescriber's order. Aggressive force should never be used to try and clear a catheter, since this may cause a clot to dislodge or a fibrin tail to break off.

110. Number 1 is correct.

Rationale: Drugs requiring peak and trough levels, such as vancomycin, require precise timing in order to obtain accurate results. The peak dose should be drawn 1 – 2 hours after infusion, when drug levels are at their highest. Troughs are drawn when the drug is at its lowest level, which is right before the next dose is due. Options 2, 3, and 4 reflect inaccurate draw times.

111. Number 1 is correct.

Rationale: The nurse should give the next dose as ordered. The therapeutic range for a vancomycin trough is 10 – 20 mcg/mL, so this client is within range. There is no need to wait and redraw the trough. Since the trough level is therapeutic, there is no need to hold the medication and notify the health care provider.

112. Number 1 is correct.

Rationale: Beer, anchovies, and liver are high in purine and should be avoided in clients prone to gout. Options 2 and 3 may be included in the diet, unless there are other reasons to avoid these foods. Option 4 lists food high in tyramine, which should be avoided by clients taking certain medications, such as MAOI. Unless the client is on one of these medications, there is no need to avoid those foods.

113. Number 2 is correct.

Rationale: Stage II ulcers present with partial thickness loss of dermis and a red-pink wound bed. No slough is present. Stage I ulcers have intact skin with a red area. The area may be firm, painful, soft, or cooler or warmer compared to adjacent tissue. Stage III ulcers have full-thickness skin loss and may contain slough. The wound may have visible subcutaneous tissue, and tunneling and undermining may or may not be present. Stage IV ulcers present with full-thickness skin loss and exposed bone, muscle, or tendons. Eschar and slough may be present, and tunneling and undermining may develop. Unstageable wounds cannot be staged due to eschar or slough covering the wound. The wound bed must be visualized in order to stage the wound.

114. Number 3 is correct.

Rationale: The maximum recommended dose for acetaminophen is 4 g/day. The client ingested 9 g as a one-time dose, which is sufficient to induce liver impairment. The priority action is to remove as much of the medication from the stomach as possible. The second action would be activated charcoal. IV fluids will not affect the metabolism of acetaminophen by the liver yet may be used to maintain hydration. Acetylcysteine is effective in third-stage liver injury; given the time interval of ingestion, it would be premature to administer this pharmaceutical.

115. Number 3 is correct.

Rationale: Loss of protein in wound drainage requires high-calorie intake for proper healing. Heat directly applied to the wound will be ineffective to promote healing. Antibiotic therapy is not indicated as the ulcer is not considered infected. Wet to dry dressings are appropriate for stage III wounds.

116. Number 1 is correct.

Rationale: The surgical permit must be signed before a preoperative medication is administered. Other actions follow this initial step in this sequence: 2, 3, and 4.

117. Number 4 is correct.

Rationale: Quality improvement involves identifying areas and developing guidelines and policies to improve the quality of nursing practice. Advocacy is the process by which nurses inform clients of treatment options, side effects, and risks, and respect client choices even if they do not agree with them. The nurse is acting in the client's best interest. Client rights give the client the right to refuse treatment or care. HIPAA is another example of client rights. Consultation involves communicating with other health care professionals or disciplines to provide needed care for a client.

118. Number 1 is correct.

Rationale: Measles is highly infectious and travels via droplets in the air. Clients with measles should be isolated in negative-pressure rooms that conform to current CDC guidelines for controlling airborne infectious diseases. The client with a broken femur is just as susceptible to measles as the client with diabetes, unless he has been vaccinated, has laboratory-confirmed evidence of immunity, or was born before 1957. Optimal client safety requires the use of the negative-pressure room, regardless of the immune status of other clients. All staff and visitors entering the negative-pressure room should don appropriate personal protective equipment and follow universal precautions, in addition to airborne precautions. A private room at the end of the hall is not isolated enough to be safe without the negative-pressure room designation.

119. Number 2 is correct.

Rationale: Lifting the urinary catheter bag above the client's bladder allows backflow of urine and increases the risk of a urinary tract infection. The bag should be passed around the end of the bed, not up and over the client. Stopping a tube feeding to check residual is a correct action. Scanning the armband and medication prior to administration is the correct and safe technique to ensure client safety. Recording vital signs and observing other nurses in the blood administration process is educational for the student nurse and demonstrates proper procedure for blood administration.

120. Number 3 is correct.

Rationale: The client experiencing the MI should be seen first, as this is a potentially life-threatening event. The client with dull abdominal pain and constipation should be seen and his pain assessed, but this is not as urgent as the client experiencing an MI. Pain due to sickle cell crisis must be addressed as soon as possible, but the client with an MI takes priority. The client with mild incision pain from a laparoscopic appendectomy needs to be assessed, but the client with an MI takes priority. When prioritizing care for multiple clients in pain, the nurse should first consider pain caused by a potentially life-threatening event before seeing other clients.

121. Number 3 is correct.

Rationale: C. diff is highly contagious, and soiled linens require special handling. The nurse should bag all linens in a red biohazard bag and place in the designated area for biohazard bags in the soiled utility area. Linens do not need to be thrown in the trash can, as the laundry process requires very hot water and specific detergents to kill microorganisms for hospital settings. Dirty linens should never be left in the client's room, as this increases the risk of contamination to health care givers in the client's room. The linens should never be placed in with regular dirty linen.

122. Numbers 1, 3, and 4 are correct.

Rationale: Gloves should be worn when in contact, or potential contact, with blood, body fluids, secretions, or excretions.

123. Numbers 2 and 3 are correct.

Rationale: When a medication error is discovered, the nurse should immediately notify the health care provider and inform her of the dose ordered, the dose actually given, follow-up vital signs, and any adverse effects noted. The client with chest pain and atrial fibrillation will be on telemetry, so the nurse should run more frequent rhythm strips to chart the client's tolerance of the dose. An incidence report should be completed, but these reports are *never* mentioned in the chart. The nurse should not delay notifying the health care provider, regardless of how well the client seems to tolerate the dose. The nurse should not blame the dosing error on the pharmacy, as it is up to the nurse to verify that the dose in the package is correct. Also, there is no indication that the pharmacy loaded the wrong dose in the medication dispenser. If that were the case, a diligent nurse would catch it before the medication was given and could notify the pharmacy that the loaded doses were incorrect. In that case, the nurse should wait until the proper doses are loaded before giving the medication. The nurse is the last safety point between the medication and the client and carries the ultimate responsibility for verifying any medication before administering.

124. Numbers 2, 3, and 5 are correct.

Rationale: To avoid injury, the nurses should use proper lifting techniques when pulling a client up in the bed or turning. A nurse should never attempt to pull a client up alone, no matter how small the client is. This places the client at risk for skin shear and skin breakdown. If the client is alert and can follow commands, having her fold her arms over her chest helps streamline the body and makes pulling easier. For larger clients or clients who have no motor control, lifting devices may need to be used. All staff should be educated on the proper use of lift devices. If the client can tolerate it, placing the bed flat or slightly Trendelenburg makes it easier to pull the client up. The bed should be in a comfortable position at approximately waist height. Extending the elbows away from the body strains the arms; elbows should be held close to the sides of the body.

125. Number 4 is correct.

Rationale: Metallic items including shrapnel cannot go into an MRI because they can become dislodged. If a client has past military duty, further questioning should be done to determine if he served in combat and was exposed to any shrapnel. Caution should also be used with anyone who may have had a gunshot wound in the past. Vertigo, atrial fibrillation, and allergy to contrast dye do not affect an MRI. Clients with allergy to contrast dye may require prophylactic treatment before undergoing a CT with contrast.

126. Number 2 is correct.

Rationale: Establishing therapeutic communication by sitting quietly with the client demonstrates compassion. A referral may be warranted, but the test question seeks the correct action to be taken by the nurse. Arranging for a hemodialysis client to speak with her does not allow the client to explore her feelings with the nurse. Leaving the client alone fails to establish a therapeutic relationship with the nurse.

127. Number 1 is correct.

Rationale: Raising new issues during the ending phase of a relationship is counterproductive. The other actions are consistent with appropriate termination of a therapeutic relationship.

128. Number 1 is correct.

Rationale: A disturbed body image is most common in adjusting to a colostomy. The client should not have panic attacks, although he may not be comfortable caring for the colostomy. Mobility is not impaired after a colostomy. The client should be having less pain postoperatively.

129. Number 3 is correct.

Rationale: Cisplatin is contraindicated and should not be given to clients with a creatinine clearance below 30 mL/min. The iron level is within normal limits and is not a contraindication of administering cisplatin. The ammonia level is also within normal limits, which is important to monitor as cisplatin should be used cautiously with hepatic impairment. BNP is used to measure the severity of heart failure; this value is within the normal range.

130. Number 4 is correct.

Rationale: Ramipril is a category C drug during the first trimester of pregnancy; it is a category D drug in the second and third trimesters. Captopril is a category D drug in pregnancy. The health care provider must be notified and the medications discontinued immediately. ACE inhibitor therapy may increase exercise tolerance in clients once hypertension is controlled. Dizziness upon standing is a common side effect of ACE inhibitors, and clients should be reminded to stand up slowly from a sitting position. Improved blood pressure control decreases shortness of breath in many clients.

131. The nurse will give 1.3 mL.

Solution:

0.25 g × 1000 = 250 mg	Convert 0.25 g to mg.
$\dfrac{250 \text{ mg}}{400 \text{ mg}} \times 2$ mL	Set up a proportion to solve. Recall that the concentration is 400 mg streptomycin per 2 mL of solution.
= 1.25 mL	Solve.
= 1.3 mL	Round up to find the quantity in milliliters.

132. The nurse will give 0.7 mL.

Solution:

$\dfrac{350 \text{ mg}}{500 \text{ mg}} \times 1$ mL	Set up a proportion to solve. Recall that the concentration is 500 mg ampicillin per 1 mL of solution.
= 0.7 mL	Solve.

133. Number 5 is correct.

Rationale: Unstageable wounds cannot be staged due to eschar or slough covering the wound. The wound bed must be visualized in order to stage the wound. Stage I ulcers have intact skin with a red area. The area may be firm, painful, soft, or cooler or warmer compared to adjacent tissue. Stage II ulcers present with partial thickness loss of dermis and a red-pink wound bed. No slough is present. Stage III ulcers have full-thickness skin loss and may contain slough. The wound may have visible subcutaneous tissue, and tunneling and undermining may or may not be present. Stage IV ulcers present with full-thickness skin loss and exposed bone, muscle, or tendons. Eschar and slough may be present, and tunneling and undermining may develop.

134. Numbers 2, 3, and 4 are correct.

Rationale: With viral hepatitis, lab findings include increased AST and ammonia levels. Serum albumin and ALT levels decrease. Prothrombin time is prolonged in viral hepatitis.

135. Number 2 is correct.

Rationale: *Gravida* refers to any pregnancy, including the current one, regardless of length. *Para* refers to birth after 20 weeks' gestation whether the infant is born dead or alive.

136. Number 4 is correct.

Rationale: Chemotherapy administration and monitoring must be performed by nurses who have been certified in chemotherapy. This nurse is not certified and is not familiar with side effects or complications to be aware of. The nurse may care for another client who is not receiving chemotherapy. Client safety is always a priority, and though the nurse may observe other nurses administering chemotherapy as a learning moment, she is still prohibited from providing care that lies outside her area of training and expertise. Assessing pain and assessing the IV site are important, but not as important as ensuring that the nurse is familiar with chemotherapy administration. Asking about drug side effects is beneficial for the nurse who is not familiar with the drug, but does not address the fact that the nurse must be chemotherapy certified.

137. Numbers 1, 2, and 4 are correct.

Rationale: Cognitive delays and low levels of literacy are more common in clients in the lower socioeconomic groups than in higher income groups. Lower socioeconomic groups tend to suffer from lack of access to health resources, whether it is transportation to get to the doctor or access to a computer to look up information about their condition. Having adequate health insurance is an advantage, not a barrier to learning. A lack of interest in learning about the condition is not related to income; the client may simply be in denial about the diagnosis or not be ready to learn due to pain or fatigue.

138. The infusion rate is 9 mL/hr.

Solution:

$\dfrac{20{,}000 \text{ units}}{250 \text{ mL}}$	Divide the total units of heparin by milliliters (bag size).
= 80 units/mL $\dfrac{750 \text{ units}}{80 \text{ units}}$	Set up a proportion using the quotient, 80, and solve for units per hour, using the directive of 750 units.
= 9.38	Divide and solve.
9 mL/hr	Round down to find the infusion rate.

139. Number 1 is correct.

Rationale: The nurse has a duty to protect the client when self-harm or suicidal behavior is present. Self-harm could lead to suicide, and the nurse must inform the parents immediately. HIPAA and client privacy take a back seat to client safety. Asking the student to inform the nurse if the friend attempts suicide delays seeking help and allows the self-destructive behavior to continue. Calling the hospital and asking for a psychiatric consult is not the appropriate way to manage the situation. Telling the student that the nurse will just run into the friend in the hall is not feasible and delays getting appropriate care for the friend.

140. The correct order is 3, 1, 2, 4.

Rationale: The gown front and sleeves are considered contaminated, requiring the stated order of removing the gown (per Centers for Disease Control guidelines).

141. Number 3 is correct.

Rationale: Metformin should be held before and up to 48 hours afterward when radiologic studies require the use of IV contrast dye due to the increased risk of acute renal failure or lactic acidosis. None of the other medications are contraindicated with IV contrast dye.

142. Number 1 is correct.

Rationale: A side effect of levothyroxine is weight loss. Weight gain and light sensitivity are not side effects of this medication. Levothyroxine can cause insomnia, not excessive sleepiness.

143. Answers:

Position	Reason
1. Fowler's	nasogastric tube in place
2. lithotomy	gynecological procedures
3. prone	post neck surgery
4. reverse Trendelenburg's	prevent pulmonary aspiration
5. Sim's	administering an enema

144. Number 2 is correct.

Rationale: In an effort to maintain client safety with the least restrictive method, the nurse may apply a vest restraint device to subtly remind the client to not get out of bed. As a mild sedative, Xanax dosage would begin at 0.25 mg two to three times daily. The stated dosage of 6 mg is an excessive amount of medication. Requesting a family member to stay around the clock would inappropriately relegate the responsibility for safety from the hospital to the family. Moving the client closer to the nurses' station will not promote client safety.

145. Numbers 1 and 3 are correct.

Rationale: Adequate dietary nutrition is essential to provide necessary nutrients to both the baby and the mother. Medications should be taken as directed to help keep blood glucose in control. Exercise should be done regularly before, during, and after pregnancy. Blood sugar should be monitored as symptoms warrant since pregnancy causes the body's need for energy to change.

146. Number 1 is correct.

Rationale: Crossing the legs when sitting decreases blood flow, which may lead to clot formation. If the client is bed-bound, the nurse should tell the client to avoid crossing one leg over another while lying in bed. Telling the client to avoid car rides longer than two hours may not be practical; longer car rides can be done safely if regular breaks are taken to walk around for a few minutes. Putting a pillow under the knees restricts blood flow to the lower extremities and increases the risk of a clot. Not all clients are candidates for blood thinners; the nurse should focus on actions that the client can do to prevent clots. This engages the client in managing her own care.

147. Numbers 3, 4, and 5 are correct.

Rationale: Following a hypophysectomy, the client is at increased risk of bleeding and increased intracranial pressure. To minimize the risk of increased pressure and bleeding, the client should avoid bending the head down and putting pressure on the nose. Blowing the nose should be avoided until approved by the health care provider. The client will need to mouth breathe while the nasal packing is in place. Brushing the teeth can increase intracranial pressure, which delays healing. The drip pad should remain in place for 2 or 3 days and be removed by the surgeon or by the client following the surgeon's guidelines.

148. The infusion rate is 72 mL/hr.

Solution:

$\dfrac{500 \text{ mg dopamine}}{500 \text{ mL}}$	Find the drug concentration.
= 1 mg/mL	
1 mg (1,000) = 1,000 mcg	Convert mg to mcg.
20 mcg/kg/min × 60 kg × 60 min/hr	Multiply medication amount by client's weight and time, and solve.
= 72,000	
$\dfrac{72,000}{1,000 \text{ mcg/mL}}$	Divide quotient by 1,000 for final drop rate.
= **72 mL/hr**	

149. Number 1 is correct.

Rationale: The client returning from surgery is the priority here, especially since an open appendectomy was performed. A client with an open procedure is at greater risk of bleeding than clients who have laparoscopic surgeries. The nurse should view the dressing and verify that it is dry and intact, or note and mark any staining. The client due for lisinopril would be expected to have a higher blood pressure; the nurse can assess the client and then administer the medication early if needed. The client on the non-rebreather mask has an expected oxygen saturation level of 96%, which is in the acceptable range. The client with COPD tends to have lower oxygen saturation levels, even on oxygen. Too much oxygen can compromise breathing, as the drive to breathe is caused by being slightly hypoxic in COPD clients.

150. 7 mL

Solution:

$\dfrac{665 \text{ mg}}{95 \text{ mg/mL}} = 7$	Divide 665 mg of Claforan by 95 mg/mL.
7×1 mL	Multiply the quotient, 7, by 1 mL.
= 7 mL	Solve.

The nurse will administer 7 mL of solution.

TWO: Practice Test Two

READ THE QUESTION, AND THEN CHOOSE THE MOST CORRECT ANSWER.

1. The nurse is at the nurses' station charting when a physician comes up and says, "Since you are already logged into the computer, I need you to look up some labs on a client." The client is not cared for by this nurse. Which response by the nurse is **most** appropriate?

   1. "Let me check that for you in a moment."
   2. "Why don't you call the lab? That will be quicker."
   3. "That is not my client, but I will get his nurse for you."
   4. "I can't do that because of HIPAA, but I will let the charge nurse look it up."

2. A new nurse has just completed orientation and is working on the medical unit. The new nurse is shadowing the charge nurse as they both care for a client with a potassium level of 6.3 mEq/L. Which action by the new nurse requires intervention by the charge nurse?

   1. The nurse prepares to administer spironolactone (Aldactone) 25 mg PO.
   2. The nurse delivers the client's morning meal tray for a low-potassium diet.
   3. The nurse administers sodium polystyrene sulfonate (Kayexalate) 15 g PO.
   4. The nurse teaches the client the importance of ambulating, coughing, and deep-breathing.

3. The nurse has rounded on all the assigned clients. While rounding, several health care providers have written orders on the nurse's clients. Which order would be the **priority** for the nurse to address?

   1. furosemide (Lasix) 80 mg IV push STAT for a client with fluid overload
   2. a new insulin sliding scale for a client with a glucose level of 242
   3. perform a dressing change on a client with a stage 2 diabetic foot ulcer
   4. discharge a client who was admitted for removal of an abdominal abscess

4. An RN notices an LPN in the medication room drawing up morphine. The RN asks the LPN who it is for. The LPN states that one of her clients needs pain medication. The RN offers to administer the dose, but the LPN says, "It's ok. I can give it. I've had this client for several days and she is stable." Which is the correct response by the nurse?

    1. "Let me double-check the dose with you."

    2. "OK, but let me know if you need help with anything."

    3. "I am going to report this to the charge nurse immediately."

    4. "You shouldn't do that. Let me chart it while you give it to save time."

5. The nurse is caring for a client who has agreed to sign a HIPAA release so that her medical records can be released to her primary health care provider. The client's pen is malfunctioning, and the nurse hurriedly takes the form with her, intending to return with another pen. The nurse then becomes involved in a code and forgets about the form. The next day, the nurse returns to work and finds the form in her clipboard. Since the client started signing just as the pen quit, the nurse decides that there is enough of a signature on the form to release the information. She sends the medical records to the primary health care provider's office. Which violation has the nurse committed?

    1. released information to the wrong provider

    2. missing signature on form

    3. released the wrong client's information

    4. There is no violation.

6. The nurse is precepting a student nurse on the postsurgical floor. The student nurse needs to draw a potassium level. Which of the following statements by the student nurse is correct regarding blood draws from venous catheters?

    1. "I can obtain the sample from the short peripheral catheter if I flush it well."

    2. "I should flush with 10 to 20 mL of sterile normal saline after drawing blood from any catheter."

    3. "Drawing blood from a central venous line is less risky than sticking the client if he is afraid of needles."

    4. "I should use a syringe with a large needle to transfer blood into the test tube to avoid hemolyzing the sample."

7. A client in restraints is assigned to a newly graduated nurse. The nurse understands that which of the following are true regarding restraints? **Select all that apply.**

    1. Restraints can be chemical, mechanical, or physical.

    2. Children under 9 years of age have a 30-minute time limit in restraints.

    3. Bed rails are a form of restraint if used to prevent the client from leaving the bed.

    4. Restraints must be assessed every 2 hours for proper application and continued need.

    5. Once released, the client may be placed back in restraints for up to 24 hours if needed.

    6. Active listening, diversionary techniques, and reducing stimulation are alternatives to restraints.

8. The nurse is preparing to teach about poisonous snake bites to community members at the local recreational department. What information should the nurse provide regarding prehospital care? **Select all that apply.**

    1. Attempt to kill or capture the snake for identification purposes.

    2. Apply ice to the wound and elevate the affected extremity to the level of the heart.

    3. Immobilize the affected extremity with a splint and maintain the extremity at the level of the heart.

    4. Move the person to a safe area away from the snake and encourage rest to decrease venous circulation.

    5. Apply ice to the wound and place a tourniquet before elevating the affected extremity to the level of the heart.

9. The nurse is caring for a client with dementia who tends to wander. Which of the following actions can help with this behavior? **Select all that apply.**

    1. providing frequent toileting or incontinence care as needed

    2. assessing client for pain and treat with appropriate medications

    3. reorienting the client and use validation therapy, as appropriate

    4. allowing the client to sit in a recliner at the nurses' station for close monitoring

    5. using chemical or physical restraints to prevent the client from exiting the bed

10. The nurse is performing a neurological assessment on a client. She asks the client to smile, close both eyes, and frown. Which cranial nerve (CN) is the nurse testing?

    1. CN V

    2. CN VII

    3. CN VIII

    4. CN XI

11. The nurse is calculating the Apgar score for a newborn. Findings are as follows:

> **Heart rate:** 110
> **Respiratory effort:** good cry
> **Muscle tone:** some flexion of extremities
> **Reflex irritability:** grimace
> **Color:** completely pink

What is the Apgar score for this neonate?

    1. 7

    2. 8

    3. 9

    4. 10

12. The wife of a client with colorectal cancer (CRC) is talking to the nurse about prevention and screening of the disease. Which statement should the nurse make to the wife?

    1. "A diet low in fat and high in fiber can help lower the risk, along with eating more fruit such as oranges."

    2. "When an adult turns 40 years of age, a colonoscopy should be done to screen for CRC, regardless of family history."

    3. "Those with average risk at age 50 and up should have a colonoscopy and fecal occult blood test every five years."

    4. "Those with average risk at age 50 and up should have a colonoscopy and fecal occult blood test every 10 years."

13. A client is admitted with possible appendicitis. Which finding by the nurse would be expected in assessment of this client?

    1. a positive psoas sign

    2. a positive Murphy's sign

    3. a positive Homan's sign

    4. a positive Chadwick's sign

14. The nurse is caring for a client with end-stage kidney disease. The client says, "I have decided that I don't want any more dialysis or treatments. This is just prolonging the inevitable." The nurse responds, "You have every right to do so. I will notify the nephrologist of your wishes." Which ethical principle is being demonstrated by the nurse?

    1. justice

    2. fidelity

    3. autonomy

    4. beneficence

15. The nurse is caring for a 10-year-old client who states, "I am really good at soccer because I practice every day." According to Erikson's eight stages of development, which psychosocial crisis does this statement reflect?

    1. initiative vs. guilt

    2. industry vs. inferiority

    3. generativity vs. self-absorption

    4. autonomy vs. shame and doubt

16. The nurse is caring for a client with depression over the recent death of her father from cancer. The client states, "It's my fault. I should have insisted he get regular checkups instead of letting him put it off." The nurse responds, "You feel like it's your fault?" Which therapeutic communication technique is the nurse using?

    1. exploring

    2. reflecting

    3. restating

    4. focusing

17. Which task is included in the working phase of the nurse-client relationship?

    1. identifying the client's strengths and limitations

    2. establishing rapport and creating an environment of trust

    3. continuously evaluating progress toward the client's goals

    4. exploring feelings about the termination phase of the relationship

18. The nurse is reflecting on the client-nurse relationship. Which statement is correct regarding the orientation (introductory) phase of the relationship?

    1. identifying the client's strengths and limitations

    2. promoting the client's insight and perception of reality

    3. continuously evaluating progress toward the client's goals

    4. exploring feelings about the termination phase of the relationship

19. The nurse is caring for a client after an open reduction to the left ulna. The client's left arm is in a plaster cast with an Ace wrap for reinforcement. Which intervention by the nurse can offer nonpharmacological comfort to this client?

    1. elevate the left arm on a pillow and apply an ice pack over the approximate location of the surgical incision

    2. call the physician and obtain an order for acetaminophen (Tylenol) 650 mg PO PRN q6 hours as needed for pain

    3. advise the client that if he starts to itch under the cast, he can use a wire coat hanger or an ink pen to gently scratch up under the cast

    4. perform range-of-motion exercises twice a shift, including bending the fingers, opening and closing the hand, and lifting the arm up to shoulder level

20. A client is on bed rest following surgery for a fractured femur. The nurse is teaching the client about what to expect while on bed rest. Which dietary choice would the nurse advise the client to avoid while on bed rest?

    1. high-fiber fruits

    2. grapefruit juice

    3. goods high in fat

    4. milk or milk-based products

21. The nurse is caring for a client who is intubated and on the ventilator. The client is alert but cannot talk while intubated. Which method of communication would be the **best** choice for this client?

    1. a clipboard with pen and paper

    2. a picture board that the client could point to

    3. asking the client to mouth words while a family member interprets the meaning

    4. telling the client to blink once for yes and twice for no while asking close-ended questions

22. The nurse is precepting a student nurse who is helping to care for a client with a hip fracture. The client has Buck's traction applied. Which statement by the student nurse indicates a need for further explanation by the primary nurse?

    1. "The weight on Buck's traction should be between 5 and 7 pounds."
    2. "Buck's traction is a type of skeletal traction that helps in bone realignment."
    3. "The weights should hang freely and be checked regularly for correct positioning."
    4. "Diligent pin site care is crucial to prevent infection in clients with skeletal traction."

23. The nurse is caring for a client with a Foley catheter. While rounding on the client, the nurse notices that the client's urinary output has suddenly stopped over the last 2 hours. The client's kidney function is within normal limits. Which intervention would the nurse expect to perform? **Select all that apply**.

    1. check the tubing for any kinks or to see if it is under the client
    2. attempt to gently flush the Foley with 30 cc of sterile saline
    3. perform a bladder scan, record the results, and notify the health care provider
    4. pull back on the catheter about 6 inches, then reinsert it to see if urine flow begins
    5. assess the client for bladder distention and discomfort if the client is alert and oriented

24. The nurse is preparing a client with type 2 diabetes for a CT with contrast to evaluate diverticulitis with a possible mass. Which of the following medications on the client's medication list would be of concern to the nurse?

    1. fish oil
    2. warfarin (Coumadin)
    3. fluoxetine (Prozac)
    4. metformin (Glucophage)

25. The nurse is teaching a client on the proper technique to use an inhaler with a spacer for asthma management. Which action by the client would require intervention by the nurse?

    1. The client shakes the unit vigorously 3 or 4 times.
    2. The client places the inhaler over his tongue and seals his lips tightly around it.
    3. The client administers the next puff immediately after exhaling.
    4. After administering the dose, the client keeps his lips closed and holds his breath for at least 10 seconds before exhaling.

26. The nurse is caring for a client with cancer who is exhibiting signs and symptoms that death is near. The client's daughter says that she does not want her mother to receive morphine because it will hasten her death. What response by the nurse is **most** appropriate?

    1. "We always give morphine to clients at the end-of-life stage."
    2. "We can give oxygen instead of morphine to help with breathing and distress."
    3. "Morphine will reduce anxiety and reduce the sensation of air hunger in your mother."
    4. "We will wait until the very end to give the morphine and use nonpharmacologic measures instead."

27. The nurse is preparing to administer blood to a client with anemia. Which signs and symptoms of transfusion reaction should the nurse monitor for during the first 30 minutes? **Select all that apply.**

   1. The client has a respiratory rate of 18 breaths/minute.
   2. The client's blood pressure increases from 104/56 to 164/92.
   3. The client has an oxygen saturation level of 97% on 2L of oxygen.
   4. The client becomes restless and confused with distended jugular veins.
   5. The client complains of low back pain and a sense of impending doom.

28. The nurse is reviewing medication orders for his clients. Which order would necessitate contacting the health care provider?

   1. Paxil (paroxetine) 20 mg PO daily for a 57-year-old client with social anxiety disorder
   2. Phenergan (promethazine hydrochloride) 12.5 mg PR q12h prn for a child with Reye's syndrome
   3. Diflucan (fluconazole) 150 mg × 1 dose PO for a 24-year-old client with vaginal candidiasis
   4. Lopressor (metoprolol tartrate) 50 mg PO daily for a 48-year-old client with hypertension

29. Which statement by the client regarding sickle cell disease indicates a need for further teaching?

   1. "I should avoid strenuous exercise."
   2. "I can enjoy one glass of red wine per day."
   3. "I will avoid cigarettes and all tobacco products."
   4. "I should avoid traveling to places at high altitudes such as Denver."

30. A client with hyperkalemia is admitted to the telemetry unit. Which of the following would require notification of the health care provider? **Select all that apply.**

   1. The telemetry strip shows spiked T waves.
   2. The client has a heart rate of 53 beats per minute.
   3. The client has a heart rate of 84 beats per minute.
   4. The client does not eat the cantaloupe on his meal tray.
   5. The client's urinary output is 30 cc per hour via urinary catheterization.

31. The nurse is caring for a client with a small-bowel obstruction. A Salem sump nasogastric tube (NGT) is in place. Which finding by the nurse requires corrective action? **Select all that apply.**

   1. There is a sudden decrease in output.
   2. The NGT is set to low continuous suction.
   3. The NGT is set to medium intermittent suction.
   4. The patient is positioned in the semi-Fowler's position.
   5. The client dislodges the tube and the nurse replaces it, confirming placement by X-ray before use.

32. The nurse is caring for a client with suspected meningitis who will be having a lumbar puncture. Which statement regarding aftercare is correct?

    1. Specimen jars should be labeled and numbered and taken to the laboratory immediately and refrigerated.

    2. The nurse should position the client with the head of the bed up 20 degrees so the client can drink fluids to replace CSF removed during the procedure.

    3. The nurse should put the client in the low semi-Fowler's position with a pillow under her abdomen to increase intraabdominal pressure.

    4. The nurse should assess for numbness, tingling, pain at injection site, movement of the extremities, any drainage at the site, and the ability to void.

33. The nurse receives an order from blood cultures and sensitivity for a client. Which statement is correct concerning this test?

    1. Preliminary test results are available 36 hours to allow the organisms time to grow.

    2. Growth and identification of the organism often takes 48 to 72 hours to complete.

    3. If the client has IV antibiotics infusing, stop the infusion before drawing blood cultures.

    4. If catheter sepsis is suspected, culturing the catheter tip is more accurate for identification.

34. The nurse is teaching the parents of a client with iron deficiency anemia about administering a liquid oral iron supplement. Which statement by the parents indicates that teaching was successful?

    1. "We will give the iron through a straw."

    2. "The iron should be given just before breakfast."

    3. "We will give it with food to decrease stomach upset."

    4. "We will mix the iron with a milkshake so it will taste better."

35. The nurse is providing discharge teaching for an 8-year-old client with hemophilia. Which activity should the nurse suggest for this child?

    1. soccer

    2. field hockey

    3. piano lessons

    4. skateboarding

36. A nurse is caring for a client with Parkinson's disease who takes an MAOI as part of the medication regimen. Which item on the lunch tray would the nurse remove?

    1. cheese

    2. an apple

    3. bread with butter

    4. a cup of whole milk

37. The nurse is caring for a client with a long history of taking magnesium hydroxide for managing symptoms of peptic ulcer disease. Which finding in the client's medical history would be of concern to the nurse?

   1. asthma
   2. arthritis
   3. heart failure
   4. enlarged prostate

38. The nurse is caring for a client with a digitalis level of 2.1 ng/mL. Which signs would the nurse be alert for in this client?

   1. tinnitus
   2. flushed skin
   3. easy bruising
   4. anorexia, nausea, or diarrhea

39. The charge nurse on a surgical unit incorporates an authoritative style of leadership. Which characteristics describe this style of leadership? **Select all that apply.**

   1. involves little planning
   2. motivates staff by coercion
   3. motivates staff by supporting their achievements
   4. involves communication flow down the chain of command
   5. includes group members in the decision-making process

40. The nurse is caring for a client on the oncology unit. Which nursing activity is appropriate to delegate to the unit LPN?

   1. obtaining vital signs
   2. administering blood
   3. administering IV pain medication
   4. administering chemotherapy if the nurse is busy with another client

41. The nurse is caring for a client with advanced heart failure and cardiomyopathy. The nurse understands that involving nursing, nutritional services, cardiology, and pharmacy in the client's care team is an example of which approach?

   1. peer review
   2. team nursing
   3. multidisciplinary
   4. community nursing

42. The nurse is admitting a client with acute liver failure. According to the Patient's Bill of Rights, which responsibilities does the nurse understand to be the client's duty? **Select all that apply.**

   1. providing her own translator if she does not speak English
   2. screening and stabilization from emergency services as needed
   3. providing proof of insurance or ability to pay before care begins
   4. accepting responsibility for refusing treatments and medications that may alter health outcomes
   5. providing truthful and accurate information regarding medical history, medications, and lifestyle habits, such as drug abuse or smoking, that might affect care

43. The nurse is caring for a homeless client diagnosed with right-sided heart failure. The nurse anticipates that upon discharge the client will need assistance regarding medications, locating a shelter, and follow-up to ensure that the client can obtain transportation to the next appointment with the cardiologist. The nurse understands that this is an example of which content area of care management?

   1. advocacy
   2. delegation
   3. ethical practice
   4. continuity of care
   5. advance directive

44. The nurse is providing instruction to a client's family regarding home safety with thrombocytopenia. Which statement by the client's family indicates a need for further education?

   1. "He should use an electric razor for shaving instead of a razor."
   2. "We will use soft-bristled toothbrushes or tooth sponges for oral care."
   3. "He can no longer take aspirin or aspirin-containing products for a headache."
   4. "We should put rugs down on the hardwood floors to prevent his feet from getting cold."

45. The nurse is caring for a client with a retained placenta following a noneventful vaginal birth of a full-term infant. The nurse understands which of the following is true regarding a retained placenta?

   1. Placental fragments may be detected on an MRI or CT scan.
   2. Nitroglycerin IV may be given to promote uterine relaxation.
   3. Removing the remaining fragments helps lower the risk of postpartum infection.
   4. If placental fragments remain, the uterus will feel firm due to retained fragments.

46. The nurse is preparing to admit a client from the emergency department with tuberculosis. Which of the following should the nurse anticipate in caring for this client? **Select all that apply.**

1. fall precautions
2. droplet precautions
3. airborne precautions
4. standard precautions
5. placement in a negative airflow room
6. use of PPE, including an N95 mask or powered air purifying respirators (PAPRs)

47. The nurse is teaching safe client handling techniques to a group of student nurses. Which action by a student nurse would require intervention?

1. placing the bed at waist level while providing direct client care
2. using a mechanical lift to transfer a weak, obese client to a recliner
3. placing the bed supine and at waist level to move the client up in the bed
4. providing the client with a gait or transfer belt to assist in ambulating to toilet

48. The nurse is seeing a client and her 11-month-old baby in the clinic for a wellness checkup. Which comment by the mother would prompt the nurse to notify the health care provider?

1. "She loves to play peekaboo."
2. "She loves to look at herself in the mirror."
3. "She does not like to be around strangers."
4. "She does not try to crawl when I put her down."

49. The nurse is caring for a client who is 14 weeks pregnant. The client is asking about vaccinations that can be given during pregnancy. Which of the following vaccines does the nurse tell the client that are safe during pregnancy?

1. mumps
2. measles
3. smallpox
4. influenza

50. The nurse is caring for a pregnant client who is Rh negative. A nursing student asks the nurse for more information about the Rh factor. Which is the correct response by the nurse?

1. "If the mother and father are both Rh-negative, the mother should be given RhoGAM in the 28th week."
2. "If the mother is Rh-negative and the father is Rh-positive, the client should receive an injection of RhoGAM in the 28th week."
3. "If the mother is Rh-negative and the father is Rh-positive, the client should receive an injection of RhoGAM in the 24th week."
4. "If the mother is Rh-positive and the father is Rh-negative, the client should receive an injection of RhoGAM in the 24th week."

51. The nurse is preparing to educate a 17-year-old male about testicular cancer at a yearly physical. What information would the nurse include in her teaching?

    1. Testicular cancer is more common in men over 50.

    2. Testicular cancer has one of the highest cancer death rates.

    3. Self-examination of the testicles should be done after bathing.

    4. Self-examination of the testicles should be done before bathing.

52. The nurse is performing discharge teaching to a client newly diagnosed with hypertension and high cholesterol. Which statement by the client indicates that the nurse's teaching was effective?

    1. "I need to buy canned foods that are low in sodium."

    2. "I can substitute lean sirloin for my homemade fried chicken."

    3. "I will take a can of soup to work for lunch instead of eating a burger."

    4. "Frozen dinners are better for me than eating in the cafeteria at work."

53. The nurse is caring for a client with end-stage kidney disease and multiple organ failure. Which action by the nurse indicates an understanding of end-of-life care? **Select all that apply.**

    1. The nurse explains signs and symptoms that indicate death is near.

    2. The nurse explains to the client and family what to expect during the final phase of the illness.

    3. Cultural beliefs are acknowledged, but priority is placed on life-lengthening treatment options.

    4. The nurse avoids talking to the client about impending death to avoid upsetting him and the family.

    5. The nurse asks the client and family what their goals and wishes are regarding care, pain management, and emergency resuscitation.

54. The nurse is talking in the lounge with other nurses about grief and loss. The nurse understands which to be true regarding grief and loss? **Select all that apply.**

    1. The process of grief is detrimental to physical and emotional health.

    2. Age, gender, and culture are a few factors that influence the grieving process.

    3. The nurse must explore his own feelings about death before he may effectively help others.

    4. The nurse should discourage expression of grief and loss because it may upset other clients nearby.

    5. The nurse can help the family develop ways to relieve loneliness and depression following the death of a loved one.

55. The nurse has assessed the assigned group of clients. Which client would the nurse identify as being at the **greatest** risk for alterations in sensory perception?

    1. a client in a halo vest following an automobile accident
    2. a child with severe autism who is having a tonsillectomy
    3. a teenager who broke her leg during cheerleader practice
    4. a schoolteacher who was hospitalized for shortness of breath

56. The nurse is caring for a client who is having surgery the next morning. The client says, "I'm really scared about surgery. I've never been put to sleep before and I'm afraid I might not wake up." Which response by the nurse is the **most** therapeutic?

    1. "Why are you worried about such a minor procedure?"
    2. "We can call the doctor and cancel the surgery if you would prefer."
    3. "It's normal to be afraid of something new like surgery. Tell me how you feel."
    4. "Don't worry, you have a really good doctor and he will see to it that nothing goes wrong."

57. The nurse is caring for a client who has just been diagnosed with ovarian cancer. The nurse is using silence as an effective therapeutic response. How is silence an effective therapeutic response?

    1. It is not therapeutic; it implies that the nurse is not listening.
    2. It encourages the client to keep her feelings to herself.
    3. It allows the client time to think and reflect and lead the conversation.
    4. It allows the nurse to think about other tasks she needs to tackle to provide efficient care to all of her clients.

58. The nurse is caring for an adult who had an appendectomy 6 hours ago. Which intervention would the nurse expect to perform to promote rest and sleep? **Select all that apply.**

    1. provide a substantial meal of meatloaf, mashed potatoes, corn, and milk
    2. offer Ambien 5 mg as ordered
    3. lower the temperature of the room
    4. change bed linen

59. The nurse is taking care of an elderly client with congestive heart failure. Which of the following are the **most** appropriate nursing interventions to reduce the workload of the heart and to promote comfort and rest? **Select all that apply.**

    1. obtain daily weight
    2. provide assistance with self-care activities
    3. provide sensory stimulation
    4. check vital signs after activity

60. The nurse is preparing an adult male for a transurethral resection of the prostate (TURP). Which statement by the client indicates a need for further teaching by the nurse?

   1. "My urine may change color because of bleeding."
   2. "I will need to drink water frequently."
   3. "I will have a dressing where the surgeon cuts."
   4. "I will have a catheter in place after surgery."

61. The nurse is assisting a client who has experienced a left-sided cerebral vascular accident. The client requires assistance with personal hygiene. Which intervention should the nurse do **initially**?

   1. provide positive feedback
   2. place hygiene items on the client's left side
   3. provide assistive devices
   4. assess abilities and level of deficit

62. The nurse is preparing a middle-aged female for a total knee replacement (TKR) surgery on her left leg tomorrow. Which statement by the nurse is incorrect?

   1. "Have you had a cold within the past 2 weeks?"
   2. "You will receive a dose of an antibiotic before surgery."
   3. "When you need to urinate the first night you'll need to use a fracture pan."
   4. "You should ask for medication when you are in pain."

63. The nurse is preparing to administer levofloxacin (Levaquin) 400 mg orally to a client with a urinary tract infection. Which statement by the client requires further teaching by the nurse?

   1. "I will need to wear sunscreen if I am outdoors."
   2. "I need to finish all the medication, even if my symptoms go away."
   3. "I should take my antacid right before my pill so I don't get heartburn."
   4. "I need to check my pulse twice daily and call my doctor if I have new-onset irregular heartbeats."

64. The nurse is reviewing a new client's medication orders. Which order would prompt the nurse to notify the health care provider?

   1. allopurinol 300 mg PO daily
   2. potassium chloride 20 mEq PO daily
   3. warfarin (Coumadin) 50 mg PO daily
   4. metoprolol (Lopressor) 50 mg PO daily

65. The nurse is caring for a client with congestive heart failure who is scheduled for the morning dose of digoxin 0.125 mg PO. The client's apical pulse is 54. Which is the **priority** nursing action?

    1. place the client on 2L of oxygen via nasal cannula

    2. hold the drug and notify the health care provider

    3. wait an hour and recheck the pulse; then administer the drug

    4. administer the drug and ask the unlicensed assistive personnel (UAP) to recheck the pulse in 30 minutes

66. The nurse is caring for a client who has an order for Diuril. Directions say to reconstitute with 20 mL of sterile water. This will provide a concentration of _____mg/mL.

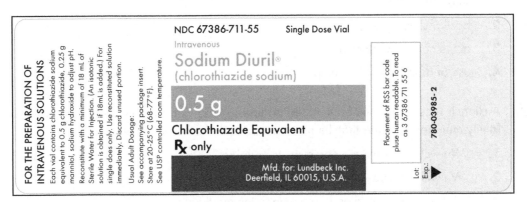

67. A 34-year-old client is receiving an IM injection of ceftriaxone (Rocephin) for a urinary tract infection. Which is correct regarding IM injections?

    1. A 1-inch-long 25-gauge needle should be used.

    2. The injection should be given at a 45-degree angle.

    3. The injection should be given at a 90-degree angle.

    4. A bleb should form on the skin's surface following injection.

68. A client with an upper GI bleed is about to undergo gastric lavage by the nurse. Which action by the nurse is correct in performing this procedure?

    1. instill 200 to 300 mL of a prewarmed solution

    2. instill 400 to 600 mL of a room-temperature solution

    3. position the client on the right side during the procedure

    4. manually withdraw the solution until clear or light pink with no clots

69. The nurse is caring for a client with a wound with purulent, foul-smelling drainage. A wound culture is ordered. Which describes the correct collection technique?

    1. clean the wound with normal saline before obtaining specimen

    2. allow 24 hours for antibiotic therapy to take effect before sampling

    3. obtain the specimen from the drainage at the bottom of the wound

    4. culture the outer surface around the wound before collecting exudate

70. In caring for a critically ill client with a nasogastric tube (NGT) for enteral feeding, which action by the nurse demonstrates competency in NGT care? **Select all that apply.**

   1. The nurse checks gastric residual every 4 hours for continuous feedings.
   2. The nurse maintains the client in a low Fowler's position during feeding.
   3. The nurse checks gastric residual before each bolus or intermittent feeding.
   4. The tubing is changed every 48 hours or when the bag appears visibly soiled.
   5. The nurse returns the residual to the stomach unless the volume is greater than 250 mL.

71. A client has orders for placing a small-bore nasoenteric tube. Which finding in the health history would prompt the nurse to notify the prescriber before placing tube?

   1. small-bowel lesion
   2. basilar skull fracture
   3. acute coronary syndrome
   4. use of diabetic insulin pump

72. A client is receiving patient-controlled analgesia following surgery. Which statement by a family member indicates that the nurse needs to do further teaching?

   1. "We will call you if the pump starts beeping."
   2. "We will call you if she becomes oversedated."
   3. "Nausea is not an allergic reaction to the medication."
   4. "If she is asleep, we will press the button for her so she won't wake up in pain."

73. The nurse is assigned a male client with a long-term in-dwelling catheter for incontinence. The nurse plans on performing which of the following to prevent complications?

   1. perform perineal care using sterile technique
   2. irrigate daily with 60 cc normal saline
   3. restrict fluids to 1,500 cc/day
   4. stabilize the catheter on the abdomen

74. A 54-year-old female is brought into the ED by her spouse. The client's spouse tells the nurse the client has been experiencing muscle stiffness, increased perspiration, and anxiety. The nurse obtains bloodwork as ordered by the physician, including a complete blood count and a comprehensive metabolic panel. For which result should the nurse immediately notify the physician?

   1. calcium 7.2 mg/dL
   2. alkaline phosphatase 120 IU/L
   3. sodium 143 mEq/L
   4. creatinine 0.8 mg/dL

75. The nurse knows which of the following body systems is responsible for the production of somatostatin?

   1. endocrine system
   2. gastrointestinal system
   3. lymphatic system
   4. cardiac system

76. The nurse is auscultating the apical pulse over the PMI (point of maximum impact). Which heart sounds would be audible?

   1. S2 and S3
   2. S3 and S4
   3. S4 and S1
   4. S1 and S2

77. The nurse is caring for a client in intensive care with a diagnosis of traumatic brain injury. The client is found to be restless, complains of extreme nausea, and is weak on the left arm and leg. Which is the **best** response by the nurse?

   1. check the blood pressure
   2. elevate the client's head to 30 degrees
   3. administer oxygen
   4. increase the IV rate

78. An RN is in charge of a team on a medical/surgical unit that includes an LPN. The RN understands that which of the following is an activity that falls outside the scope of practice of an LPN?

   1. administer oral medications to a client
   2. insert a nasogastric tube
   3. care for a patient with a tracheostomy
   4. develop a nursing care plan

79. The nurse has received report on the day's assigned clients. Which of the following clients should the nurse see **first**?

   1. a client who is post-op day 2 from a spinal fusion at L3-4 with a pain level of 4 on a scale of 1 – 10
   2. a client with a peripheral IV on a 6-hour infusion with 42 cc remaining
   3. a client who is 6 hours post–atrial fibrillation ablation, is agitated, has a HR of 130 with B/P at 90/50, and has a urine output of 30 cc in the last 2 hours
   4. a client with a nasogastric tube in place who is complaining of gastric distress

80. The nurse is caring for a 27-year-old female who presents to the ED with a fractured arm along with multiple bruises in various stages of healing around her left eye and chest. The client implies an intimate domestic partner inflicted her injuries. Which statement by the nurse is **most** appropriate?

    1. "Why do you stay with a person like that?"
    2. "Are you in need of an immediate place for safety?"
    3. "Why did he hit you?"
    4. "You need to report your partner to the police."

81. The nurse in a long-term care setting wants to delegate the task of ambulating an elderly client with a walker to an unlicensed assistive personnel (UAP). Before delegating a task to the UAP, the nurse should **first** ensure which of the following is accomplished?

    1. The client is comfortable with the UAP assisting them.
    2. The UAP is comfortable with performing the task.
    3. The UAP has performed the task previously.
    4. The UAP is approved to perform this task based on a credentialing process approved by the facility.

82. The nurse is precepting a student nurse on an orthopedic floor. The student nurse needs to insert an indwelling catheter into a male client. Which of the following statements by the student nurse are correct regarding insertion of the catheter? **Select all that apply.**

    1. "I need to establish an aseptic field."
    2. "I will place the client in the supine position."
    3. "I will lubricate the tip of the catheter with sterile lubricant included in the tray."
    4. "I will inflate the catheter balloon with 5 cc of sterile water."

83. The nurse is working in a cardiac care unit with an LPN. A new client has just arrived. Which task is **not** appropriate for the nurse to delegate to the LPN?

    1. manage existing IV fluid administration
    2. administer IM pain medication
    3. insert an indwelling catheter
    4. assess response to pain medication

84. The charge nurse is making assignments for the day shift. One of the nurses is 5 months pregnant. Which of the following clients is the **most** appropriate assignment for this expectant nurse?

    1. a client with shingles
    2. a client with measles
    3. a client with pneumonia
    4. a client with *Clostridium difficile*

85. The nurse is caring for a client with documented severe allergies to latex. Which item on the client's meal tray should the nurse remove?

   1. a banana
   2. a bowl of beef broth
   3. a vanilla pudding cup
   4. a cup of strawberries

86. The nurse enters a client's room and finds him lying on the floor. The client says to the nurse, "I fell because I was trying to go to the bathroom and no one answered my call light." Which of the following actions by the nurse are correct? **Select all that apply.**

   1. assist the client back to bed
   2. complete an incident report
   3. notify the health care provider
   4. assess the client for any injuries
   5. document in the medical record that the client fell

87. A tornado warning has been issued in the area surrounding the hospital. Which action by the nurse is **most** appropriate to ensure client safety?

   1. leave window blinds open so that staff can monitor the weather
   2. close blinds, roll client beds out into the hallway, and close the doors to all the rooms
   3. close window blinds and leave client doors open so the nurse can hear if a client calls out
   4. leave blinds open but turn beds away from the windows and place as far away as possible from windows

88. The nurse is caring for a 27-year-old client in active labor. After reviewing the fetal heart tone strip shown, the nurse should take which action **first**?

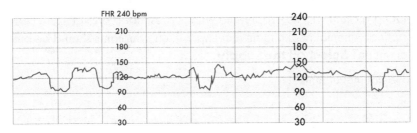
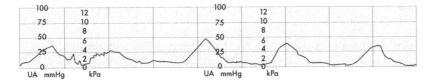

   1. reposition the client
   2. draw a potassium level
   3. notify the health care provider
   4. prepare the client for a cesarean section

89. The nurse is admitting a client with a diagnosis of severe malignant catatonia to the in-patient psychiatric unit. Under which condition would the nurse support the use of electroconvulsive therapy (ECT) as a first-line treatment?

    1. The client is in the first trimester of pregnancy.
    2. The client is gainfully employed.
    3. The client lives in an assisted living facility.
    4. The client is over 50 years of age.

90. An adolescent client is seen by the nurse at a school where a fatal shooting incident occurred on campus 3 months earlier. The nurse documents that the client is experiencing flashbacks, avoiding the location of the shooting, having angry outbursts, and experiencing a loss of interest in playing his favorite musical instrument. The nurse suspects the client is experiencing post-traumatic stress disorder. Which intervention would be the **best** for the nurse to implement?

    1. arrange private counseling sessions with the client over the next 5 school days
    2. refer the client to the multidisciplinary school crisis team that includes the nurse
    3. assure the client the campus is safe
    4. excuse the client from school for three days

91. A 17-year-old adolescent, diagnosed with schizophrenia, is admitted by the nurse to a psychiatric facility. Which behaviors would characterize this diagnosis? **Select all that apply.**

    1. flat affect
    2. fast speech pattern
    3. hallucinations
    4. feeling energized

92. The nurse is monitoring a client with schizophrenia who is prescribed aripiprazole (Abilify). During a multidisciplinary mental health team meeting, which symptoms should be brought to the psychiatrist's attention? **Select all that apply.**

    1. uncontrolled facial movements
    2. hypertension
    3. stiff muscles
    4. bradycardia

93. During the nurse's assessment of a client who has been diagnosed with anorexia nervosa, the nurse evaluates certain characteristics that accompany an intense fear of gaining weight. What characteristics are **most** applicable? **Select all that apply.**

    1. fatigue
    2. excessive exercise regime
    3. normal weight
    4. high blood pressure

94. A client is provided instructions for a low-sodium diet. Which statement by the client indicates an understanding of the diet?

    1. "I'll miss eating tomatoes."

    2. "I'll enjoy eating take-out more frequently."

    3. "I'll avoid potato chips and cheese."

    4. "I'll miss eating celery."

95. During assessment of a client, the nurse notes crackles in the lung bases and bilateral pedal edema. A common cause of fluid volume excess is which factor?

    1. excessive IV infusion

    2. short-term corticosteroid administration

    3. prolonged diarrhea

    4. high fever

96. A client with diverticulitis fills out her lunch menu after instruction from the nurse on proper diet. Which selection by the client demonstrates the need for further teaching?

    1. tuna salad on tomato with crackers and a banana

    2. egg salad on whole wheat bread and a pear

    3. creamy peanut butter and grape jelly sandwich and an orange

    4. chicken salad on pita bread and a plum

97. The nurse recognizes that if eaten by a client, which food can alter results when stool is checked for occult blood?

    1. potatoes

    2. dairy products

    3. raw fruits

    4. beef

98. A client with sleep apnea complains of leg cramps that wake him from sleep. Which instruction should the nurse provide?

    1. drink a glass of water at bedtime

    2. wear compression hose at night

    3. elevate the head of the bed at night

    4. dorsiflex the foot

99. The nurse is caring for a client receiving theophylline for asthma. In reviewing client labs, the nurse understands that the dose is therapeutic when the drug level is at what concentration?

    1. 0.8 – 2 mcg/L

    2. 10 – 20 mg/L

    3. 10 – 20 mcg/mL

    4. 0.8 – 12 mmol/L

100. The nurse is caring for a client receiving pantoprazole. The nurse understands that long-term use of proton pump inhibitors increases the risk of which serious side effects? **Select all that apply.**

1. nausea
2. depression
3. constipation
4. rhabdomyolysis
5. long bone fractures

101. The nurse is observing a student nurse administer a client's medications via a nasogastric (NG) tube. The nurse understands that the student nurse needs further teach if the student nurse performs which action?

1. aspirates and checks the residual
2. places client in the semi-Fowler's position
3. verifies that the medications may be given via NG tube
4. stops the tube feeding before medication administration
5. flushes tubing with 15 – 30 cc of water after administering meds

102. The nurse is caring for a client with chronic kidney failure who is receiving Epoetin alfa. The nurse understands which statement to be true regarding this medication?

1. Side effects include joint pain and hypotension.
2. It stimulates the production of white blood cells.
3. Side effects include bloody urine and headaches.
4. It is given once a week either via the IM route or subcutaneously.

103. The nurse is working on the cardiac unit with a client scheduled to receive digitalis. The nurse understands that which finding is a contraindication for this medication? **Select all that apply.**

1. AV block
2. atrial flutter
3. atrial fibrillation
4. sick sinus syndrome
5. Wolff-Parkinson-White syndrome

104. The nurse is caring for a client receiving IV vancomycin. The trough level is 14 mcg/mL. The next dose is now due. What is the correct response by the nurse?

1. give the next dose as ordered
2. wait 2 hours and redraw the trough
3. wait 30 minutes and redraw the trough
4. hold the dose and notify the health care provider

105. The nurse is caring for a client taking vancomycin. The nurse anticipates drawing a peak and trough on this client. Which statement regarding peak and trough levels is correct?

   1. The peak is drawn 1 hour after the infusion, and the trough is drawn right before the next scheduled dose.
   2. The peak is drawn 2 hours after the infusion, and the trough is drawn 1 hour before the next scheduled dose.
   3. The peak should be drawn immediately after infusion, and the trough is drawn right before the next scheduled dose.
   4. The peak should be drawn 30 minutes before the next scheduled dose, and the trough drawn immediately after the infusion.

106. The nurse is preparing to discharge a client diagnosed with gout. Which statement by the client indicates understanding of dietary restrictions while managing gout?

   1. "I should avoid beer, anchovies, and liver."
   2. "I should avoid bananas, grapefruit, and oranges."
   3. "I should avoid dairy products such as milk and ice cream."
   4. "I should avoid red wine, dark chocolate, and aged cheeses."

107. The nurse is assessing a client who has a sacral pressure ulcer. The wound has partial thickness, loss of dermis, and a red-pink wound bed. No slough is present. How would the nurse chart this wound?

   1. Stage I
   2. Stage II
   3. Stage III
   4. Stage IV
   5. unstageable

108. The nurse is caring for a client with a wound that presents with full-thickness tissue loss and eschar covering the wound bed. The nurse would record this wound as which stage?

   1. Stage I
   2. Stage II
   3. Stage III
   4. Stage IV
   5. unstageable

109. Nurses must be familiar with the American Nurses Association (ANA) Code of Ethics for Nurses. The nurse understands that which ethical principle is defined as the nurse's duty to do no harm? **Fill in the blank.**

_____

110. The nurse is reviewing a rhythm strip of a client on the telemetry unit. There are no discernible P waves, and a sawtooth pattern of waves is present. The atrial rate is regular, and the PR interval is not measurable. The nurse would chart which rhythm for this client?

   1. atrial flutter
   2. atrial fibrillation
   3. torsades de pointes
   4. normal sinus rhythm
   5. ventricular fibrillation

111. The nurse is caring for a client with a diagnosis of fluid overload caused by congestive heart failure. Which findings would the nurse expect to find when reviewing client labs? **Select all that apply.**

   1. decreased BUN
   2. increased hematocrit
   3. increased sodium levels
   4. decreased sodium levels
   5. increased serum osmolality

112. The nurse is caring for an elderly client who presents to the ED with poor appetite, confusion, and weakness. Lab work is ordered for the client. The nurse should immediately notify the health care provider for which lab result?

   1. chloride 99 mEq/L
   2. calcium 9.4 mg/dL
   3. sodium 118 mEq/L
   4. potassium 4.2 mEq/L

113. The nurse is precepting a student nurse on the cardiac floor and reviewing the cardiac cycle. The nurse knows that the student nurse understands ventricular systole when the student nurse states that blood enters which vessels during ventricular systole?

   1. the aorta and vena cava
   2. the aorta and pulmonary vein
   3. the aorta and pulmonary artery
   4. the pulmonary vein and vena cava
   5. the pulmonary artery and vena cava

114. The nurse is reviewing a client's PRN pain medications. There is an order for acetaminophen 1,000 mg PO q4 hours as needed for pain. How should the nurse proceed?

   1. call the health care provider to clarify the order
   2. administer the medication as ordered if needed for pain
   3. give other PRN medications for pain and ignore the order
   4. avoid giving pain medication every 4 hours and give it every 6 hours

115. The nurse has an order to administer 100 units of regular insulin in 500 mL of 0.9% NS to infuse at 12 units per hour. The nurse should program the IV pump to deliver how many mLs per hour?

_____

116. The ED nurse is caring for a client whose native tongue is not English. The client speaks Korean and only understands a few words of English. The nurse understands that which response is **best** regarding how to communicate with this client?

   1. ask a bilingual family member to tell the client to point to where the pain is

   2. call the oncology unit and ask for the nurse who is a native Korean to come and translate

   3. show the client the equipment before using it, such as indicating that an IV line will be placed in the arm

   4. call for an official Korean interpreter on the facility's translator hotline to communicate with the client, family, and health care provider

117. A nurse manager and a case manager are talking to a group of new nurses about the differences of case management and care coordination. The nurse manager understands which to be true regarding the differences?

   1. With care coordination, the stakeholder can be an insurance company or a hospital.

   2. The main goal of case management is to promote a better quality of life for the client.

   3. Case management is based on a holistic approach and an understanding of client-family dynamics.

   4. In care coordination, the client defines the scope of work based on a plan that is created with input from the client.

118. The newly graduated nurse is caring for an elderly client on the medical-surgical floor. The nurse recalls learning about client advocacy. Which actions by the nurse indicate an understanding of client advocacy? **Select all that apply.**

   1. The nurse speaks to the daughters regarding care-making decisions, since the client is elderly and may not understand.

   2. The nurse tells the family that they should really consider making the client an organ donor in case something happens.

   3. The nurse makes sure the client understands treatment options, including possible outcomes if the client refuses treatment.

   4. The nurse obtains an interpreter for the client if her native language is not English and she only understands her native language.

   5. The nurse asks the client for a copy of advance directives or a living will, or provides information if the client does not have one.

119. A nurse manager is educating a group of nursing students about the Patient's Bill of Rights. The nurse knows that the student nurses have an understanding of the bill when one of the nurses makes which statement?

    1. "Clients have the right to view their medical records but may not copy any of the information contained in the records."

    2. "Clients may be declined care at an emergency department or need preauthorization for care if they do not have premium-level insurance."

    3. "Clients have the right to a quick and objective review of any claim that they levy against a health care facility, physician, or health care plan."

    4. "It is the admitting nurse's job to verify the client's past medical history, medications, and treatments, even if the client refuses to cooperate in giving the information."

120. Nurses are expected to understand the principles of triage when caring for multiple clients. The ICU charge nurse is reviewing assignments. Based on the principles of triage, to which client would the charge nurse give priority for treatment? **Select all that apply.**

    1. a client on a ventilator who has an alarm sounding

    2. a client who has just returned from an open appendectomy

    3. a client ready to transfer to the floor after the nurse calls report

    4. a client who has been talking with family and is now unresponsive

    5. a client receiving a new antibiotic who complains of tingling in the mouth

    6. a client who has not eaten yet and is a type 2 diabetic with a morning blood sugar of 90

121. A nurse asks an unlicensed assistive personnel (UAP) to help admit a 22-year-old female client with ulcerative colitis. Which activity is appropriate for the nurse to assign the UAP?

    1. obtain a stool sample

    2. obtain abbreviated history of symptoms for the past 30 days

    3. instruct the client on the reason for undergoing a lower gastric X-ray exam

    4. obtain a sample of gastric contents from nasogastric tube

122. The nurse is caring for a client who was admitted for chest pain. The client is oriented to person and place, but is often confused about the month of the year or what season it is. A family member tells the nurse, "I'd like for you to sign as a witness on my mother's living will, in case something happens to her and we need to make health care decisions for her." Which is the **best** response by the nurse?

    1. "Let me have a copy so my attorney can look at it."

    2. "My unit manager will need to come witness with me."

    3. "Do you think your mother understands what is going on right now?"

    4. "I'm sorry, but it is against policy for staff members to witness client forms."

123. The nurse is caring for a client who is disoriented. To avoid using restraints, the nurse chooses alternative methods to help keep the client oriented. Which interventions would the nurse use for this client? **Select all that apply.**

    1. maintain normal toileting routines

    2. minimize visitation so that the client may rest

    3. evaluate the client's medications for side effects

    4. keep familiar items such as family pictures near the bedside

    5. use calendars and clocks to orient the client to the date and time

    6. place the client in a room near the end of the hall to minimize noise

124. The nurse has just administered morphine 4 mg IV to a client with severe pain from a kidney stone. The client then asks to get up to the toilet. Which is the correct nursing action for this client?

    1. assist the client to the toilet

    2. offer the client a bedpan or urinal

    3. obtain an order for a Foley catheter

    4. place a bedside commode in the room

125. The nurse is educating a group of student nurses about fire safety. Which statement by a student nurse indicates a need for further teaching by the facility nurse?

    1. "Oxygen near the vicinity of the fire should be turned off if it is safe to do so."

    2. "Bedridden clients may be moved in their beds or in a wheelchair if they are able to sit in it safely."

    3. "Clients who are ambulatory may walk to a safe area but cannot assist in evacuating other clients due to HIPAA laws."

    4. "Clients on a ventilator should be manually bagged with an Ambu bag until the fire threat is over and they can be placed back on the ventilator."

126. The nurse is preparing to discharge a 60-year-old woman on warfarin (Coumadin) after mitral valve replacement. Which dietary restriction should the nurse advise the client to make?

    1. avoid green tea

    2. avoid cauliflower

    3. avoid green beans

    4. avoid asparagus

127. A non-immune nurse should not be assigned a client who has which of the vaccine-preventable airborne diseases? **Select all that apply.**

    1. tuberculosis

    2. influenza

    3. smallpox

    4. pertussis

128. A client is admitted for deep vein thrombosis and is receiving 5,000 units of heparin subcutaneously every 8 hours. In case of a serious bleeding reaction, the nurse has which of the following drugs readily available?

    1. warfarin

    2. potassium chloride

    3. vitamin K

    4. protamine sulfate

129. The nurse finds that a client receiving digoxin (Lanoxin) 0.25 mg orally has an apical pulse of 54. Which of the following should the nurse do **first**?

    1. withhold the medicine and contact the prescribing physician

    2. ask another nurse to verify the apical pulse

    3. administer the medication and recheck the pulse in 30 minutes

    4. order a stat ECG

130. A client with pulmonary edema is ordered IV hydrocortisone (Solu-Cortef) 40 mg b.i.d. Which laboratory value would the nurse expect to see as a result of this therapy?

    1. elevated magnesium

    2. lowered magnesium

    3. elevated glucose

    4. lowered glucose

131. The nurse is preparing to teach a client about the prescribed furosemide (Lasix). The nurse should instruct the client about which adverse effect?

    1. increased appetite

    2. leg cramps

    3. anorexia

    4. dry mouth

132. The nurse has an order to administer a heparin drip at 12 units/kg/hr. The client weighs 178 pounds. The heparin is available as 25,000 units in 500 mL D5W. At which rate should the nurse program the pump?

    _____

133. The nurse is caring for a female client following the removal of the parathyroid glands. The client complains of a "pins and needles" sensation and difficulty swallowing lunch. The nurse would expect which laboratory value to be abnormal?

    1. calcium

    2. potassium

    3. magnesium

    4. blood glucose

134. The nurse is reviewing labs on a group of adult clients. Which lab value would prompt the nurse to **immediately** notify the health care provider?

1. hemoglobin 4.8 g/dL
2. troponin T 0.04 ng/mL
3. phosphorus 3.8 mg/dL
4. bilirubin (total) 0.7 mg/dL

135. The nurse has a client complaining of chest pain. Where should the nurse place the V5 lead for a 12-lead EKG?

1. in the left midaxillary line
2. in the fifth intercostal right midclavicular line
3. in the fourth intercostal space to the left of the sternum
4. in the fourth intercostal space to the right of the sternum

136. The nurse is caring for a client who will have a pulmonary function test (PFT) performed as an outpatient following hospital discharge. Which should the nurse include in his teaching on the procedure? **Select all that apply.**

1. have a driver accompany the client to the test site
2. limit activity in the days leading up to the test
3. remain NPO after midnight the day before the test
4. do not smoke for at least 6 – 8 hours before the test
5. withhold bronchodilators for 4 – 6 hours prior to the test
6. increase aerobic activity as much as possible in the days before the test

137. The nurse is caring for a client with marked clubbing of the fingers and toes. The nurse understands which to be true regarding clubbing? **Select all that apply.**

1. It is a permanent condition.
2. Clients on dialysis often have clubbing.
3. Sickle cell disease may cause clubbing.
4. It is caused by acute oxygen deprivation.
5. It can be caused by right-sided heart failure.
6. It is common in clients with congenital heart defects.

138. The charge nurse is making an assignment for an LPN on an upcoming shift. Which assignment would be appropriate?

1. a client with a recent head injury and active seizures
2. a post-operative patient requiring vital sign monitoring every hour
3. a post-operative patient receiving a blood transfusion
4. a client with diabetes requiring discharge instruction on insulin injection

139. On the diagram, identify the location where the client would present with acute abdominal pain for the specified diagnosis.

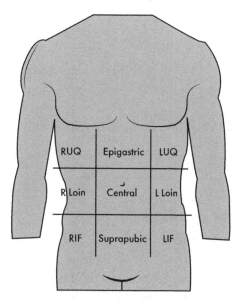

Diagnosis   **Abdominal Location**

1. acute cholecystitis   _____

2. acute appendicitis   _____

3. acute cystitis   _____

4. acute peptic ulcer   _____

5. splenic infarction   _____

140. The nurse is providing discharge instructions to the parents of a 6-month-old child with surgical repair for cryptorchidism. Which instruction would NOT be stressed?

1. observe surgical site for bleeding

2. enforce bed rest for 2 – 3 days

3. palpate scrotum to check testicle location

4. avoid strenuous activity for at least one month

141. A local politician is admitted to the emergency department. The nurse notices a staff member not involved with the care of this client reading his medical record. The nurse knows this is a violation of which of the following?

1. the Patient's Bill of Rights

2. the Patient Self-Determination Act

3. the Health Insurance Portability and Accountability Act (HIPAA)

4. the Uniform Anatomical Gift Act

142. The nurse begins administration of blood to a client on a medical unit. The nurse knows that which of the following activities is inappropriate to delegate to the unlicensed assistive personnel (UAP)?

1. assist with bathing
2. obtain a snack from the kitchen
3. explain to the client the reason for the transfusion
4. obtain the client's blood pressure

143. Which statement is incorrect regarding the Federal Nursing Home Reform Act from the Omnibus Budget Reconciliation Act of 1987 (OBRA '87)?

1. the right to be free of unnecessary chemical restraints
2. the right to choose a personal physician
3. the right to access medical records
4. the right to organize hospital personnel within a union

144. The nurse is preparing to do a 12-lead ECG on a client. Which of the following shows where the V1 lead should be placed?

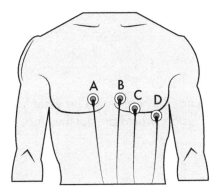

1. site A
2. site B
3. site C
4. site D

145. The nurse is making a home visit to an elderly client during the summer. Upon arrival, the nurse notices the refrigerator and freezer doors are open as the client is using both for air conditioning. Which of the following actions by the nurse are **most** appropriate?

1. instruct the client to place a fan in front of the freezer to enhance circulation of cool air
2. hold a meeting with the client and family to advise them of the safety risks of this practice
3. note this observation in the client's medical record, but do not discuss with the client
4. report the incident to the nursing supervisor

146. Upon entering the client's room the nurse discovers a dose of amoxicillin at the bedside. Which of the following should the nurse do?

   1. file an incident report and document the finding in the client's medical record

   2. document the finding in the client's medical record only

   3. report the incident to the nursing supervisor

   4. file an incident report but do not document the finding in the client's medical record

147. A student nurse is assigned to care for a client in a protective environment room. The nurse knows to intervene upon observing which of the following deliveries by the nursing student?

   1. indwelling catheterization kit

   2. flower bouquet

   3. tray of food containing disposable plate and utensils

   4. oral medication

148. The nurse is reviewing labs for a client whose potassium level is 5.3 mEq/L. Which order should the nurse anticipate from the health care provider?

   1. an order for K-Dur

   2. an order for Pradaxa

   3. an order for Namenda

   4. an order for Kayexalate

149. The nurse is caring for a client diagnosed with glaucoma. The health care provider has ordered timolol maleate. Which finding in the client's history would prompt the nurse to notify the health care provider?

   1. asthma

   2. migraines

   3. atrial fibrillation

   4. urinary tract infection

150. The nurse is caring for a laboring client who is on an oxytocin infusion. The client experiences seven contractions in a 10-minute time period. The fetal heart rate tracing is a category III. Which action should the nurse take?

   1. discontinue the oxytocin infusion

   2. increase the oxytocin infusion rate

   3. decrease the oxytocin infusion rate by half

   4. reposition the client into a high-Fowler's position

PRACTICE TEST TWO ANSWER KEY

1. Number 3 is correct.

Rationale: The only personnel who should access the client's medical record are those providing direct care to the client. HIPAA guidelines do not permit nurses to look up labs on another client, even if requested by the physician. By calling the client's nurse to the nurses' station, the appropriate nurse can look up the labs. Also, the client's nurse may need to speak to the physician about the client. Suggesting the physician call the lab himself is confrontational and does not expedite transmission of necessary information about the client to the physician. The charge nurse is also prohibited by HIPAA from looking up data on a client unless she is caring for that client.

2. Number 1 is correct.

Rationale: Spironolactone is a potassium-sparing diuretic, which is inappropriate for this client. Furosemide (Lasix) is a better choice for this client, because it helps remove excess potassium. Delivering a low-potassium meal tray is an appropriate action. Sodium polystyrene sulfonate (Kayexalate) helps remove excess potassium from the body, and is often prescribed for clients who have elevated potassium levels. All clients should be ambulating, coughing, and deep-breathing as their condition permits.

3. Number 1 is correct.

Rationale: STAT orders should always be performed first, unless there is another eminently life-threatening event in progress. The priority is to administer the Lasix for the client in fluid overload. Untreated fluid overload can lead to crackles and other adventitious lung sounds, making breathing more laborious. Additional fluid also places strain on the heart, which must pump more effectively against the extra fluid. Edema develops, and the extra fluid to be excreted places a burden upon the kidneys. Blood pressure also increases. The next task would be to administer insulin to the client with an elevated blood sugar. It is important to get the blood sugar under control to prevent damage to the body's cells. The client should then be discharged to avoid any delay in allowing her to return home. The dressing change will be time consuming and should be performed last, after the more time-sensitive tasks have been completed.

4. Number 3 is correct.

Rationale: In most states, LPNs are not permitted to administer IV medications such as morphine. The nurse must immediately report this to the charge nurse and nursing supervisor. The LPN is acting outside the scope of practice and is at risk of losing her license. This is especially concerning because the LPN states that she has done this before. Offering to double-check the dose does not negate the fact that the LPN is still violating the law by administering the medication. Offering to help the LPN is not a constructive way to handle the situation. The nurse should not offer to chart it while the LPN administers it because this still violates the LPN's scope of practice. Additionally, this places the RN in the position of knowingly aiding the LPN in violating the state nursing practice law. The RN is required by law to report any instances in which another nurse is breaking the law or practicing nursing in a manner that could cause harm to the client.

5. Number 2 is correct.

Rationale: An incomplete signature (for instance, if the ink of a pen ran out) is considered a missing signature. The nurse should get another form and pen and have it filled out. The information was released to the proper provider; it was just provided with legal authorization in the form of a signed HIPAA form. The wrong client's information was not released. Although the client wants the information released, the nurse has still violated HIPAA due to the missing signature.

6. Number 2 is correct.

Rationale: Flushing the catheter with 10 to 20 mL of sterile normal saline is necessary to ensure a patent line. Short peripheral catheters should not be used for routine blood sampling because manipulation can cause vein irritation and necessitate removal of the catheter. Obtaining blood samples from central venous lines carries a much greater risk of infection and may interfere with test results depending on the types of fluids that have been infused recently. Transferring blood into test tubes should be done without using exposed needles, for example, by using a vacutainer system.

7. Numbers 1, 3, and 6 are correct.

Rationale: A restraint is any mechanical, chemical, or physical device, equipment, or material that prevents or limits movement of any part of the client's body. Bed rails are also a form of restraint, and many facilities have implemented policies barring the use of all four bed rails to keep clients in bed. Alternatives to restraints include active listening, diversionary techniques, reducing stimulation, and verbal interventions or asking the client for cooperation. Children under 9 years of age have a 1-hour time limit in restraints. Assessment of restraints and offering food, hydration, and toileting must be done regularly every 15 to 30 minutes. Many facilities mandate a trial release for clients in restraints. If restraints are removed, a new order must be obtained before replacing them. The use of restraints requires careful and complete documentation by the nurse.

8. Numbers 3 and 4 are correct.

Rationale: Immobilizing and splinting the affected extremity may help limit the spread of the venom. The extremity should be maintained at the level of the heart. Safety is the first priority, so the person should be moved to a safe area and encouraged to rest quietly to decrease venous circulation of venom. Community members should not attempt to kill or capture the snake; if feasible, a digital photograph can be taken at a safe distance for identification. Applying ice is ineffective and may worsen the person's outcome.

9. Numbers 1, 2, and 3 are correct.

Rationale: Offering frequent toileting or incontinence care can prevent client wandering in search of the bathroom. All clients should be assessed for pain per agency protocols and treated with appropriate medications to prevent wandering to the nurses' station or other areas in search of pain medications. Reorientation therapy and validation can help reorient the client and reduce wandering. While the client may remain in an area where she can be closely monitored, it is not appropriate for the client to remain at the nurses' station due to HIPPA and privacy concerns. Chemical or physical restraints should never be used for the nurse's convenience and may increase agitation and the propensity to wander.

10. Number 2 is correct.

Rationale: CN V is the trigeminal nerve responsible for sensory function. The nurse tests the nerve by asking the client to close his eyes and then randomly touching the client's face with a cotton ball. The client indicates whenever she feels the sensation. Motor function of CN V is tested by asking the client to clench her teeth and open and close her mouth several times. CN VII is the facial nerve and is tested by asking the client to smile, close both eyes, frown, puff cheeks, raise eyebrows, or show teeth. CN VIII is the vestibulocochlear nerve. Hearing loss or tinnitus is indicative of deficits with the cochlear branch of the nerve. Vertigo indicates a deficit of the vestibular branch. CN XI is an accessory nerve and is tested by asking the client to shrug her shoulders.

11. Number 2 is correct.

Rationale: The Apgar score provides a rapid assessment of how well the newborn is tolerating life outside the womb based on five signs that indicate the physiologic state. This newborn scored as follows:

Heart rate > 110 = 2 points

Respiratory effort: good cry = 2 points

Muscle tone: some flexion of extremities = 1 point

Reflex irritability: grimace = 1 point

Color: completely pink = 2 points

Scores of 0 to 3 indicate severe distress requiring immediate intervention, such as suctioning the airway. Scores of 4 to 6 indicate moderate difficulty and may require less emergent interventions. Scores of 7 to 10 indicate minimal or no distress and show that routine newborn care is appropriate.

12.   Number 4 is correct.

Rationale: Regular screening should begin at age 50 for those without a family history of CRC. Fecal occult blood testing and a colonoscopy should be done every 10 years or a double-contrast barium enema every 5 years. Screening should begin earlier and more frequently for those who have a personal or family history of CRC. Dietary guidelines include lowering fat and refined carbohydrates and eating high-fiber foods. At age 40, the client should discuss the need for screening with the health care provider.

13.   Number 1 is correct.

Rationale: A positive psoas sign indicates inflammation of the psoas muscle associated with peritoneal inflammation or appendicitis. A positive Murphy's sign indicates cholecystitis. A positive Homan's sign may indicate a blood clot in one of the deep veins in the leg. Chadwick's sign is a normal finding in pregnancy.

14.   Number 3 is correct.

Rationale: Autonomy is respecting the rights of others to make their own decisions regarding care. Justice is the duty to distribute resources or care equally without regard to personal attributes (e.g., the nurse devotes equal attention to a homeless client who attempted suicide and to the client with a stroke). Fidelity or non-maleficence is maintaining loyalty and commitment to the client and doing no wrong to the client. The concept of fidelity includes keeping promises made to the client (e.g., the client asks the nurse not to reveal a cancer diagnosis to the family because he is concerned that his family will insist on aggressive treatment). Beneficence is the duty to act to promote the good of others (i.e., spending extra time to talk with a lonely, elderly client).

15.   Number 2 is correct.

Rationale: The client at this age is in the industry vs. inferiority stage. Successful resolution results in competence and the ability to work. Initiative vs. guilt is the stage of the preschool (ages 3 – 6) child. The desired outcome is a sense of purpose and ability to initiate one's own activities. Middle adulthood (ages 35 – 65) is a period of generativity vs. self-absorption. Success at this stage results in the ability to give and care for others. The child in early childhood (ages 1 1/2 – 3) is experiencing autonomy vs. shame and doubt. Successful resolution of this stage gives the child willpower and a sense of self-control.

16.   Number 3 is correct.

Rationale: Restating repeats the main idea expressed by the client. It allows the client to clarify the message if it has been misunderstood. Exploring examines certain ideas or experiences more fully. If the client chooses not to elaborate, the nurse does not probe further. Reflecting turns the question back to the client for recognition and acceptance. Focusing concentrates on one point and is useful when the client is jumping from one topic to another.

17.   Number 3 is correct.

Rationale: Continuously evaluating progress toward the client's goals is part of the working phase of the relationship. During this phase the therapeutic work of the relationship is accomplished. Identifying the client's strengths and limitations occurs during the orientation (introductory) phase. Exploring feelings about the termination phase of the relationship is accomplished during the termination phase itself. The main task of this phase is bringing a therapeutic conclusion to the relationship.

18.   Number 1 is correct.

Rationale: Identifying the client's strengths and limitations occurs during the orientation (introductory) phase. Promoting the client's insight and perception of reality and continuously evaluating progress toward the client's goals are part of the working phase of the relationship. During this phase the therapeutic work of the relationship is accomplished. Exploring feelings about the termination phase of the relationship is accomplished during the termination phase itself. The main task of this phase is bringing a therapeutic conclusion to the relationship.

19. Number 1 is correct.

Rationale: Elevating the arm and applying ice packs over the approximate location of the incision can help minimize swelling and pain. Option 2 is incorrect because the goal of the intervention is to use nonpharmacological comfort measures. Option 3 is incorrect because no foreign objects should ever be inserted into a cast. If the client is itching, suggest blowing cool air into the cast with a blow dryer. The air must be cool in order to avoid burning the skin or increasing the pain. While range-of-motion exercises are important to maintain mobility, this intervention will not promote comfort and may in fact temporarily increase client discomfort.

20. Number 4 is correct.

Rationale: Consuming large amounts of milk or milk-based products places demand on the kidneys to excrete excess calcium and can cause kidney stones. High-fiber fruits provide needed fiber to prevent constipation while immobile. There is no need to avoid grapefruit juice while on bed rest. While high-fat foods may be a poor dietary choice for health reasons, they are not contraindicated on bed rest.

21. Number 2 is correct.

Rationale: A picture board has pictures of common client needs while in the hospital. Pointing to a picture of a toilet or a pained face requires the least effort on the client's part. A clipboard with pen and paper is not the best choice because it is difficult to write lying down while trying to hold a clipboard firmly. Some clients may use one, but often the handwriting is illegible, leading to frustration for the client when the request can't be read. The client will not be able to mouth words properly while intubated, and involving the family in a guessing game is nonproductive and can increase frustration. Asking the client to blink to indicate answers is ineffective communication because the client may be tired or unable to blink on demand.

22. Number 2 is correct.

Rationale: Buck's traction is a type of skin traction used mainly to reduce painful muscle spasms. A Velcro boot is placed around the affected limb, with the weights attached via a single pulley and the leg elevated. The weight range for skin traction is from 5 to 7 pounds. Using a heavier weight increases the risk of severe skin irritation. Skeletal traction uses heavier weights (15 – 30 pounds) and surgical screws that attach directly to the bone. The weights should hang freely and not be moved unless ordered by the health care provider. Pin site care should be done regularly and the skin checked for signs of infection such as redness, swelling, or pus.

23. Numbers 1, 2, 3, and 5 are correct.

Rationale: The first step is to be sure the tubing has not become kinked or lodged under the client. The next step is to gently flush the Foley with 30 cc of sterile saline. Sometimes there may be a blood clot or sediment blocking the flow of urine. Avoid aggressive interventions in order to prevent trauma to the urethra. If the client is alert and oriented, ask the client if he feels pain or pressure or a sense of urinary urgency. The client may not show signs of discomfort, especially if mental function is impaired. A bladder scan is a noninvasive manner in which to determine how much urine is in the bladder. The results should be recorded and the health care provider notified. Joint Commission guidelines encourage minimal use of Foley catheters for the minimum time possible in order to prevent infection. Facility protocols may not allow the nurse to automatically place a new Foley, so the health care provider should be notified to obtain an order for a new Foley. The bulb of the Foley may be lodged against the urethral opening. In this case, the nurse may attempt to reinsert about 2 inches of the catheter *after* cleaning it with soap and water. This will move the bulb far enough to see if the bulb is blocking urine outflow. However, removing a substantial amount of the tubing and reinserting it increases the risk of infection, even if it has been cleaned.

24. Number 4 is correct.

Rationale: Metformin must be discontinued at least 24 hours before studies with contrast media because of the risk of lactic acidosis, which can be life-threatening. Hold metformin for at least 48 hours post-procedure and do not resume therapy until kidney function has been evaluated. Fish oil is a supplement and does not pose a risk for clients undergoing CT with contrast. Coumadin is an anticoagulant and does not pose a risk with contrast. Prozac is an antidepressant and does not pose a risk with contrast.

25. Number 3 is correct.

Rationale: Options 1, 2, and 4 describe the proper technique for use of an inhaler with a spacer. The client should wait at least 1 minute between puffs.

26. Number 3 is correct.

Rationale: Option 1 is a nontherapeutic response and devalues the client's dignity. Oxygen therapy for dyspnea in clients near death has not been established as a standard of care for all clients. Morphine and other opioids are the standard treatment and should be given early in the course of dyspnea. Nonpharmacologic interventions may be used concurrently with medication to enhance comfort but should not substitute for pharmacological treatment.

27. Numbers 2, 4, and 5 are correct.

Rationale: The respiratory rate is within normal limits. Hypertension indicates circulatory overload, which can occur when blood products are administered too quickly. The oxygen saturation level is within normal limits. Other signs of circulatory overload include restlessness, confusion, and distended jugular veins. Low back pain and a sense of impending doom indicate a hemolytic transfusion reaction caused by blood type or Rh incompatibility.

28. Number 2 is correct.

Rationale: Phenergan is contraindicated in children with Reye's syndrome. Paxil 20 mg PO daily is an appropriate dose for this client and condition. Diflucan 150 mg PO is given as a one-time dose to treat vaginal candidiasis. Lopressor 50 mg PO daily is an appropriate treatment for this client's hypertension.

29. Number 2 is correct.

Rationale: Guidelines for prevention of sickle cell crisis include avoiding strenuous exercise, avoiding alcohol and tobacco in any form, and avoiding travel to high altitude destinations.

30. Numbers 1 and 2 are correct.

Rationale: Spiked T waves are an abnormal finding. Left untreated, complete heart block or asystole can occur. Cardiovascular changes are the most serious problem in hyperkalemia. A heart rate less than 60 beats per minute is an abnormal finding and may cause cardiac compromise. The normal resting adult heart rate is 60 – 100 beats per minute. Cantaloupe is high in potassium and should not be eaten by this client. Normal urine output is 30 cc per hour.

31. Numbers 1 and 3 are correct.

Rationale: A sudden decrease in output may indicate blockage. A Salem sump tube is attached to low continuous suction. Medium intermittent suction is not appropriate for this tube. The semi-Fowler's position is most appropriate for the client with an NGT. If the NGT needs to be repositioned or replaced, confirmation of proper placement is needed before use.

32. Number 4 is correct.

Rationale: After a lumbar puncture, the nurse should assess for numbness, tingling, pain at injection site, movement of the extremities, any drainage at the site, and the ability to void. Report unusual findings to the health care provider. Specimens should not be refrigerated. The client must lie in a reclining position for up to 12 hours with the head flat to avoid a spinal headache. The client may sip through a straw to replace fluids. Positioning the client prone with a pillow under the abdomen increases intraabdominal pressure, which indirectly increases the pressure in the tissues surrounding the spinal cord. This helps slow continued CSF flow from the spinal canal.

33. Number 2 is correct.

    Rationale: Cultures normally require 48 to 72 hours to complete growing. Preliminary test results are available at 24 hours. If IV antibiotics are infusing, the nurse should draw cultures just before administering the next dose in order to avoid compromising results. If catheter sepsis is suspected, drawing cultures through the catheter is more accurate than culturing the catheter tip only.

34. Number 1 is correct.

    Rationale: Iron stains the teeth and should be given through a straw or by placing a medicine dropper in the back of the mouth. The child or parent should brush or wipe the teeth to prevent staining. Iron should be given on an empty stomach between meals to maximize absorption. Iron should not be mixed with food before administering.

35. Number 3 is correct.

    Rationale: A child with hemophilia should avoid contact sports. Piano lessons are the best option, as the others involve contact sports.

36. Number 1 is correct.

    Rationale: Clients taking MAOI should avoid foods high in tyramine, including aged or smoked foods, cheese, meats with added nitrates, and pickled foods. The other menu options are permissible for this client.

37. Number 3 is correct.

    Rationale: Clients with heart failure experience decreased kidney perfusion. Magnesium hydroxide is excreted through the kidneys, leaving the client at risk for magnesium toxicity. The other conditions listed do not affect the body's ability to clear magnesium.

38. Number 4 is correct.

    Rationale: The therapeutic range of digitalis is 0.5 to 2 ng/mL. This client is at the toxic level. Early signs of digitalis toxicity include anorexia, nausea, and diarrhea. Tinnitus, flushed skin, and easy bruising are not consistent with toxic digitalis levels.

39. Numbers 2 and 4 are correct.

    Rationale: Authoritative leadership motivates staff by coercion and employs a top-down communication style. A laissez-faire style of leadership is very laid-back and involves little planning. The democratic style of leadership motivates staff by supporting their achievements and includes group members in the decision-making process.

40. Number 1 is correct.

    Rationale: Obtaining vital signs is within the scope of practice for LPNs. They cannot administer blood but may witness signatures on the blood consent form, depending on the state and facility policies. IV pain medication cannot be given by LPNs as they are given IV push. LPNs may not administer chemotherapy in any state, regardless of the reason, as this is beyond the scope of practice.

41. Number 3 is correct.

    Rationale: The multidisciplinary approach engages members from a diverse group of health care teams to provide an individualized and comprehensive approach to treatment and management of a given disease or condition. Peer review involves evaluating and giving constructive feedback on nursing care. Team nursing involves caring for a group of clients on a floor or in a specialty care unit. Community nursing involves caring for a group of clients within a particular community. These clients may be seen in health departments and clinics, and often have limited money and resources with which to manage their health.

42. Numbers 4 and 5 are correct.

Rationale: The Patient's Bill of Rights covers the rights and responsibilities of all clients seeking health care services. The client is responsible for any outcomes if she refuses recommended treatments and medications, as long she is considered competent. A client who is not competent to make decisions, such as a child or someone mentally incapacitated, should have a responsible family member or legal caregiver make decisions for her. The client is also responsible for providing truthful information on past medical history, medications, drug abuse, smoking, or any other factors that affect the client's health. The client has a right to a translator if she does not speak English; it is not her responsibility to provide one. The client has the right to be screened and stabilized by emergency services if needed; this is not a responsibility borne by the client. Providing proof of insurance or ability to pay is not a client responsibility addressed by the Patient's Bill of Rights.

43. Number 1 is correct.

Rationale: Advocacy is the process by which nurses promote and protect the client's rights. This client will need a social services consult to identify available shelters, medication programs, and transportation to maintain optimal health. A nurse advocates for the client by knowing when to seek help from other disciplines. Delegation involves identifying a task to be handed off and the appropriate person to whom the task should be delegated. Ethical practice guides nurses in making choices regarding right versus wrong, as well as American Nurses Association guidelines for ethical practice. Continuity of care provides high-quality, cost-effective care by cooperation among health care providers. Transferring a client to another department and giving concise handoff reports to an oncoming shift are examples of continuity of care. An advance directive is a legal document in which the client specifies the kind of care and specific care actions he does or does not want if he becomes unable to speak for himself.

44. Number 4 is correct.

Rationale: Injury prevention is important for this client. Throw rugs should be avoided because of the potential to trip and fall. Options 1, 2, and 3 are appropriate safety measures for the client with thrombocytopenia.

45. Number 2 is correct.

Rationale: Tocolytics such as nitroglycerin IV may help relax the uterus. Ultrasonography is used to detect remaining fragments. After the removal of a retained placenta or fragments, the client is at continued risk of postpartum hemorrhage and infection. Retention of fragments causes the uterus to feel boggy due to uterine atony.

46. Numbers 3, 4, 5, and 6 are correct.

Rationale: Airborne precautions are used for infections caused by organisms that may remain airborne for extended periods, such as tuberculosis and measles. Standard precautions apply to all clients as all body fluids, moist membranes, and excretions are potentially infectious. Negative airflow rooms exchange air and discharge room air to the outside or through HEPA filters. N95 masks or PAPRs prevent inhalation of contaminated air. Fall precautions may or may not be needed for this client. Droplet precautions are used for infections caused by organisms that travel 3 feet but are not suspended for long periods of time, such as mumps and influenza.

47. Number 3 is correct.

Rationale: The bed should be at hip level when moving clients. Waist level is appropriate bed positioning for providing direct client care. Proper use of mechanical or electric transfer equipment can safely move the client who is weak or obese without compromising client safety or placing other caregivers at risk. Gait or transfer belts are useful for clients who may be unsteady on their feet when ambulating.

48. Number 4 is correct.

Rationale: While all babies achieve milestones at slightly different times, a child should be crawling by 8 – 12 months. The nurse should notify the health care provider for further assessment. The other options are expected developmental milestones that are achieved before age 8 – 12 months.

49. Number 4 is correct.

Rationale: The influenza vaccine is safe for pregnant women. The other vaccines have been found to harm the developing fetus and are contraindicated in pregnancy.

50. Number 2 is correct.

Rationale: RhoGAM is given in the 28th week if the mother is Rh-negative and the father is Rh-positive. If both mother and father are Rh-negative, the mother does not need RhoGAM, as her child will not be Rh-positive. Option 3 is incorrect because RhoGAM is given in the 28th week, not the 24th. Option 4 is incorrect because if the mother is Rh-positive and the father is Rh-negative, RhoGAM is not needed since the mother is already positive.

51. Number 3 is correct.

Rationale: Self-examination of the testicles should be done after bathing because the scrotum is more relaxed. A lump or swelling should be reported to the health care provider. Testicular cancer is more common in men ages 15 – 35 and is one of the most curable cancers.

52. Number 1 is correct.

Rationale: Canned foods tend to be high in sodium, so low-sodium or no-salt-added versions are a better diet choice for this client. Red meat is high in saturated fat, so it is not a better substitute than fried chicken. Red meats and fried foods should be eliminated from the diet or eaten sparingly. Canned soup is high in sodium unless labeled otherwise; the client needs to select low-sodium varieties. Frozen foods are another sodium-rich category unless otherwise labeled. The client needs to understand that processed foods (frozen foods, canned goods, and boxed items such as crackers) should be avoided as much as reasonably possible. Learning to read labels will help the client lower sodium intake.

53. Numbers 1, 2, and 5 are correct.

Rationale: In providing end-of-life care, the nurse explains to the client and family the signs and symptoms that death is approaching. Explaining what to expect during the final phase of the illness may help alleviate fear and anxiety as the family observes their loved one transitioning through the stages of death. Addressing client and family wishes regarding care, pain management, and emergency resuscitation respects their wishes and ensures that their choices are carried out as much as possible. Cultural beliefs are acknowledged, and life-lengthening treatment options may give way to maintaining comfort. The nurse should not avoid the difficult topic about end-of-life care, but ensure that open discussion is a central part of the client's care.

54. Numbers 2, 3, and 5 are correct.

Rationale: Age, gender, and culture are a few factors that influence the grieving process. The nurse must explore his own feelings about death before he may effectively help others. Nurses can help families find ways to cope with the loneliness and depression that follows the death of a loved one. The process of grief is normal following a loss, and expression of grief is essential for physical and emotional well-being. The expression of grief should never be discouraged; family members should have a quiet room in which they may express their feelings in private.

55. Number 2 is correct.

Rationale: A child with severe autism who is having a tonsillectomy is at greatest risk for alterations in sensory perception. Clients with severe autism experience altered thought processes. Adding an unfamiliar environment (the hospital) with pain from a surgical procedure compounds the risk of altered sensory perception. The client in the halo vest may have pain and restricted mobility, but he does not have as great a risk for altered perception as the child with severe autism. A teenager who broke her leg during cheerleader practice is more likely to have a large social group and be less isolated. A schoolteacher is more likely to work in a stimulating environment and have many social contacts. Risk factors for altered perception include emotional disorders, a non-stimulating environment, acute illness, limited mobility, pain, decreased cognitive ability, and impaired hearing or vision.

56. Number 3 is correct.

Rationale: Telling the client that it is normal to be afraid and asking how he feels is the most therapeutic option. Asking the client why he is worried about such a minor procedure puts the client on the defensive and trivializes the procedure. What the nurse may see as a minor procedure may feel like major surgery to the client. Offering to call the doctor and cancel the surgery may not be an option, depending on the procedure the client is having. It also does not allow for exploration of the client's feelings and may increase the client's fear if the nurse is quick to offer canceling the procedure. Telling the client not to worry and that the doctor will be sure that nothing goes wrong offers false reassurance and dismisses the client's feelings.

57. Number 3 is correct.

Rationale: Silence allows the client time to think and reflect and lead the conversation in the desired direction. Silence does not imply that the nurse is not listening, nor does it encourage the client to keep her feelings to herself. Silence is part of listening; the nurse should be focused on the client and not thinking ahead to what else she needs to do.

58. Numbers 2, 3, and 4 are correct.

Rationale: Providing an ordered hypnotic will promote sleep. Lowering the temperature of the room will promote sleep. Fresh linens will provide comfort. A light snack rather than a large meal should be provided.

59. Numbers 1 and 2 are correct.

Rationale: Weight is the most accurate measure for volume retention that is a stress on the cardiac workload. Assistance with self-care activities should be done to avoid exertion. The environment should be comfortable and quiet to reduce stress. Vital signs should be checked before and after activity, especially if the client is taking vasodilators or diuretics.

60. Number 3 is correct.

Rationale: A TURP is done by means of a scope introduced through the urethra so there is no incision. The color of the urine will change according to how much bleeding occurs after surgery. The most common type of bleeding is from a venous source resulting in dark burgundy coloration with dark clots. This type of bleeding will typically stop on its own. Bright red urine with bright red clots is considered more aggressive and may require intervention. Drinking water will help flush the kidneys and/or bladder of bacteria and clots. A catheter is typically inserted after a TURP.

61. Number 4 is correct.

Rationale: Assessment is the first step of the nursing process and should precede all interventions. Provide positive feedback to the client when independent activity or progress occurs. Because hemiparesis typically occurs on the opposite side of the injury to the brain, hygiene items should be placed on the client's right side. As determined after assessment, assistive devices are provided for self-care activities.

62. Number 3 is correct.

Rationale: Post TKR surgery a client will be asked to ambulate the day of surgery, making a fracture pan unnecessary. Having a cold or infection of any kind up to 2 weeks prior to surgery may be a contraindication for surgery. Standard practice is to administer a preoperative antibiotic. Pain medication is routinely ordered post-op and is administered as needed by the client.

63. Number 3 is correct.

Rationale: Antacids should not be taken within 2 hours of Levaquin because they interfere with absorption of the drug, especially if they contain aluminum or magnesium. Levaquin, along with many other antibiotics, increases sun sensitivity. The client should avoid going outdoors or wear sunscreen while on therapy. Taking the complete course of medication prevents rebound infections and antibiotic resistance. Clients should be taught how to take their pulse and report any new-onset irregular heartbeats, as fluoroquinolones may cause serious dysrhythmias.

64. Number 3 is correct.

Rationale: Warfarin doses typically range from 2 to 10 mg PO daily, with dosing adjusted to maintain the PT 1.2 – 2 × the control, or an INR of 2 – 3. This is a higher-than-expected dose.

65. Number 2 is correct.

Rationale: If the client's apical pulse is below 60, the nurse should hold the medication and notify the health care provider. Placing oxygen on the client will not have any effect on the pulse. Waiting an hour to recheck the pulse means a delay in medication administration, but also allows time for the pulse to drop lower, which may worsen client outcomes. There should never be a delay when there is a need to notify the health care provider. Administering the drug may cause the client to become severely bradycardic, and the UAP is not licensed to assess the client, especially when medications have been administered. The nurse is ultimately responsible for follow-up assessments on all clients.

66. 25 mg/mL.

Solution:

0.5 g = 500 mg	Convert grams to milligrams.
$\dfrac{500 \text{ mg}}{20 \text{ mL}}$	Divide milligrams of Diuril by milliliters of sterile water for reconstitution.
= 25 mg/mL	Solve the equation.

Reconstitution with 20 mL of sterile water yields a concentration of 25 mg/mL.

67. Number 3 is correct.

Rationale: IM injections are given at a 90-degree angle. A 25-gauge 1-inch needle is suitable for IM injections in children. A 45-degree angle is used to administer subcutaneous injections. A bleb should form only when giving intradermal injections.

68. Number 4 is correct.

Rationale: When performing gastric lavage, the solution is instilled and removed until returns are clear or light pink without clots. The volume of solution is 200 to 300 mL and should be at room temperature. The client is placed on the left side during the procedure.

69. Number 1 is correct.

Rationale: The wound should be cleaned with normal saline before sampling in order to remove normal skin flora. Do not delay culturing the wound; if the client is not already on antibiotics, the culture results guide the health care provider in prescribing the appropriate therapy. Old drainage should never be used as a sample because resident bacterial colonies from the skin are present in the exudate and may not be the cause of infection. The outer surface of the wound should not be cultured.

70. Numbers 1, 3, and 5 are correct.

Rationale: With continuous feedings, residual should be checked every 4 hours to assess for delayed gastric emptying. In noncritical clients, residual should be checked every 4 to 6 hours or according to agency policy. Residual is also checked before each bolus or intermittent feeding. If the volume is less than 250 mL, the contents are returned to the stomach to prevent electrolyte imbalance. For volumes greater than 250 mL, the nurse should follow agency policy or prescriber's orders. Clients should be positioned in a high Fowler's position or with the head of bed elevated at least 30 (preferably 45) degrees to prevent aspiration. The tubing and bag are changed every 24 hours to prevent bacterial growth.

71. Number 2 is correct.

Rationale: A history of basilar skull fracture may contraindicate tube placement. Neurological injury can result from intracranial passage of the tube. The other history findings are not indicative of a need to notify the health care provider.

72. Number 4 is correct.

Rationale: No one other than the client should press the button to deliver medication, in order to avoid oversedation. Remind the family to report if anyone other than the client administers a dose. The family should call if the pump starts beeping or the client becomes oversedated. Nausea is not an allergic reaction.

73. Number 4 is correct.

Rationale: Stabilizing the catheter for a male on the abdomen prevents meatus damage and erosion. Medical asepsis is adequate for perineal care. Routine irrigation is unnecessary. Unless medically contraindicated, fluids should be encouraged to 2,000 cc/day rather than restricted.

74. Number 1 is correct.

Rationale: The normal lab value for calcium is 8.5 – 10.2 mg/dL. The symptoms of hypocalcemia include muscle stiffness/spasms, diaphoresis, and anxiety. The lab values stated are within normal range for alkaline phosphatase, sodium, and creatinine.

75. Number 2 is correct.

Rationale: While somatostatin is secreted by different tissues, of significance is the gastrointestinal system, specifically the pancreas and the intestinal tract. Somatostatin inhibits the secretion of other hormones, including insulin and glucagon.

76. Number 4 is correct.

Rationale: Heart sounds S1 (tricuspid and mitral valves close) and S2 (aortic and pulmonic valves close) are auscultated to determine the apical pulse over the point of maximal impact. The third heart sound (S3) occurs slightly after S2. The fourth heart sound (S4) is heard slightly before S1.

77. Number 2 is correct.

Rationale: The client's symptoms are consistent with increased intracranial pressure (ICP). The best immediate response is to elevate the client's head to 30 degrees to produce a drop in ICP. Checking the blood pressure is a secondary action. Oxygen administration will not impact the increased ICP. Increasing the IV rate would be contraindicated.

78.   Number 4 is correct.

Rationale: Developing a nursing care plan requires the advanced knowledge consistent with the education of a registered nurse. An LPN may update or modify a care plan based on a change in client status. The other listed responsibilities are within the scope of an LPN.

79.   Number 3 is correct.

Rationale: The client who is post–atrial fibrillation ablation is experiencing symptoms of cardiac tamponade, a serious complication seen after this procedure. Cardiac tamponade occurs when the ablation penetrates the pericardium allowing fluid to collect, preventing the heart from expanding properly. Emergency intervention is required with this client, including a pericardiocentesis up to a thoracotomy to drain fluid. The other clients may be seen after assessing the client for a cardiac tamponade. While each of these needs is important to address quickly, the nurse first addresses situations that may be life-threatening for the client.

80.   Number 2 is correct.

Rationale: Safety of the client is a primary concern. While domestic abuse of an adult female does not require reporting to a federal agency, the nurse is in a position to intervene with the client. Other responses are nontherapeutic communications that fail to promote a constructive relationship with the client.

81.   Number 4 is correct.

Rationale: Before delegating tasks to the UAP, the nurse must ensure the UAP's competency is verified by the facility. Such verification may result from an external certification authority or the facility itself. Neither the client's comfort level with the UAP nor the UAP's comfort performing the task is relevant to the appropriate delegation of the task. The task previously being performed by the UAP fails to ensure verification of competency.

82.   Numbers 2 and 3 are correct.

Rationale: Clients need to be in the supine position to allow access to the perineal area. Sterile lubricant, part of the standard catheter kit, is applied to the tip of the catheter to ease entrance through the meatus. A sterile field is maintained when inserting an indwelling catheter. The amount of sterile water used to inflate the catheter balloon depends on the size of the balloon. Typically a 5 cc balloon will be inflated with 7 – 10 cc of sterile water (part of the catheter kit) to maintain the position of the catheter within the bladder.

83.   Number 4 is correct.

Rationale: Assessment of client response to a therapeutic intervention may only be done by a registered nurse. All other tasks are within the scope of practice of an LPN.

84.   Number 4 is correct.

Rationale: The client with *Clostridium difficile* is on contact precautions. Personal protective equipment (PPE)—including gown, gloves, mask, and shoe covers—provides a barrier between the client and nurse. Meticulous hand care and hand washing are required when caring for a client with *Clostridium difficile*, regardless of pregnancy status of the health care worker. Shingles and measles pose a high risk to pregnant women, and the CDC recommends that pregnant women avoid exposure to these clients. Pneumonia requires droplet precautions, because pneumonia may be contracted without direct client contact. Therefore, pneumonia exposure is even riskier for the pregnant nurse. When possible, pregnant nurses should avoid isolation clients. Facility and CDC guidelines should be followed when assigning pregnant staff to clients on precautions.

85. Number 1 is correct.

Rationale: Latex allergies can cause what is known as a cross-reaction when bananas are consumed by someone with the allergy. Latex is made from rubber tree sap, which is a member of the same plant family as bananas. Certain clients may also be sensitive to kiwi, avocado, and other foods. Options 2, 3, and 4 contain foods that would not cause a cross-reaction with latex allergy.

86. Numbers 1, 2, 3, and 4 are correct.

Rationale: When a client is found in the floor, the nurse should first assess the client for any injuries and then obtain help to assist the client back to the bed. The health care provider should be notified immediately, as the client may need an X-ray or CT to assess for fractures or internal injuries, especially if he hit his head. An incident report must be completed to comply with Joint Commission safety standards; client falls are monitored and facilities use this information to prevent similar incidents in the future. The nurse should not state in the medical record that the client fell, even if the client reports this, because the nurse did not witness the fall. The nurse would instead note that the client was found lying on the floor, followed by a narrative documenting the nurse's interventions. Many falls can be prevented by ensuring that call lights are within reach and answered promptly, and that personal effects are close by. Confused clients may require a family member or sitter. All clients should be assessed for fall risk upon admission and wear a special "fall risk" bracelet to alert staff.

87. Number 2 is correct.

Rationale: The safest option for client safety is to move beds into the hall and close window coverings and client room doors. Leaving window coverings open increases the risk of harm by flying debris. Closing blinds and leaving clients in their rooms with the doors open is not the safest option. Option 4 may be used in critical care areas where clients are on ventilators and other equipment that would be difficult to move into the hallway, but it is not the safest option.

88. Number 1 is correct.

Rationale: The fetal heart tone strip shows variable decelerations, which are caused by umbilical cord compression. The nurse should reposition the client. Drawing a potassium level will not resolve the problem. The health care provider does not need to be notified unless decelerations worsen after repositioning. There is no indication at this time for a cesarean section.

89. Number 1 is correct.

Rationale: During the first trimester of pregnancy, a nonpharmologic biologic treatment option like ECT is a viable option. The employment status, living environment, or age of the client would not impact the decision to use ECT.

90. Number 2 is correct.

Rationale: The trauma experienced by the client would respond best to a multidisciplinary school team that includes the nurse. Private counseling sessions with the client may be beneficial, yet a holistic approach is preferable. Assuring the client the campus is safe is not within the scope of nursing practice, and it would not be beneficial. Excusing the client from school perpetuates avoidance symptoms, which is not considered therapeutic.

91. Numbers 1 and 3 are correct.

Rationale: Schizophrenia typically occurs between the ages of 16 and 30. It is considered a severe mental disorder that affects an individual's relationship with reality. Symptoms of psychotic behavior are categorized as positive (such as hallucinations), negative (such as a flat affect), and cognitive (such as limited executive functioning). The final category of symptoms is cognitive (ability to process information). Bipolar disorder signs and symptoms during a manic episode include a fast speech pattern and the feeling of being energized.

92. Numbers 1 and 3 are correct.

   Rationale: Aripiprazole (Abilify) is an atypical antipsychotic used to treat schizophrenia and bipolar disorder in both adults and adolescents. Uncontrolled body movements (including the face, tongue, or other body parts) is indicative of tardive dyskinesia, a known serious side effect of Abilify. Stiff muscles may be indicative of neuroleptic malignant syndrome, a known serious side effect of Abilify. Hypertension and bradycardia are not side effects of Abilify.

93. Numbers 1 and 2 are correct.

   Rationale: Individuals who suffer from the eating disorder anorexia nervosa usually have a distorted body image and are preoccupied with controlling their weight and shape. Common characteristics are fatigue from lack of food along with an excessive exercise regime to lose weight. Alternately, bulimia nervosa clients are typically of normal weight. Low, rather than high, blood pressure is associated with anorexia.

94. Number 3 is correct.

   Rationale: Potato chips and cheese are high in sodium and should be avoided when on a low-sodium diet. Tomatoes and celery are not high in sodium and may be consumed. Most take-out foods are high in sodium and should be avoided.

95. Number 1 is correct.

   Rationale: In a compromised client, fluid volume excess can result from excessive IV infusion. Administration of corticosteroids on a short-term basis will not affect fluid volume excess. Diarrhea and fever will result in loss of body fluids rather than accumulation.

96. Number 1 is correct.

   Rationale: Clients with diverticulitis should consume low-roughage foods, avoiding nuts, seeds, popcorn, and raw celery. Seeds and tomatoes should be avoided. Consuming high-fiber foods such as fresh fruit and whole wheat bread is encouraged. Creamy peanut butter and jelly may be consumed by persons with diverticulitis. Chicken salad may be consumed by clients with diverticulitis.

97. Number 4 is correct.

   Rationale: Red meat consumption may cause false positive readings as will foods high in iron. The other foods do not cause false-positive readings.

98. Number 4 is correct.

   Rationale: Dorsiflexion of the foot is recommended to relieve a muscle spasm. Drinking a glass of water at bedtime will improve hydration but will not address the complaint. Compression hose are recommended for wearing during the day but should be removed at night. Elevating the head of the bed at night is recommended for gastric reflex disorder and in some cardiac and respiratory disorders.

99. Number 3 is correct.

   Rationale: The therapeutic level of theophylline is 10 – 20 mcg/mL. Option 1 represents the therapeutic level of digoxin. Option 2 represents the therapeutic level of phenytoin. Option 4 represents the therapeutic level of lithium.

100. Numbers 2, 4, and 5 are correct.

   Rationale: Serious side effects caused by long-term use of proton pump inhibitors include depression, rhabdomyolysis, and long bone fractures. Serious side effects are more likely at higher doses. Nausea and constipation are minor side effects.

101. Number 2 is correct.

Rationale: The client should be in the high-Fowler's position when administering medications by NG tube to prevent aspiration. Before administration, the nurse must aspirate and check the residual, and then return it to the stomach. Not all medications may be given via NG tube. Extended release and enteric coated medications may not be given via this route. If tube feeding is in place, it must be stopped before giving medications. Following medication administration, the tubing should be flushed with 15 – 30 cc of water, or as per facility protocol.

102. Number 4 is correct.

Rationale: Epoetin alfa is usually given as a weekly injection either IM or subcutaneously. Side effects include joint pain, hypertension, and headaches. Bloody urine is not a side effect of this medication.

103. Numbers 1, 4, and 5 are correct.

Rationale: Digitalis is given to treat atrial flutter and atrial fibrillation. It is contraindicated in AV block, sick sinus syndrome, and Wolff-Parkinson-White syndrome.

104. Number 1 is correct.

Rationale: The nurse should give the next dose as ordered. The therapeutic range for a vancomycin trough is 10 – 20 mcg/mL, so this client is within range. There is no need to wait and redraw the trough. Since the trough level is therapeutic, there is no need to hold the medication and notify the health care provider.

105. Number 1 is correct.

Rationale: Drugs requiring peak and trough levels, such as vancomycin, require precise timing in order to obtain accurate results. The peak dose should be drawn 1 – 2 hours after infusion, when drug levels are at their highest. Troughs are drawn when the drug is at its lowest level, which is right before the next dose is due. Options 2, 3, and 4 reflect inaccurate draw times.

106. Number 1 is correct.

Rationale: Beer, anchovies, and liver are high in purine and should be avoided in clients prone to gout. Options 2 and 3 may be included in the diet, unless there are other reasons to avoid these foods. Option 4 lists food high in tyramine, which should be avoided by clients taking certain medications, such as MAOI. Unless the client is on one of these medications, there is no need to avoid those foods.

107. Number 2 is correct.

Rationale: Stage II ulcers present with partial thickness loss of dermis and a red-pink wound bed. No slough is present. Stage I ulcers have intact skin with a red area. The area may be firm, painful, soft, or cooler or warmer compared to adjacent tissue. Stage III ulcers have full-thickness skin loss and may contain slough. The wound may have visible subcutaneous tissue, and tunneling and undermining may or may not be present. Stage IV ulcers present with full-thickness skin loss and exposed bone, muscle, or tendons. Eschar and slough may be present, and tunneling and undermining may develop. Unstageable wounds cannot be staged due to eschar or slough covering the wound. The wound bed must be visualized in order to stage the wound.

108. Number 5 is correct.

Rationale: Unstageable wounds cannot be staged due to eschar or slough covering the wound. The wound bed must be visualized in order to stage the wound. Stage I ulcers have intact skin with a red area. The area may be firm, painful, soft, or cooler or warmer compared to adjacent tissue. Stage II ulcers present with partial thickness loss of dermis and a red-pink wound bed. No slough is present. Stage III ulcers have full-thickness skin loss and may contain slough. The wound may have visible subcutaneous tissue, and tunneling and undermining may or may not be present. Stage IV ulcers present with full-thickness skin loss and exposed bone, muscle, or tendons. Eschar and slough may be present, and tunneling and undermining may develop.

109. (Correct response: Nonmaleficence)

Rationale: Nonmaleficence is the ethical principle that states the nurse's duty is to do no harm.

110. Number 1 is correct.

Rationale: In atrial flutter, there are no discernible P waves, and a distinct sawtooth wave pattern is present. The atrial rate is regular, and the PR interval is not measurable. In atrial fibrillation, the rhythm would be very irregular with coarse, asynchronous waves. Torasades de pointes, or "twisting of the points," is characterized by QRS complexes that twist around the baseline and is a form of polymorphic ventricular tachycardia. It may resolve spontaneously or progress to ventricular fibrillation. Normal sinus rhythm is the rhythm of a healthy heart, originating from the sinus node. The heart rate is between 60 and 100 with a distinct P wave and regular QRS complexes. Ventricular fibrillation is life-threatening, as the ventricles are unable to pump any blood due to disorganized electrical activity. Untreated, it quickly leads to cardiac arrest.

111. Numbers 1 and 4 are correct.

Rationale: In fluid overload, BUN and sodium levels would be decreased due to hemodilution. Hematocrit and serum osmolality would also be decreased due to extra fluid volume.

112. Number 3 is correct.

Rationale: The normal sodium range is 135 to 145 mEq/L. Levels below 120 mEq/L are critical and may lead to death if left untreated. The values given for chloride, calcium, and potassium are within the normal range and do not require treatment.

113. Number 3 is correct.

Rationale: During ventricular systole, blood enters the aorta and the pulmonary artery. The other options do not correctly explain which vessels the blood enters during the ventricular systole phase of the cardiac cycle.

114. Number 1 is correct.

Rationale: The nurse should notify the health care provider and ask for another order. At this dose, the client may potentially receive 6,000 mg of acetaminophen in 24 hours, which far exceeds current FDA recommendations of a maximum dose of 4,000 mg per day. This dose can cause liver damage, especially in clients with decreased liver function. Administering the medication as ordered exposes the client to the risk of an excessive dose. Giving other PRN medications and ignoring the order may potentially harm the client if another nurse follows the order as written. Giving the medication on a different schedule than ordered places the nurse in the position of practicing medicine without a license. Client safety is always a priority in administering medication.

115. The nurse should set the IV pump to 60 mL/hr.

Solution:

$\dfrac{100 \text{ units}}{500 \text{ mL}} = \dfrac{12 \text{ units}}{x \text{ mL}}$	Set up a proportion to solve for milliliters per hour.
$100x = 500(12)$	Solve for x.
$100x = 6{,}000$	
$x = 60$ mL/hr	The IV pump should deliver 60 mL per hour.

116. Number 4 is correct.

Rationale: The client has a legal right to receive communications in her native language regarding care. Most facilities have twenty-four hour telephone interpretation services for almost all spoken languages. The interpreter is fluent in medical terminology in all relevant languages and can accurately relay information from the health care provider to the client and/or family. Asking a bilingual family member for assistance is of limited help. The family member may not be able to accurately communicate instructions on describing pain (dull, sharp, radiating) or using the pain scale. Calling another nurse within the facility to translate is problematic. Not only is a nurse being removed from another unit, leaving her clients in the care of other staff, but there is the potential for a lawsuit if she fails to properly translate information. Facility interpreters, including those for deaf clients, should be certified in their language and have ongoing training. They are responsible if information is not properly translated or conveyed to the client. Showing the client equipment to be used and indicating where it will be used may not be effective in cases of elderly clients, those with altered mental status, or those who have not received care in a facility setting prior to the ED admission.

117. Number 4 is correct.

Rationale: Care coordination is limited in that the scope of work is based on a plan that is created with input from the client. The stakeholder in case management is an insurance company or a hospital. The main goal of care coordination is to promote a better quality of life for the client, while case management's goal also includes legal and financial issues that may involve stakeholders. Additionally, eliminating noncompliance and overutilization of resources is addressed. Care coordination is based on a holistic approach and an understanding of client-family dynamics, with less emphasis on issues that affect stakeholders. Advocating for client needs is emphasized over stakeholder interests.

118. Numbers 3, 4, and 5 are correct.

Rationale: Responses 3, 4, and 5 are examples of how a nurse keeps the client's interest at the focus of care and maintains the role of client advocate. One of the duties is making sure that the client understands treatment options, including possible outcomes if the client refuses treatment. The nurse must also ensure that the client receives instruction in her native tongue if she does not speak English. This is especially important when obtaining consent for surgery and other invasive procedures. Copies of living wills, advance directives, and other legal health care documents should be placed in the client's chart if available. Only speaking to family members regarding the client's care is rude and does not show consideration for the client's wishes for her care. The nurse should not insist that any client become an organ donor. The nurse's opinion is secondary to the client's wishes. The nurse serves as a client advocate by following the client's wishes, not pushing what he thinks is best for the client.

119. Number 3 is correct.

Rationale: The Patient's Bill of Rights gives all clients the right to a quick and objective review of any claim that they levy against a health care facility, physician, or health care plan. Clients also have the right to view and receive copies of their medical records. Anyone presenting to an emergency department, whether insured or not, has the right to receive life-saving treatment and stabilization, or be transferred to another, more appropriate facility if required. It is against the law for an emergency department to refuse treatment to anyone, regardless of ability to pay. The client is responsible for providing correct information regarding past medical history, medications, and treatments. While the nurse is expected to make all reasonable efforts to corroborate client reports, the ultimate responsibility lies with the consumer of health care.

120. Numbers 1, 2, 4, and 5 are correct.

Rationale: Principles of triage include treating the least stable clients first. In this scenario, there are four clients requiring immediate attention. When a piece of equipment alarms, the first course of action is to check the client, and then troubleshoot the alarm. The nurse should never ignore any alarm for any reason. Clients who have just returned from surgery, especially an open surgical approach, are at risk for loss of airway due to anesthesia, bleeding from the site, and other potential surgery-specific risks. A sudden change in level of consciousness requires immediate action to determine the cause. Tingling in the mouth is a sign of a possibly serious allergic reaction and may occur if the client receives a new medication for the first time. This client is at high risk of anaphylactic shock. A client who is ready to transfer to the floor is stable and therefore not a priority situation. The client with diabetes who has a blood sugar of 90 is within a safe range and does not require emergent treatment or monitoring.

121. Number 1 is correct.

    Rationale: Obtaining a stool sample from the client is within the scope of practice of the UAP, making the assignment of this task appropriate. Compiling the history of symptoms requires the nurse's level of knowledge. Educating the client on diagnostic testing is outside the scope of acceptable UAP tasks as is obtaining a sample of gastric contents from a nasogastric tube.

122. Number 4 is correct.

    Rationale: It is never in the nurse's best interest to sign legal documents with clients that are not part of the admissions or informed consent process. The nurse knows the client is not fully oriented to person, place, and time; therefore, the nurse is not acting in the best interest of the client as a client advocate. The nurse may also face disciplinary action from the state board of nursing, or could become involved in a legal case if anything happens to the patient. Most facilities would not allow nurses to sign as a witness on these types of documents. Asking for a copy of the document implies that the nurse will witness it, which is incorrect. Having a copy of the document in the nurse's possession away from the facility would be a HIPAA violation. The unit manager may not serve as a witness in this situation. Asking the daughter if the client is aware of what is going on incorrectly implies that the nurse might sign the document. The nurse has the clinical training and expertise to determine when a client is not fully oriented—not a family member.

123. Numbers 1, 3, 4, and 5 are correct.

    Rationale: Maintaining normal toileting routines and frequent checks for toileting needs helps reassure the client that her needs are being met. Many medications cause further confusion, so the nurse should note any medications that might need to be reviewed with the health care provider. Having pictures and other familiar objects reinforces that the room belongs to the client during her stay. Clocks and calendars help orient the client and give her a sense of time and place. Family members and visitors should be encouraged, not discouraged, to visit as they can help alert the nurse to client needs. Companionship is important to the client's self-esteem and may prevent boredom, which can lead to getting up unassisted or wandering. The client should be as close to the nurses' station as possible so that frequent checks by multiple staff are quicker and easier.

124. Number 2 is correct.

    Rationale: The nurse should offer the client a bedpan or urinal. The client who has been medicated with morphine is at high risk for falls and should not get up. Assisting the client to the toilet increases the risk of falls. Foley catheters should not be used simply for client or nurse convenience, due to the risk of infection. Placing a bedside commode still allows the client to get up from the bed, and the client is unlikely to require assistance if the bedside commode is within close reach.

125. Number 3 is correct.

    Rationale: Ambulatory clients may assist in moving clients in wheelchairs during a fire emergency without fear of HIPAA violations. Clients should not overexert themselves, however. Doing so may render them needing aid as well. Oxygen sources near a fire should be shut off if safe to do so. Bedridden clients who can sit safely in a wheelchair may be evacuated in wheelchairs, and the weakest or most needy clients can be moved in their beds. Less staff is required to move a wheelchair compared to a bed. Clients on ventilators must be manually bagged with an Ambu bag until they can be placed back on the ventilator.

126. Number 1 is correct.

Rationale: Foods high in vitamin K, including green tea, will lessen warfarin's effectiveness and should be avoided. The vegetables listed are not contraindicated when taking warfarin (Coumadin).

127. Numbers 2, 3, and 4 are correct.

Rationale: A nonimmune nurse should refrain from being assigned to care for a client with a vaccine-preventable airborne disease such as measles, chicken pox, smallpox, influenza, and pertussis. While tuberculosis is an airborne disease, the vaccine for prevention is rarely used in the United States.

128. Number 4 is correct.

Rationale: Protamine sulfate is needed to neutralize the effects of heparin. Warfarin is the generic name for Coumadin, which is used to prevent blood clot formation. Potassium chloride is used to treat or prevent low amounts of potassium. Vitamin K is the antidote in case of Coumadin overdose.

129. Number 1 is correct.

Rationale: Unless otherwise ordered, a client's apical pulse needs to be 60 for digoxin administration. The nurse should withhold the medicine and contact the prescribing physician. Having another nurse verify the apical pulse is not the correct first action as there is no indication that the digoxin should be administered regardless or that the first nurse made an error. A stat ECG is unnecessary.

130. Number 3 is correct.

Rationale: Solu-cortef (hydrocortisone sodium succinate) is a corticosteroid hormone (glucocorticoid) used as an anti-inflammatory agent for numerous diseases. It is known to elevate (not lower) glucose level. The effect on magnesium is insubstantial.

131. Number 4 is correct.

Rationale: Furosemide (Lasix) is a diuretic that inhibits the absorption of sodium and chloride from the loop of Henle and distal renal tubule. This action increases renal excretion of water, sodium, chloride, magnesium, potassium, and calcium. This reduction of body fluid and electrolytes may produce a dry mouth. Appetite is not affected by furosemide. Leg cramps are an adverse effect of hypokalemia.

132. The nurse should set the IV pump to 19mL/hr.

Solution:

$\dfrac{178 \text{ lbs}}{2.2 \text{ kg}} = 80.90 = 81$ kg	Convert the client's weight to kilograms.
12 units/kg/hr (81 kg)	Calculate the infusion rate.
= 972 units/hr	
$\dfrac{500 \text{ mL}}{25{,}000 \text{ units}} = \dfrac{x \text{ mL}}{972 \text{ units}}$	Set up a proportion to solve for milliliters per hour.
500(972) = 25,000x	Calculate and solve for x.
486,000 = 25,000x	
x = 19.44 mL = **19 mL/hr**	Round down to find the rate.

133. Number 1 is correct.

Rationale: Hypocalcemia indicates hypoparathyroidism. Symptoms include paresthesias and dysphagia. Hypoparathyroidism does not alter potassium, magnesium, or blood glucose levels.

134. Number 1 is correct.

Rationale: The normal range for hemoglobin is 14 – 18 g/dL in males and 12 – 16 g/dL in females. This client's hemoglobin value is critically low, which places him at increased risk for stroke, heart attack, congestive heart failure, and angina. The troponin, phosphorus, and bilirubin levels given are within normal limits.

135. Number 1 is correct.

Rationale: The V5 lead should be placed in the left midaxillary line. The V4 lead is placed in the fifth intercostal right midclavicular line. The V2 lead is placed in the fourth intercostal space to the left of the sternum. The V1 lead is placed in the fourth intercostal space to the right of the sternum.

136. Numbers 4 and 5 are correct.

Rationale: In preparing for a PFT, the nurse should teach the client to avoid smoking at least 6 to 8 hours before the test. Bronchodilators should be withheld for 4 to 6 hours before the test. There is no need for the client to take a driver with her because she will not be sedated. The client should maintain normal activity levels, neither limiting nor increasing activity before the test. Maintaining normal activity levels gives a truer picture of the client's lung function. There is no need to be NPO for the test.

137. Numbers 3, 5, and 6 are correct.

Rationale: Clubbing may be found in clients with sickle cell disease and right-sided heart failure. It is common in clients with congenital heart defects. Clubbing can be reversible if the underlying cause is resolved. It is caused by chronic, not acute, oxygen deprivation.

138. Number 2 is correct.

Rationale: The LPN is able to monitor vital signs and report the findings to the charge nurse. A client with a recent head injury and active seizures requires assessment skills consistent with an RN. LPNs are not licensed to administer blood products. Client education must be conducted by an RN.

139. Answers:

Diagnosis	Abdominal Location
1. acute cholecystitis	RUQ
2. acute appendicitis	RIF
3. acute cystitis	suprapubic
4. acute peptic ulcer	epigastric
5. splenic infarction	LUQ

140. Number 3 is correct.

Rationale: Repair for undescended testicles, an orchiopexy, is performed on infant males aged 5 – 15 months using laparoscopy via an inguinal approach. The procedure is performed under general anesthesia. Two incisions are made, one in the groin and another in the scrotum. The surgical site should be monitored for bleeding. Bed rest for several days is advisable to allow for recovery from anesthesia. As well, strenuous activity should be avoided to prevent trauma to the surgical site. Palpation of the scrotum to check testicle location will be done by the surgeon at the regular follow-up visit.

141. Number 3 is correct.

Rationale: HIPAA protects personal information that should be shared only with personnel directly involved in client care. The Patient's Bill of Rights states an individual's right to health care. The Patient Self-Determination Act addresses the individual's right to make decisions about his health care. The Uniform Anatomical Gift Act addresses the donation of body parts by the individual for the purpose of education, science, and medicine.

142. Number 3 is correct.

Rationale: Explaining the reason for the transfusion requires the knowledge base of a nurse. As such, this activity may not be delegated to a UAP. In contrast, the other stated activities are within the scope of practice of a UAP.

143. Number 4 is correct.

Rationale: OBRA '87 provides the right for residents to organize and participate in a resident or family council. The act does not address organizing hospital personnel. The other stated rights are included in the act.

144. Number 1 is correct.

145. Number 2 is correct.

Rationale: The nurse has an obligation to promote safety of the client in the home. Leaving the refrigerator and freezer door open for extended periods of time may lessen the temperature of perishable food items. Instructing the client to place a fan in front of the freezer serves to encourage risky behavior. The nurse has an obligation to intervene when an unsafe practice is observed in the house. In a reasonable period of time the nurse should inform the nursing supervisor, but this is not the most appropriate action to address a potential safety hazard.

146. Number 1 is correct.

Rationale: Both an incident report and documentation of the finding in the client's medical record should occur. The incident report is an internal communication mechanism meant for performance and quality improvement. Reporting the incident to the nursing supervisor fails to adequately communicate a medication administration error. Filing an incident report addresses internal notification of a potential area for improvement yet fails to document a potential problem in the client's medical record.

147. Number 2 is correct.

Rationale: Of the items listed, only delivery of flowers (fresh or dried) is not allowed in a protective environment. The remaining items are acceptable for delivery.

148. Number 4 is correct.

Rationale: The nurse would anticipate an order for Kayexalate, which lowers elevated potassium levels. K-Dur is given for hypokalemia. Pradaxa is an anticoagulant given to prevent stroke in clients with nonvalvular atrial fibrillation. Namenda is used to manage moderate to severe Alzheimer's.

149. Number 1 is correct.

Rationale: Timolol maleate treats glaucoma by reducing intraocular pressure. It should be used with caution in clients with asthma because the beta-adrenergic effects can worsen asthma exacerbations. Migraines, atrial fibrillation, and urinary tract infection are not contraindications to prescribing timolol maleate.

150. Number 1 is correct.

Rationale: Oxytocin is a high-alert medication used to induce or augment labor. The presence of more than five contractions in a 10-minute time period indicates uterine tachysystole. The nurse should immediately discontinue the infusion and reposition or maintain the client in the side-lying position. A bolus of 500 mL of lactated Ringer's should be administered. If the preceding measures do not resolve the fetal heart rate tracing, the nurse may administer 10 L/min of oxygen. If there is still no response, the nurse may give 0.25 mg of terbutaline based on standing orders or facility protocols. The health care provider should be notified. Increasing the oxytocin infusion rate will worsen the client's condition, while merely decreasing the rate will not be effective enough. The client does not need to be in a high-Fowler's position, but may be positioned on either side.

THREE: Practice Test Three

READ THE QUESTION, AND THEN CHOOSE THE MOST CORRECT ANSWER.

1. A child with a known peanut allergy is eating lunch at summer camp and develops an anaphylactic reaction from accidentally ingesting peanut butter–flavored cookies. The nurse's first intervention should be to

   1. have the child lie down on the ground.
   2. take the child's blood pressure.
   3. verify the child has stopped eating and has no more cookies in his mouth.
   4. ask the child how many cookies he ate.

2. A post-operative client with an abdominal wound tries to reach over and take a book off the bedside table. He immediately screams and calls for the nurse. The nurse notices serosanguineous drainage coming from the incision on the abdomen. The first action the nurse should take is to

   1. cover the incision with a sterile cloth or dressing.
   2. lower the head of the bed to less than 10 degrees.
   3. check the client's vitals to assess for drop in blood pressure.
   4. call and alert the surgeon.

3. A nurse has been hired by a company to educate employees on health risks. Which of the following may suggest substance abuse by certain employees in the workplace? **Select all that apply.**

   1. frequent call-ins and tardiness
   2. taking only the allocated two 15-minute breaks per shift
   3. increasingly poor performance evaluations
   4. meeting coworkers for dinner after work
   5. eating lunch alone at the desk instead of in the breakroom

4. A nurse assessing a client charts his blood pressure as 134/86. The pulse pressure would be
   1. 48.
   2. 86.
   3. 220.
   4. 96.

5. The nurse is assessing for abdominal pulsations in a client with a visible mass below the umbilicus. The nurse should use which technique?
   1. light palpation
   2. inspection
   3. percussion
   4. deep palpation

6. A physician orders 1,000 units of IV heparin to be infused over 2 hours. The pharmacy sends 10,000 units in 500 mL of 0.9% NaCl. The nurse would set the pump to administer how many mL/hr?
   1. 50 mL/hr
   2. 25 mL/hr
   3. 75 mL/hr
   4. 15 mL/hr

7. During her yearly exam, a woman's blood pressure is recorded as 146/90. She tells the nurse that her mother and grandmother had hypertension, so it likely runs in her family. Which of the following is the nurse's **best** response?
   1. "This indicates prehypertension and is nothing to worry about yet. Please come back in a few months and we will check it again."
   2. "Since hypertension runs in your family, this reading is within normal limits."
   3. "This shows that you have stage 2 hypertension. You will likely be prescribed medication today and will also need to see the nutritionist."
   4. "This shows that you have stage 1 hypertension. You may need to take medication and will need to make lifestyle changes as well."

8. After a cardiac catheterization procedure, the nurse should ask the client to remain in which position?
   1. on the left side, with both knees bent slightly
   2. semi-Fowler's position
   3. supine with a small pillow under the head
   4. high-Fowler's position

9. A woman comes to the clinic for a well-woman exam. The nurse charts her height as 5 feet, 3 inches and weight as 146 pounds. Her body mass index (BMI) would be

   1. 25.9.
   2. 19.6.
   3. 24.2.
   4. 28.5.

10. During a pre-op assessment, the nurse would chart which finding(s) as subjective data? **Select all that apply.**

    1. The client is sweating and wringing his hands.
    2. The client states, "I am having second thoughts about my surgery."
    3. The client reports he has lost 6 pounds in the last 2 months.
    4. The client's blood pressure is 128/82.
    5. The client rates his pain as a 3 on a scale of 0 – 10.

11. Which of the following would be considered a sensible type of fluid loss?

    1. sweat
    2. respiratory excretions
    3. vomit
    4. water loss in feces

12. Which of the following actions does NOT require the use of standard precautions?

    1. contact with blood
    2. contact with urine
    3. contact with sweat
    4. contact with vomit

13. A client diagnosed with gout 10 years ago admits she has never treated her gout and hoped it would just go away. The nurse knows all of the following are potential complications from untreated gout EXCEPT

    1. kidney stones.
    2. nodules of uric acid under the skin.
    3. deformed joints.
    4. peripheral neuropathy.

14. Which of the following is NOT a component of evidence-based practice?

    1. outcomes of research studies
    2. culturally competent care
    3. patient values
    4. clinical expertise

15. The nurse is caring for a 72-year-old female who must remain on bed rest after a hip fracture. The client has become confused and disoriented over the past 2 days. Which of the following is the **best** nursing intervention?

   1. placing familiar objects such as family photos, a clock, and a personal calendar on the wall

   2. asking the physician to order restraints so the client does not try and get up

   3. asking the client's daughter to stay overnight so the client is comforted by a familiar face

   4. moving the client to a better staffed floor, so she can be watched more carefully

16. Which of the following is NOT considered a risk factor for developing breast cancer?

   1. early menarche

   2. nulliparity

   3. early menopause

   4. previous history of uterine cancer

17. A client in ICU has a chest tube, and the nurse is assessing the chest tube drainage system. The nurse notices intermittent bubbling in the water seal chamber. What action should the nurse take?

   1. clamp the chest tube and call for help

   2. document the findings in the client chart

   3. document an air leak and notify the physician

   4. call the physician to report the findings

18. Which of the following tasks would an RN NOT delegate to an LPN?

   1. changing a sterile dressing on a stage 3 decubitus ulcer

   2. assessing a 30-year-old female's ability to ambulate after surgery

   3. administering a tube feeding for a 36-year-old male with ALS

   4. inserting a Foley catheter for a 79-year-old male with prostate cancer

19. Someone sees a nursing assistant yell at an elderly client and throw his lunch tray off the table. The nursing assistant could likely be charged with

   1. negligence.

   2. assault.

   3. malpractice.

   4. battery.

20. Which of the following is a core measure set developed by the Joint Commission?

   1. genetics

   2. lymphoma

   3. nosocomial infections

   4. heart failure

21. Which of the following would be considered a tertiary prevention? **Select all that apply.**

    1. The nurse administers a PPD test for a travel visa clearance.

    2. The nurse administers vancomycin to a client with a bacterial infection.

    3. The nurse works with a stroke patient to implement assistive devices in activities of daily living.

    4. The nurse presents information about smoking cessation at a health fair.

    5. The nurse administers an influenza vaccine to a 60-year-old male.

22. A 20-year-old woman who has been laboring at home for several hours has been admitted to the labor and delivery unit at the hospital. The nurse has come in to assess her progress. Which of the following is indicative of being in the active phase of labor?

    1. contractions lasting 45 seconds, 4 minutes apart, with cervical dilation of 4 cm

    2. contractions lasting 30 seconds, 6 minutes apart, with cervical dilation of 3 cm

    3. contractions lasting 60 seconds, 1 minute apart, with cervical dilation of 7 cm

    4. contractions lasting 90 seconds, 2 minutes apart, with cervical dilation of 8 cm

23. A student nurse is developing a care plan for a 23-year-old woman with Meniere's disease. Which of the following would NOT be an expected intervention?

    1. administer narcotic pain medication PRN as ordered

    2. refer client to dietician to plan meals with reduced sodium levels

    3. assist client out of bed to shower and to toilet

    4. encourage client to eat several, similarly sized meals throughout the day

24. A young woman experiencing a flare-up of Crohn's disease is confused about what kinds of foods she should eat and asks the nurse for a sample menu. Which of the following is the nurse's **best** suggestion for a breakfast meal?

    1. grits with margarine, sliced banana, and apple juice

    2. whole grain cereal with raisins, and one-half cup of coffee

    3. breakfast sandwich with bacon, fresh tomato, and onion on wheat bread, and a cup of tea

    4. bran waffles with crunchy peanut butter spread, and prune juice

25. Which laboratory finding would indicate a 62-year-old male client is at risk for ventricular dysrhythmia?

    1. magnesium 0.8 mmEq/L

    2. potassium 4.2 mmol/L

    3. creatinine 1.3 mg/dL

    4. total calcium 2.8 mmol/L

26. A client in ICU is being closely monitored after a fall. The nurse notices a slight increase in intracranial pressure (ICP). The nurse should intervene by

    1. increasing oxygen flow.
    2. elevating the head of the bed to 90 degrees.
    3. turning and repositioning the patient on his side.
    4. suctioning the patient at least hourly.

27. A patient is rushed to the emergency room after being found unconscious at home. His blood pressure is 70/35. The nurse anticipates an order for what medication?

    1. atropine sulfate (Atropine)
    2. amiodarone (Cordarone)
    3. magnesium sulfate
    4. adenosine (Adenoscan)

28. Place the steps for an abdominal assessment in the correct order.

    ___ auscultation

    ___ palpation

    ___ inspection

    ___ percussion

29. A 32-year-old woman comes into the clinic for a well-woman exam and asks for information on an intrauterine device (IUD) for contraception. The nurse should explain that all of the following are potential risks EXCEPT

    1. stroke.
    2. pelvic infections.
    3. abnormal menstrual bleeding.
    4. ectopic pregnancy.

30. Which of the following are true statements regarding peripherally inserted central catheter (PICC) lines? **Select all that apply.**

    1. requires sterile technique during insertion
    2. can be inserted by any LPN or RN
    3. lower risk of infection compared to other central lines
    4. increased risk of pneumothorax
    5. can be inserted at the patient bedside

31. A client taking furosemide (Lasix) comes into the clinic for routine bloodwork. Which of the following findings indicates an adverse effect of Lasix?

   1. chloride 102 mg/dL

   2. ammonia 36 µmol/L

   3. uric acid 13.5 mg/dL

   4. ferritin 176 ng/mL

32. An 82-year-old woman is being admitted to a long-term care facility. Her assigned nurse completes a full assessment, including calculating the risk for skin breakdown based on the Braden Scale. To determine a Braden Scale score, the nurse evaluates all of the following EXCEPT

   1. nutritional status.

   2. sensory perception.

   3. past history of skin breakdown.

   4. activity level.

33. A nurse receives an order to dilute ceftriaxone sodium powder in a vial prior to administration. The nurse should ensure the powder is fully diluted by

   1. shaking the vial for at least 60 seconds.

   2. rolling the vial between the palms of the hands.

   3. allowing vial to sit for at least 10 minutes before administering.

   4. asking the pharmacy to dilute the mixture.

34. A nurse is assessing a 33-year-old patient who underwent a cholecystectomy 18 hours prior. The nurse notes 500 mL of greenish-brown fluid has drained from the T-tube postoperatively. The nurse should

   1. chart these findings and reassess on the next rounding.

   2. call the physician and report the drainage.

   3. flush and irrigate the tube.

   4. chart these findings and indicate an infection is suspected.

35. All of the following are parts of the middle ear EXCEPT the

   1. pinna.

   2. incus.

   3. stapes.

   4. malleus.

36. A client has been admitted to the floor with suspected infective endocarditis. The nurse knows to look for which signs and symptoms that would indicate infective endocarditis? **Select all that apply.**

    1. weight gain
    2. fever
    3. Roth's spots
    4. murmur
    5. anemia

37. A 28-year-old woman with Guillain-Barre syndrome has been intubated and is on mechanical ventilation due to ascending paralysis. She has become increasingly worried and upset as the day has gone on. What would be the **best** response by the nurse to help the woman cope?

    1. "I am going to keep you heavily sedated so you will not have to be scared. When you wake up, you won't remember ever being sick."
    2. "I know this is overwhelming; this is a very complicated syndrome and it's too hard for you to understand. Just trust the health care providers."
    3. "I am going to hang a 'no visitors' sign on your door. You do not want your family to see you this way."
    4. "I know you are worried, and I am here to answer any questions you have. It is good to have your family here visiting to offer some distraction from being in bed."

38. A neonatal nurse assesses a premature newborn baby using the Apgar score. All of the following assessments are given a score EXCEPT

    1. grimace.
    2. pulse.
    3. activity.
    4. rooting.
    5. appearance.

39. A nurse must record daily liquid intake and output for a client with heart failure. The daily liquid intake includes 16 ounces of water, 12 ounces of apple juice, 1 pint of strawberry ice cream, and 0.75 L of normal saline IV. What would the nurse chart as daily intake in milliliters? Calculate and fill in the blank.

    _____

40. The nurse reviews a 21-year-old female's bloodwork from the lab. Which result would be charted as an abnormal finding?

    1. platelets 129
    2. RBC 4.2
    3. WBC 15.6
    4. hematocrit 38%

41. According to Maslow's hierarchy of needs, order the following needs from most basic to most advanced (bottom of the pyramid to the top):

___ safety and security

___ esteem

___ physiological

___ love and belonging

___ self-actualization

42. A child with a history of seizures begins to seize suddenly in his hospital room. The nurse would do all of the following interventions EXCEPT

    1. loosen the child's clothing and remove the pillow from his bed.

    2. administer lorazepam rectally.

    3. roll the child on his side.

    4. restrain the child's arms and legs.

43. A 37-year-old postpartum client explains to the nurse she had a deep vein thrombosis (DVT) after the birth of her last child. To help prevent a DVT during this hospital stay, the nurse should encourage the client to do all of the following EXCEPT

    1. wear thigh-high anti-embolism stockings as much as possible.

    2. increase daily fluid intake.

    3. avoid ambulating except to get up to use the restroom.

    4. prop legs up on pillows while sitting in bed.

44. A 19-year-old male was prescribed sertraline (Zoloft) 3 weeks ago for depression. He calls the clinic today and tells the nurse that he has been feeling increasingly anxious and wants to stop taking the medication because it is not working. The **best** response for the nurse is

    1. "You can stop taking the Zoloft, but let's make another appointment with your provider so you can try a different medication."

    2. "Increased anxiety is a normal side effect for the first few weeks of taking this medication. It will take several weeks to determine if it is working. Please keep taking it as prescribed."

    3. "Increased anxiety is not a normal side effect of Zoloft. What day this week can you come to the clinic to discuss this with your provider?"

    4. "Try taking half the prescribed dose for the next week and see if that helps the feelings of anxiety."

45. The nurse administers 6 units of Humalog (lispro) insulin sub-q to a client at 8:30 a.m. The nurse knows to reassess the client and check for a possible hypoglycemic reaction at

    1. 8:45 a.m.

    2. 9:30 a.m.

    3. 11:30 a.m.

    4. 12:00 p.m.

46. The transverse plane

    1. divides the body into superior and inferior sections.

    2. divides the body into right and left halves.

    3. divides the body into four sections cut diagonally.

    4. divides the body into ventral and dorsal sections.

47. A 10-year-old girl has been diagnosed with scabies. There are three other children and two adults living in the household. The nurse can **best** educate caregivers by stating,

    1. "Scabies is only transmitted through person-to-person contact."

    2. "Everyone in the household needs to receive treatment."

    3. "If anyone shows symptoms, come into the clinic for treatment."

    4. "Since the child has started treatment, she is no longer contagious."

48. A client is receiving gentamicin sulfate (Gentamicin) injections as part of her treatment regimen for a pseudomonas infection. The nurse knows to assess for what potential adverse reaction to this medication?

    1. orthostatic hypotension

    2. occult bleeding

    3. torsades de pointes

    4. ototoxicity

49. All of the following are common symptoms seen in clients diagnosed with tuberculosis (TB) EXCEPT

    1. nail clubbing.

    2. night sweats.

    3. weight gain.

    4. fever.

50. A client at a psychiatric hospital tells the nurse that he does not want to join the others for dinner in the dining room because he already ate. The nurse is aware this client has been diagnosed with avoidant personality disorder. The **best** response from the nurse is to

    1. ask the client what would make group dinners more enjoyable so he will participate in the future.

    2. allow the client to skip the group dinner this time only.

    3. ask the client why he ate dinner so early.

    4. state clearly that the client is expected in the dining room and then walk with the client to the dining room.

51. On the oncology floor, a client has just received a bone marrow transplant. The nurse would expect to see which drug prescribed to prevent graft versus host disease?

    1. etoposide (Etopophos)
    2. cytarabine (Ara-C)
    3. metoclopramide (Reglan)
    4. sandimmune (Cyclosporine)

52. A nurse is working at a summer camp for teenagers. Before the camp hiking trip, the nurse creates a presentation about how to prevent Lyme disease. The nurse would include which of the following in the presentation? **Select all that apply.**

    1. rinse clothing worn on the hike in cool water at the end of the day
    2. wear dark colors during the hike to repel ticks
    3. use insect repellent containing DEET on skin, clothing, and gear
    4. cover any ticks found on skin with petroleum jelly to suffocate them
    5. keep pants legs tucked into socks to prevent ticks from contacting skin

53. A 19-year-old male with type 1 diabetes has the flu. The nurse expects what insulin changes may be required during the illness?

    1. stopping all insulin
    2. needing more insulin
    3. needing less insulin
    4. using the same amount of insulin

54. A 28-year-old woman comes into the clinic for her first prenatal appointment. She tells the nurse the first day of her last menstrual period was October 10, 2015. The nurse uses Naegele's Rule and calculates the client's estimated date of confinement as

    1. June 10, 2016.
    2. June 17, 2016.
    3. July 10, 2016.
    4. July 17, 2016.

55. Cefaclor (Ceclor) is prescribed for a child with an infection. The order states to give 20 mg/kg/day in divided doses every 8 hours. The child weighs 86 pounds. The nurse would administer how many milligrams per dose?

    1. 260 mg
    2. 68 mg
    3. 780 mg
    4. 204 mg

56. The nurse is doing hourly rounds when he finds a 73-year-old female client unconscious on the floor next to the bed. An incident report must be filled out. What is the **best** statement for the nurse to write on the incident report?

    1. "Client fell out of bed at some point between 0700 and 0800."
    2. "Client was found unresponsive on floor next to the bed."
    3. "Client likely slipped on the floor and hit her head."
    4. "Client attempted to ambulate without assistance and fell."

57. A nurse needs to draw a blood sample from a patient's central line. The line is currently infusing Ringer's lactate. In which order should the nurse take the following steps to draw the blood sample? Number the steps below.

    ___ attach the flush syringe and flush catheter with normal saline
    ___ stop the infusion and disconnect Ringer's lactate
    ___ withdraw a blood sample and discard
    ___ scrub the catheter hub
    ___ withdraw the blood sample for the lab

58. The nurse recognizes which of the following as a dual diagnosis?

    1. major depressive disorder and hypertension
    2. schizophrenia and depression
    3. bipolar disorder and alcoholism
    4. depression and obsessive-compulsive disorder

59. An end-of-life client receiving home hospice care states he no longer wants to eat. The nurse should

    1. speak with the health care provider about inserting a feeding tube.
    2. encourage the client to eat small, nutritious meals.
    3. accept the client's decision and work to make the client comfortable.
    4. ask the client's family to bring the client's favorite foods.

60. A client has surgery scheduled in 2 weeks. He decides to donate his own blood ahead of time to be stored and used in case he needs a blood transfusion during his surgery. This type of blood donation is referred to as

    1. an allogeneic donation.
    2. an xenogeneic donation.
    3. an autologous donation.
    4. a directed donation.

61. A 3-year-old boy is diagnosed with plumbism. Which of the following information in his chart does the nurse associate with his diagnosis?

    1. The child's family follows a strict vegetarian diet.
    2. The child lives in a 70-year-old farmhouse with his grandparents.
    3. The child was strictly bottle fed.
    4. The child required phototherapy after birth.

62. A teenage client tells the nurse about her plans to be a lifeguard this summer. The nurse would be concerned if she saw the client was taking which medication? **Select all that apply.**

    1. tetrahydrozoline (Tetryzoline)
    2. isotretinoin (Accutane)
    3. levonorgestrel (Levora)
    4. sulfamethoxazole (Bactrim)

63. The nurse recognizes all of the following as common physical characteristics of a child with Down syndrome EXCEPT

    1. small, low-set ears.
    2. downward slanting eyes.
    3. hyperflexibility.
    4. enlarged tongue.

64. A 28-year-old woman pregnant with twins comes in for her prenatal appointment. She tells the nurse that she has two children at home (ages 4 years and 16 months), and she had one abortion 6 years ago when she was 8 weeks along in the pregnancy. The nurse charts

    1. gravida 4, para 2.
    2. gravida 4, para 3.
    3. gravida 5, para 2.
    4. gravida 5, para 3.

65. A client has been diagnosed with glossopharyngeal neuralgia. The nurse will expect the client to

    1. experience episodes of vertigo.
    2. experience difficulty moving the tongue.
    3. experience double vision.
    4. experience episodes of pain in the throat, ears, tongue, and tonsils.

66. A client is prescribed aspirin gr. V. Each aspirin tablet is 300 mg. How many tablets does the nurse administer? Fill in the blank.

_____

67. A mother brings in her 9-month-old son for a routine checkup. She asks the nurse what developmental milestones to expect by 12 months of age. All of the following are correct responses by the nurse EXCEPT

   1. "Your son should be able to imitate a kiss or wave."

   2. "Your son should be able to hold a bottle independently."

   3. "Your son should be able to point to an object when named."

   4. "Your son should respond to his own name."

68. A client on a 72-hour psychiatric hold experiences a panic attack while getting ready for the day. The nurse should provide the following interventions ranked by priority:

   ___ stay with the client until the panic attack is over

   ___ incorporate physical activity into the client's daily routine

   ___ instruct the client to take slow, deep breaths

   ___ reduce external stimuli in the immediate area

   ___ work with the client to develop coping mechanisms

69. A school nurse is administering a hearing test for college students. Which of the following is included in the correct administration of a hearing test?

   1. The nurse should stand 6 feet away from the student.

   2. The student should cover both ears during the test.

   3. The nurse should turn away from the student and whisper a phrase.

   4. The nurse should stand 1 – 2 feet away from the student.

70. A 20-year-old male has recently been diagnosed with schizophrenia. The nurse knows which of the following are classic signs and symptoms of this disorder? **Select all that apply.**

   1. social withdrawal

   2. agitation

   3. auditory hallucinations

   4. disorganized speech

   5. obsession with personal hygiene

71. All of the following are risk factors for sudden infant death syndrome (SIDS) EXCEPT

   1. low birth weight.

   2. placing the child on his back to sleep.

   3. young maternal age.

   4. maternal smoking during pregnancy.

72. The nurse is creating a discharge plan for a client with cholecystitis. The nurse should encourage the client to follow

    1. a diet low in potassium.
    2. a diet low in fat.
    3. a diet with increased vitamin B12.
    4. a diet low in phosphorus.

73. Raynaud's disease is most commonly found in

    1. children under 10.
    2. middle-aged males.
    3. adults over the age of 65.
    4. young women.

74. Which of the following signs and symptoms would a nurse expect when examining a 22-year-old female with secondary syphilis?

    1. chancre sore near the vagina
    2. no noticeable symptoms
    3. non-itchy rash on palms and soles of the feet
    4. skin tumors

75. A client's blood pressure is 132/84. What is the mean arterial pressure?

    1. 79 mmHg
    2. 48 mmHg
    3. 92 mmHg
    4. 100 mmHg

76. A client has been prescribed tetracycline (Sumycin) for Lyme disease. All of the following statements indicate successful client teaching regarding this medication EXCEPT

    1. "I may need to take an antacid to protect my stomach."
    2. "I will need to tell my doctor right away if I suspect I am pregnant."
    3. "I need to wear sunscreen at all times."
    4. "I cannot take this medicine with any dairy products."

77. A 57-year-old male with a history of vasculitis has purple discolorations on his legs, each approximately 0.3 cm to 1 cm in size. He asks the nurse what these discolorations are called, and the nurse correctly calls them

    1. ecchymosis.
    2. purpura.
    3. petechia.
    4. bruises.

78. A client pushes his call light and tells the nurse his chest is hurting. The nurse sees his oxygen saturation is 88%. The nurse's first intervention is to

    1. perform an ECG.

    2. administer oxygen.

    3. administer morphine IV.

    4. call the Rapid Response Team.

79. A nurse has delegated care of a client in wrist restraints to a nursing assistant. The nursing assistant should check the skin circulation under the restraints at least

    1. every 15 minutes.

    2. every 30 minutes.

    3. every hour.

    4. every 2 hours.

80. The nurse receives an order to administer 1,500 mL D5W IV over 12 hours. The drop factor is 15 drops/1 mL. The IV flow rate should be set at how many drops per minute? Round to the nearest whole number.

_____

81. A tornado touched down in a large community, and the hospital is anticipating many casualties will be sent to the facility within the next few hours. The nurse should **first**

    1. activate the emergency disaster response plan.

    2. obtain any extra supplies from the supply closet.

    3. prepare a triage staging area.

    4. call in extra staff, even if they are not scheduled to work.

82. A client has been undergoing treatment for an aggressive cancer. The physicians have stated the chance of recovery is very unlikely. The client states that she prefers to cease all treatments and start palliative care. The nurse supports this decision based on which ethical principle?

    1. fidelity

    2. confidentiality

    3. justice

    4. autonomy

83. A public health nurse is preparing an educational handout about rubella, commonly known as measles. All of the following statements should be included in the informational handout EXCEPT

    1. "Rubella can be spread by coughing and sneezing."

    2. "The incubation period for rubella is 3 – 7 days."

    3. "Signs and symptoms include high fever, runny nose, and cough."

    4. "Rubella can be spread by skin-to-skin contact."

84. A home health nurse visits a 48-year-old male client who has a fear of leaving his home because the space outside is too overwhelming. He has not gone anywhere in the past 2 months. The client has likely been diagnosed with

   1. sociophobia.
   2. anthropophobia.
   3. xenophobia.
   4. agoraphobia.

85. A patient is rushed to the ER after overdosing on benzodiazepines. The nurse anticipates an order for

   1. lorazepam (Ativan).
   2. flumazenil (Romazicon).
   3. naloxone (Narcan).
   4. alprazolam (Xanax).

86. A 19-year-old female is admitted to the psychiatric floor after a suicide attempt 3 days ago. With client safety a priority, the nurse should

   1. assign the patient to the room closest to the nursing station.
   2. assign the patient to an open room with a roommate.
   3. assign the patient to a secluded, isolated room.
   4. assign a staff member to stay with the client at all times.

87. A student nurse is assigned to change a patient's dressing. The soiled bandage is saturated with bright red blood. How should the student nurse dispose of the bandage?

   1. in the hallway sharps container
   2. in a labeled or color-coded biohazard bag
   3. in the trash, but it must be double bagged
   4. in the trash can in the patient's room

88. A 14-year-old boy comes in for a yearly exam and confides in the nurse that he feels embarrassed he is shorter than most of the girls in his class. He asks if he will catch up in height. The **best** therapeutic response from the nurse is

   1. "There is no reason to be embarrassed. Everyone feels awkward at this age, not just you."
   2. "Puberty is a difficult time, but everyone grows at a different rate. In a few years, you will likely be taller than many of the girls."
   3. "So you feel embarrassed just because you are short? You shouldn't care about what the girls think."
   4. "I'm sure there are other kids in your class shorter than you. Don't worry about it too much."

89. A nurse is working in a residential facility when a fire breaks out in one hallway. The nurse and an elderly client are trapped in the client's room and cannot get out. The nurse should

1. crawl in the closet with the client and shut the door.

2. open a window in the client's room.

3. instruct the client to crawl under the bed.

4. leave the door to the room open.

90. A client has been diagnosed with renal insufficiency, which has led to pronounced fluid volume excess. The nurse would expect which of the following signs and symptoms? **Select all that apply.**

1. decreased urine output

2. hypotension

3. jugular vein distention

4. weak, thready pulse

5. tachycardia

91. In the team nursing model of client care,

1. each staff member receives different task assignments to complete for a group of clients.

2. the RN leads a team consisting of an LPN and UAP, and they all care for a client together.

3. the RN completes all care for a client on a particular shift.

4. the client assignments are determined by geographic location on the unit.

92. The charge nurse considers both patient-related and staff-related factors when making daily assignments. All of the following are patient-related factors EXCEPT

1. mechanical ventilation use.

2. complex medication regimen.

3. isolation precaution requirements.

4. nurse-to-client ratio.

93. The clinical triad of abnormalities seen in serotonin syndrome includes all of the following EXCEPT

1. cognitive effects.

2. autonomic effects.

3. somatic effects.

4. behavioral effects.

94. A child with thrush has been prescribed fluconazole (Diflucan). The child's mother asks what this medication is used for, and the nurse correctly replies,

    1. "This is an antiviral medication used to treat your child's viral infection."

    2. "This medication is used to treat yeast infections."

    3. "This medication is an analgesic that will ease your child's pain while eating."

    4. "This is an antibiotic for your child's bacterial infection."

95. A nurse performing a newborn assessment would expect what respiratory rate and heart rate as a normal finding?

    1. RR 15 breaths/minute, HR 72 beats/minute

    2. RR 35 breaths/minute, HR 96 beats/minute

    3. RR 46 breaths/minute, HR 153 beats/minute

    4. RR 68 breaths/minute, HR 137 beats/minute

96. A nurse reviews a client's lab values and sees the BUN is 18 mg/dL and the creatinine is 0.7 mg/dL. If the physician asks the nurse for the BUN-to-creatinine ratio (rounded to the nearest whole number), the nurse would answer

    1. 25:2.

    2. 26:2.

    3. 26:1.

    4. 25:1.

97. All of the following clients are at an increased risk for aspiration pneumonia EXCEPT

    1. a client receiving nasogastric tube feeding.

    2. a client receiving total parenteral nutrition.

    3. a client on mechanical ventilation.

    4. a client with dysphagia.

98. A 35-year-old male comes into the clinic after he strains his back at work. The nurse anticipates the physician may suggest which topical anesthetic?

    1. aloe

    2. zinc oxide

    3. hydrocortisone

    4. capsaicin

99. Due to a natural progression of aging, elderly clients have the **most** difficulty discerning between which two colors?

    1. yellow and green

    2. red and green

    3. blue and green

    4. yellow and red

100. A nurse is caring for a client who has just undergone an ileostomy procedure. The nurse expects how much drainage from the ileostomy during the first 24 hours post-op?

   1. 650 mL
   2. 800 mL
   3. 1,500 mL
   4. 3,500 mL

101. Which client is at the greatest risk of developing colon cancer?

   1. a 83-year-old Hispanic female with a past history of cholecystectomy
   2. a 62-year-old African American male with a past history of diabetes
   3. a 70-year-old Caucasian male with a past history of cancer treated with chemotherapy
   4. a 42-year-old Asian female who follows a high-fiber diet

102. A 19-year-old male has been experiencing vomiting and diarrhea for 3 days due to food poisoning. The nurse expects a urine specific gravity of

   1. 0.850.
   2. 1.005.
   3. 1.020.
   4. 1.041.

103. After a discharge, there is a private room available on the floor. The nurse should move which client to the private room?

   1. a 28-year-old female with Cushing's disease
   2. a 15-year-old male with pityriasis rosea
   3. a 56-year-old male with diabetes mellitus
   4. a 40-year-old male with heterochromia iridium

104. A 13-year-old female has been diagnosed with celiac disease. Which of the following dinner trays would be acceptable?

   1. baked chicken breast, carrots, baked potato with cheese
   2. turkey and cheese sandwich on wheat bread, cabbage slaw, apple slices
   3. spaghetti with meatballs, Caesar salad, banana
   4. pulled pork on flour tortillas, wild rice, black beans

105. A child with achondroplasia will likely have which of the following physical characteristics?

   1. alopecia, failure to thrive, small face, recessed jaw
   2. enlarged hands and feet, skull expansion at fontanelle, enlarged tongue
   3. poor muscle tone, slanted eyes, single palmar crease
   4. dwarf stature, short fingers and toes, short proximal limbs

106. A 62-year-old female with osteoarthritis asks the nurse how she can ease her pain and discomfort. The nurse should include which of the following in the discharge plan for the client? **Select all that apply.**

   1. maintain a healthy weight
   2. take an aspirin as needed to relieve pain
   3. incorporate high-impact exercise daily
   4. use warm compresses to relieve stiffness
   5. incorporate moderate exercise at least three times per week

107. A client diagnosed with hepatitis B asks the nurse how the virus is transmitted. Which of the following is the correct response?

   1. by infectious blood or needles
   2. by infectious blood, sexual contact, and needles, and from mother to newborn
   3. by contaminated food and water
   4. by contaminated water only

108. The school nurse recognizes that meningitis can be caused by which of the following? **Select all that apply.**

   1. fungal infections
   2. noninfectious causes
   3. parasites
   4. bacterial infections
   5. viral infections

109. A pediatric nurse would be concerned by which of the following sets of vital signs?

   1. newborn: BP 70/50, RR 47, HR 135
   3. 12-month-old: BP 65/55, RR 50, HR 130
   2. 10-year-old: BP 110/70, RR 16, HR 89
   4. 13-year-old: BP 120/82, RR 15, HR 80

110. According to Erikson's stages of physical development, school-age children 5 – 12 years old typically face which psychological crisis?

   1. ego integrity versus despair
   2. industry versus inferiority
   3. trust versus mistrust
   4. ego identity versus role confusion

111. A 62-year-old male in septic shock suddenly develops acute respiratory arrest syndrome. The nurse immediately places the client on a non-rebreather mask, but oxygenation does not improve. The nurse anticipates which of the following?

　　1.　The physician will ask the nurse to place a venturi mask on the client.

　　2.　The physician will ask the nurse to administer 5L oxygen via a nasal cannula.

　　3.　The physician will ask the nurse to place a simple face mask over the client's nose and mouth.

　　4.　The physician will ask the nurse to prepare the client for intubation.

112. An RN is supervising a team of LPNs on the med-surg floor. All of the following tasks can be delegated to a competent LPN EXCEPT

　　1.　collecting a sputum sample to be sent to the lab.

　　2.　performing a sterile straight catheterization on a 58-year-old male.

　　3.　administering a metered dose inhaler medication to a 23-year-old asthmatic.

　　4.　completing an admissions assessment for a client transferred from a long-term-care facility.

113. Which of the following medication orders requires clarification before the nurse can administer the order?

　　1.　epinephrine (EpiPen) 0.25 mg IM STAT

　　2.　heparin 30 units/kg/hr IV infusion for 24 hours

　　3.　ampicillin (Omnipen) 500 mg PO bid

　　4.　lorazepam (Ativan) 1.0 mg PO prn

114. Which client is at the highest risk for a cerebrovascular accident CVA?

　　1.　a 67-year-old Hispanic male

　　2.　a 75-year-old African American female

　　3.　a 60-year-old Caucasian male

　　4.　an 82-year-old East Asian female

115. A 51-year-old client received a kidney transplant. Which of the following signs and symptoms indicates possible rejection of the kidney? **Select all that apply.**

　　1.　increased urine output

　　2.　increase in blood pressure

　　3.　weight gain

　　4.　pain in lower back

　　5.　decreased creatinine

116. All of the following statements regarding scarlet fever are true EXCEPT

    1. rheumatic fever is a possible complication of scarlet fever.

    2. scarlet fever can be treated with antibiotics.

    3. a vaccine is available to protect against scarlet fever.

    4. scarlet fever is caused by an erythrogenic toxin.

117. The nurse is caring for a 36-year-old female recently diagnosed with Addison's disease. The nurse recognizes further teaching is needed if the client states,

    1. "I will need to limit my salt intake and use a salt substitute from now on."

    2. "I will have to take hormones for the rest of my life."

    3. "My husband is helping me pick out a medical alert bracelet to wear."

    4. "I have to watch for symptoms of adrenal failure."

118. The nurse would recognize which symptom as the most likely early indication of pneumonia in an elderly client?

    1. chest pain

    2. fever

    3. dyspnea

    4. altered mental status

119. A 19-year-old female comes into the women's clinic for an STD test. The nurse explains all of the following confirmed cases of STDs must be reported to the Centers for Disease Control (CDC) EXCEPT

    1. genital herpes.

    2. chlamydia.

    3. hepatitis B.

    4. gonorrhea.

120. A client requires long-term use of corticosteroids. The nurse explains which of the following is associated with chronic corticosteroid therapy?

    1. chronic fever

    2. inability to gain weight

    3. orthostatic hypotension

    4. osteoporosis

121. A nurse is preparing to administer a MMR vaccine to a 35-year-old male. The nurse should

    1. swab and clean an area of skin over the dorsogluteal muscle.

    2. prepare a 25-gauge, 1 1/2-inch needle.

    3. pinch and hold the skin while injecting the needle.

    4. inject the needle at a 90-degree angle.

122. The nurse is working with a client who experiences orthostatic hypotension. Which suggestion would benefit the client?

   1. "Sleep completely flat and do not use any pillows to prop your head."
   2. "Wear your support stockings when you sleep."
   3. "Take your blood pressure medicine immediately before trying to stand up."
   4. "Do not drink any liquids after 8 p.m."

123. A 62-year-old female comes to the clinic with the complaint that her vision seems cloudy. What other signs and symptoms may the client mention that are suggestive of cataracts? **Select all that apply.**

   1. nausea and vomiting
   2. seeing double out of one eye
   3. difficulty seeing at night
   4. pain in eyes
   5. halos seen around lights

124. A homeless client has been admitted to the hospital for observation, and he does not speak any English. The nurse does not know any of the client's medical history, but he is grimacing and looks to be in pain. The nurse should

   1. use nonverbal communication such as pointing and gestures.
   2. call for the hospital interpreter services.
   3. give the client pen and paper and encourage him to draw.
   4. wait to see if any friends or family visit the client who may be able to help.

125. A nursing instructor is preparing a lesson on the dangers of using drugs and alcohol during pregnancy. She would include which of the following as a **primary** disability associated with children diagnosed with fetal alcohol syndrome?

   1. poor motor skills
   2. promiscuous behavior
   3. future drug and alcohol dependency
   4. diagnosis of clinical depression

126. A nurse is teaching a pregnant woman about healthy nutrition during pregnancy. Which are the **best** food sources to add to the diet to help prevent neural tube defects?

   1. tuna fish, string cheese, whole milk
   2. chicken breast, eggs, applesauce
   3. sausage patties, banana slices, carrots
   4. strawberries, spinach and lettuce salad, avocado

127. A 15-year-old client is rushed to the ER after taking an entire bottle of acetaminophen (Tylenol) in a suicide attempt. The nurse's priority is obtaining which lab results?

   1. aspartate transaminase and alanine transaminase
   2. BUN and creatinine
   3. brain natriuretic peptide
   4. arterial blood gas

128. The nurse recognizes all of the following as type IV hypersensitivity reactions EXCEPT

   1. allergic contact dermatitis.
   2. Crohn's disease.
   3. graft versus host disease.
   4. penicillin allergy.

129. A 34-year-old male client underwent a vasectomy one week ago and is at the clinic for a checkup. He asks the nurse how long it will be until he no longer needs to use a backup method of birth control. The nurse explains azoospermia usually occurs

   1. 1 month after a vasectomy.
   2. 1 year after a vasectomy.
   3. 3 – 4 months after a vasectomy.
   4. 6 – 8 weeks after a vasectomy.

130. A schizophrenic client has been taking haloperidol (Haldol) for 20 months and has developed moderate extrapyramidal symptoms (EPS). The nurse anticipates the physician will likely prescribe what medication for EPS?

   1. flumazenil (Anexate)
   2. donepezil (Aricept)
   3. naloxone (Narcan)
   4. benztropine (Cogentin)

131. A 52-year-old female had a hysterectomy 3 days ago and is recovering on the post-op floor. She is scheduled for an oral pain medication every 4 hours. She received her scheduled dose 1 hour ago but pushes the call light and complains of unrelenting and severe pain. The nurse should **first**

   1. perform a full head-to-toe assessment on the client.
   2. work with the client on alternate methods to relieve pain, such as guided imagery.
   3. explain to the client it is not time to administer more pain medication.
   4. call the physician and report the current plan for pain management is not working.

132. All of the following are examples of secondary disease prevention EXCEPT

   1. leading a support group for people who suffer from depression.

   2. mammogram screenings.

   3. testing and treatment of babies born to mothers with syphilis.

   4. developing a daily exercise program to prevent a second MI.

133. The hospital conducts an information and education session on anthrax. The nurse learns the methods of anthrax transmission include which of the following? **Select all that apply.**

   1. cutaneous

   2. ocular

   3. inhalation

   4. fomite

   5. gastrointestinal

134. The nurse observes a 2 1/2-year-old toddler in the waiting room. Based on expected child development, the nurse expects to see the child engaged in which type of play?

   1. playing alone, with no interaction with other children

   2. playing cooperatively in a single-sex group

   3. playing parallel to other children, but not playing together

   4. playing and interacting cooperatively in a mixed-sex group

135. The nurse recognizes all of the following as part of the Cushing reflex triad EXCEPT

   1. cardiac arrhythmia.

   2. increased blood pressure.

   3. irregular respirations.

   4. decreased heart rate.

136. Cardiac muscles follow a certain order of electrical conduction in order for the heart to contract. What is the correct sequence of electrical impulse?

   ___ bundle of His

   ___ atrioventricular node

   ___ bundle branches

   ___ sinoatrial node

   ___ Purkinje fibers

137. A new graduate nurse completes her first full shift with her preceptor. It was a long, overwhelming day and the new nurse takes a deep breath and says to herself, "You can do this! Nursing will be a challenge but you are up for it and tomorrow is a new day." This type of communication is

    1. intrapersonal.

    2. horizontal.

    3. interpersonal.

    4. vertical.

138. A nurse from the dialysis unit floats to the med-surg floor. He is doing afternoon rounds and medication administration. He brings a client her oral medications, but the client states, "What is this? Where is my yellow pill? This big white one is not mine." The **best** action from the nurse is to

    1. take the medication out of the room and verify with the MAR and pharmacy.

    2. explain to the client this is the correct prescribed medication she is ordered.

    3. report to the nursing supervisor there has been a medication error.

    4. explain to the client that sometimes medication comes from other manufacturers and the pills may look different.

139. A nurse wants to develop a therapeutic relationship with an anxious new client. Which of the following is an open-ended question?

    1. "Do you think your anxiety medication has been helping?"

    2. "Does anyone in your family have anxiety or depression?"

    3. "How is your anxiety on the weekends when you are off work?"

    4. "So you are saying that your trouble sleeping started right around the time you started a new job?"

140. The nurse recognizes which of the following as a Category A biological agent that may be used in terroristic acts?

    1. typhoid

    2. smallpox

    3. malaria

    4. Ebola

141. A 24-year-old female agreed to participate in an 8-week research study for smoking cessation. After participating for 5 weeks, the woman tells the nurse she wants to withdraw from the study. The nurse's **best** response is

    1. "You only have 3 weeks left in the study. Please don't quit now."

    2. "Unfortunately, you are obligated to complete the study."

    3. "You have the right to stop at any time."

    4. "I will speak with your physician and see if you can be released from the study early."

142. As the nurse hangs a bag of 3-in-1 total parenteral nutrition (TPN) for a client, a family member asks what is in the bag. The nurse explains a 3-in-1 TPN solution includes

    1. lipids, proteins, and amino acids.
    2. lipids, amino acids, and electrolytes.
    3. dextrose, amino acids, and lipids.
    4. dextrose, lipids, and electrolytes.

143. A client diagnosed with hemophagocytic lymphohistiocytosis requires multiple blood transfusions. One of his family members wishes to donate blood. Which of the following conditions would DISQUALIFY someone from donating blood?

    1. current medical condition of hyperthyroidism
    2. new mother, 10 weeks postpartum
    3. currently ill with common cold
    4. past medical history of tuberculosis; completed treatment and recovered 3 years ago

144. A 24-month-old boy has been diagnosed with Duchenne muscular dystrophy (DMD). The parents come to speak with the health care team about having other children. This is an X-linked recessive disorder, and the mother is a carrier. The nurse correctly explains,

    1. "There is a 50% chance a male child will have DMD."
    2. "There is a 100% chance a female child will have DMD."
    3. "There is a 25% chance a female child will be a carrier for DMD."
    4. "There is a 100% chance a male child will have DMD."

145. A mother asks the home health nurse for guidance on what foods are safe to give her child, who is on strict neutropenic precautions. The nurse looks at the mother's grocery list and advises her to avoid

    1. canned peaches.
    2. pasteurized whole milk.
    3. the fresh veggie tray.
    4. fresh bananas.

146. A client in cardiac arrest is given 40 units of vasopressin (Pitressin) IV push. The nurse knows the desired action of this medication in a cardiac arrest is to

    1. raise blood pressure.
    2. stop cardiac arrhythmia.
    3. lower blood pressure.
    4. reset the electrical cardiac conduction system.

147. All of the following are modifiable risk factors for coronary artery disease (CAD) EXCEPT

    1. high stress.

    2. obesity.

    3. smoking.

    4. family history.

148. A 45-year-old female comes into the clinic for a yearly physical. The nurse calculates her body mass index (BMI) as 32. The nurse would chart this as

    1. obese.

    2. underweight.

    3. overweight.

    4. healthy weight.

149. A nurse is caring for an 84-year-old client who is malnourished. The nurse is concerned about all of the following complications of malnutrition EXCEPT

    1. increased risk for falls.

    2. poor wound healing.

    3. chronic heart failure.

    4. increased risk of infections.

150. An AIDS patient has developed a fungal Fusarium infection. The nurse anticipates the physician will order

    1. lamivudine/zidovudine (Combivir).

    2. famciclovir (Famvir).

    3. ciprofloxacin (Cipro).

    4. voriconazole (Vfend).

PRACTICE TEST THREE ANSWER KEY

1.   Number 3 is correct.

     Rationale: The nurse's first intervention is to stop exposure to the allergen (peanuts) by verifying the child has stopped eating the food. Once the client is safe from further exposure, the nurse can then assess for the priorities of airway, breathing, and circulation and intervene as necessary.

2.   Number 1 is correct.

     Rationale: The client likely inadvertently opened the sutures and caused the wound area to separate (wound dehiscence). The nurse's first priority is to immediately cover and protect the open wound. Then the nurse should call for help and make any other necessary interventions.

3.   Numbers 1, 3, and 5 are correct.

     Rationale: Some possible signs of substance abuse in the workplace include frequent absenteeism, poor performance at work, and isolation. Other signs may include increased workplace accidents and frequent breaks.

4.   Number 1 is correct.

     Rationale: Pulse pressure is found by calculating the difference between the systolic pressure and diastolic pressure. Here, 134 – 86 = 48, so the pulse pressure is 48.

5.   Number 1 is correct.

     Rationale: The nurse should use light palpation when assessing for pain, possible mass, or pulsations in the abdomen. Deep palpation is used for assessing organs such as liver and spleen. Inspection is a visual assessment, and percussion may be used to determine if abdominal fluid or organ enlargement is present.

6.   Number 2 is correct.

     Solution:

order/units available × amount of fluid in bag/ number of hours	To determine the amount of mL per hour, use the formula.
= 1,000 units/10,000 units × 500 mL/2 hrs	Substitute values and solve.
= 0.1 × 250 mL/hr	
= 25 mL/hr	

7.   Number 4 is correct.

     Rationale: Stage 1 hypertension is defined by a systolic level between 140 and 159 mmHg or a diastolic level between 90 and 99 mmHg. A blood pressure reading of 146/90 would be considered stage 1 hypertension and would require further blood pressure monitoring and probable lifestyle changes or medication management. Prehypertension is defined by a systolic reading between 120 and 139 mmHg or diastolic reading between 80 and 89 mmHg. Stage 2 hypertension is noted when systolic pressure is over 160 mmHg and a diastolic level is over 100 mmHg. Even if hypertension runs in the patient's family, the reading indicates she must address the issue through lifestyle changes and/or medication.

8.   Number 3 is correct.

     Rationale: After a cardiac catheterization, the client should remain flat on his back to avoid any pressure or tension on the femoral artery, which could cause bleeding from the site where the catheter was inserted. Lying on the side with knees bent places tension on the femoral artery. In the semi-Fowler's position, the client is not fully supine. In the high-Fowler's position, the client is sitting up.

9. Number 1 is correct.

Rationale: BMI is calculated by dividing the weight in kilograms by height in meters squared.

146 lbs/2.2 = 66.4 kg	Convert pounds to kilograms by dividing pounds by 2.2.
meters = number of inches/39.37 63 in./39.37 = 1.6 m 1.6 squared = 2.56	Convert inches (63) into meters and square.
kg/m^2 $66.4 \ kg/2.56 \ m^2$ = 25.9 **BMI = 25.9 (overweight)**	Calculate BMI.

10. Numbers 2, 3, and 5 are correct.

Rationale: Subjective data is information or symptoms provided by the client: his opinions, feelings, or statements. Objective data is something nurses can measure or observe by their own senses.

11. Number 3 is correct.

Rationale: Sensible fluid loss can be measured as daily output and includes gastric drainage, urine, and vomit. Insensible fluid loss from the lungs, feces, skin, and respiratory tract cannot be accurately measured as output.

12. Number 3 is correct.

Rationale: Standard precautions are recommended whenever the nurse comes in contact with blood or body fluids that could transmit blood-borne pathogens. Contact with sweat or intact skin does not require use of standard precautions.

13. Number 4 is correct.

Rationale: Untreated gout is associated with health risks such as kidney stones, nodules of hardened uric acid under the skin, and deformed joints. Other complications include heart disease and bone damage. Neuropathy is nerve damage often associated with uncontrolled diabetes.

14. Number 2 is correct.

Rationale: The three components of evidence-based practice are research outcomes, patient values, and clinical expertise.

15. Number 1 is correct.

Rationale: It is common for some patients (especially the elderly) to become disoriented during a hospital stay. The nurse's best intervention is to provide cues around the room that can reorient the client, such as familiar personal objects. Restraints are a measure of last resort, and it is inappropriate to ask the client's family to stay so the staff does not have to intervene. Transferring the client to another floor before other interventions have been attempted is also inappropriate and abdicates professional responsibility.

16. Number 3 is correct.

Rationale: Possible risks for breast cancer include early menarche, nulliparity, and previous history of breast, ovarian, or uterine cancer. Other risk factors include late menopause (not early menopause), family history of breast cancer, and having the first child after age 30.

17. Number 2 is correct.

Rationale: Intermittent bubbling in the water seal chamber is an expected finding that indicates the system is working correctly and that air is being successfully removed from the pleural space. The nurse should document and reassess again later. Constant bubbling is indicative of an air leak, and the nurse would immediately report this to the physician so it can be corrected.

18. Number 2 is correct.

Rationale: Initial assessment, such as a post-op client, is the responsibility of an RN and cannot be delegated. Examples 1, 3, and 4 are all tasks that an RN can delegate to an LPN as long as the client is stable.

19. Number 2 is correct.

Rationale: The nursing assistant could be charged with assault, which is an intentional act that threatens or attempts violence. Negligence is an act of omission or commission that results in harm to the client. Malpractice occurs when one fails to competently perform her job duties, resulting in harm, injury, or death to the client. Battery is intentional and unlawful offensive physical contact toward another person.

20. Number 4 is correct.

Rationale: The Joint Commission created core measure sets to improve the health care delivery process. Heart failure, stroke, prenatal care, tobacco treatment, and children's asthma care are examples of core measure sets. Genetics, lymphoma, and nosocomial infections are not core measure sets used by the Joint Commission.

21. Numbers 2 and 3 are correct.

Rationale: The goal of tertiary preventions is to decrease the negative impact of an illness or disease that has already occurred. Treating an infection with an antibiotic and working with stroke rehabilitation are examples of tertiary prevention. Secondary prevention aims to detect disease, such as a PPD test. Primary prevention aims to prevent a disease or injury from occurring. Encouraging smoking cessation and preventative vaccines are primary preventions.

22. Number 1 is correct.

Rationale: The active phase of labor is defined as having cervical dilation of 4 – 7 cm and contractions lasting approximately 45 – 60 seconds, about 3 – 5 minutes apart. This is the phase of labor in which a woman would typically come and check in at the hospital. Number 2 describes the early phase of labor, and numbers 3 and 4 describe the transition phase of labor.

23. Number 1 is correct.

Rationale: Meniere's disease is a condition of the inner ear that causes episodes of vertigo. The client will likely require dietary changes, such as reduction in sodium. Eating smaller, evenly sized meals throughout the day may help regulate body fluids. Since the client could become dizzy or lose her balance, it would be important to assist her in ambulation to avoid a potential fall. Narcotic pain management is not typically associated with Meniere's disease.

24. Number 1 is correct.

Rationale: A client experiencing a Crohn's disease flare-up should follow a low-residue diet. The client should avoid foods that are difficult to digest, such as whole-grain breads and cereals, nuts, most raw fruits and vegetables, dried fruits, and seeds. Cooked cereals such as grits, peeled fruits (banana or melon), and non-pulp juices would be examples of low-residue foods.

25. Number 1 is correct.

Rationale: Abnormalities in magnesium levels may put the client at risk for ventricular dysrhythmia. A hypomagnesemia level of 0.8 mEq/L would be of concern (normal range is 1.5 – 2.5 mEq/L). The other values listed are normal lab values.

26. Number 1 is correct.

Rationale: Increasing ICP requires nursing intervention; the nurse should increase the rate of oxygen because hypoxia can worsen ICP. Elevating the head of the bed, repositioning the patient, and suctioning the patient are not recommended interventions for patients experiencing (or at risk for) ICP because they can actually increase the pressure.

27. Number 1 is correct.

Rationale: Atropine is used for patients with pronounced bradycardia to regulate heart rate. Amiodarone and adenosine are used with tachycardic patients, and magnesium sulfate is used for ventricular tachycardia or ventricular fibrillation.

28. Abdominal inspections should be done in the following order:

1. inspection
2. auscultation
3. percussion
4. palpation

29. Number 1 is correct.

Rationale: Potential risks for IUD include pelvic infections, abnormal bleeding, and increased risk of ectopic pregnancy. Other potential risks include sepsis, perforation, and expulsion. Increased risk of stroke is associated with oral contraceptives.

30. Numbers 1, 3, and 5 are correct.

Rationale: Inserting a PICC line does require sterile technique, but it can be done at the bedside and carries a lower risk of infection compared to other central lines. RNs must have special training to intersect a PICC line. There is no risk of pneumothorax during insertion because of the placement method.

31. Number 3 is correct.

Rationale: An elevated uric acid level (hyperuricemia) is an adverse effect of furosemide (Lasix). A uric acid level of 13.5 mg/dL is high above normal range (0.18 – 0.48 mmol/L). Hypokalemia is also an adverse effect of Lasix.

32. Number 3 is correct.

Rationale: The Braden Scale assesses nutritional status, sensory perception, activity level, moisture, mobility, and friction/shear. It does not consider past history of skin breakdown.

33. Number 2 is correct.

Rationale: Rolling the vial between the palms of the hands will produce enough heat to aid in the dissolution of the powder. The rolling movement itself will also help dissolve the powder. Shaking the vial could break it, and leaving the vial to sit does not ensure the powder will dissolve. There is no need for the pharmacy to be involved in dissolving the powder.

34. Number 1 is correct.

Rationale: Normal post-operative drainage after a cholecystectomy is 500 – 1,000 mL/day. Immediately after surgery, the drainage will be sanguineous, but then turn to a greenish-brown color. The nurse's assessments of the patient's drainage are normal, expected findings. There is no need to call the physician, and an infection would not be suspected. Here, the tube does not need to be flushed.

35. Number 1 is correct.

    Rationale: The middle ear is composed of the incus, stapes, malleus, and tympanic membrane. The pinna is also known as the ear flap and is part of the outer ear.

36. Numbers 2, 3, 4, and 5 are correct.

    Rationale: Infective endocarditis is an inflammation of the inner tissues of the heart caused by an infective organism. A common mnemonic for signs and symptoms is FROM JANE, which stands for fever, Roth's spots, Osler's nodes, murmur, Janeway lesions, anemia, nail hemorrhage, and embolism. Other possible signs and symptoms include night sweats, weight loss, and an enlarged spleen. Weight gain is not a known indicator.

37. Number 4 is correct.

    Rationale: The nurse should use therapeutic communication to alleviate worry by providing factual information and encouraging distraction and relaxation. Answering any questions honestly and allowing the client to visit with family will help her feel more comfortable. Sedation is not appropriate in this situation. Nurses should not assume patients of sound mind are unable to understand their health status or address them in a patronizing manner.

38. Number 4 is correct.

    Rationale: The Apgar score stands for assessments of activity, pulse, grimace, appearance, and respirations. It is scored on a 0 – 10 scale, at 1 minute after birth and again at 5 minutes after birth. Rooting is not considered in the Apgar score.

39. Answer: 2,090 mL

    Solution:

1. Find how many milliliters of solids (ice cream) the patient consumed.	1 pt. ice cream = 500 mL ice cream	Convert pints to milliliters.
2. Find how many milliliters of fluids (water and apple juice) the patient consumed.	16 oz. of water + 12 oz. of juice = 28 oz. fluids (total)	Find the total amount of fluids consumed.
	1 oz. = 30 mL	Convert ounces to milliliters.
	= 28 oz. × 30 = 840 mL of fluids consumed	Find the total amount of fluids consumed in milliliters.
3. Find how many milliliters of saline IV the patient consumed.	1 L = 1,000mL	Convert liters to mL.
	0.75L saline IV × 1,000 = 750 mL saline IV consumed	Find the total amount of saline IV consumed in milliliters.
4. Combine the amount of solids, fluids, and saline IV (in milliliters) consumed to find the patient's total daily intake.	500 mL ice cream + 840 mL fluids + 750 mL saline IV = **2,090 mL**	Add the totals (in mL) of solids, fluids, and saline IV.

40. Number 3 is correct.

    Rationale: A normal white blood cell count in an adult is between 3.5 and 10.5. A high result such as 15.6 may indicate infection or inflammation. The other values listed are normal, expected values in an adult female.

41.

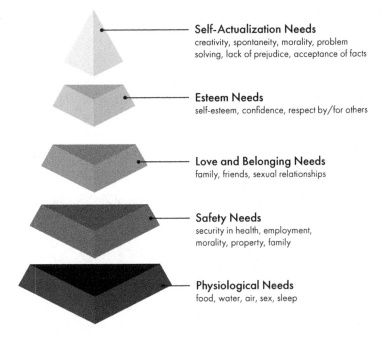

Self-Actualization Needs
creativity, spontaneity, morality, problem solving, lack of prejudice, acceptance of facts

Esteem Needs
self-esteem, confidence, respect by/for others

Love and Belonging Needs
family, friends, sexual relationships

Safety Needs
security in health, employment, morality, property, family

Physiological Needs
food, water, air, sex, sleep

Correct Response:

1. physiological
2. safety and security
3. love and belonging
4. esteem
5. self-actualization

42. Number 4 is correct.

Rationale: The nurse should never restrain a client during a seizure because musculoskeletal injury could occur. Loosening clothing and clearing the immediate area will help protect the client from injury. Lorazepam is a commonly prescribed antiseizure medication and should be administered rectally since a client in an active seizure cannot safely swallow. The client should be rolled on his side if possible to allow the tongue to return to a normal position and saliva to drain out of the mouth instead of back into the throat.

43. Number 3 is correct.

Rationale: In order to prevent a DVT, the nurse should encourage the client to wear anti-embolism stockings as much as possible, increase fluid intake, and prop legs up while sitting. The nurse should encourage the client to avoid crossing her legs while sitting and to be active and ambulate as much as possible. Inactivity increases DVT risk because the blood in the legs may pool.

44. Number 2 is correct.

Rationale: Increased anxiety is a possible side effect during the initial 4 – 6 weeks of taking sertraline. The client should continue to take the medication as prescribed and then evaluate its effect in a few weeks. The medication should not be suddenly discontinued without an order from the health care provider, and the nurse does not have the authority to change the client's dosage.

45. Number 2 is correct.

Rationale: Humalog (lispro) is fast-acting insulin, with onset of action beginning 15 minutes after injection. Humalog peaks 30 – 90 minutes after administration, and during this peak time the client is most likely to experience a hypoglycemic reaction. It would be too early to check the client at 8:45 a.m., and checking the client at 11:30 a.m. or later is too late.

46. Number 1 is correct.

Rationale: The transverse plane is also referred to the horizontal plane and divides the body into superior and inferior parts. The sagittal plane divides the body into right and left halves. The coronal plane divides the body into ventral and dorsal sections.

47. Number 2 is correct.

Rationale: Scabies is very contagious and can be transmitted from skin-to-skin contact and also by sharing towels, sheets, and bedding with an infected person. Since scabies can be transmitted before symptoms occur, everyone in the household should be treated; other members of the household may already be infected.

48. Number 4 is correct.

Rationale: Ototoxicity is a potential adverse reaction to gentamicin sulfate. Other adverse reactions include Stevens-Johnson syndrome, seizures, nephrotoxicity, and superinfection. Orthostatic hypotension, occult bleeding, and torsades de pointes are not known adverse reactions to gentamicin sulfate.

49. Number 3 is correct.

Rationale: Nail clubbing, night sweats, and fever are common symptoms of TB. Other symptoms may include weight loss, chills, and fatigue. People with TB may lose, not gain, weight.

50. Number 4 is correct.

Rationale: The nurse should not bargain with the client or ask *why* questions. The best response from the nurse is to insist that the client participate in the activity as expected. Without firm insistence to participate, a client with avoidant personality disorder is likely to continue the avoidance behavior.

51. Number 4 is correct.

Rationale: Sandimmune (Cyclosporine) is an immunosuppressive drug prescribed to prevent rejection in bone marrow or organ transplants. Etoposide and Cytarabine are anti-cancer chemotherapy drugs. Metoclopramide is an anti-nausea drug often prescribed for clients undergoing chemotherapy.

52. Numbers 3 and 5 are correct.

Rationale: The best way to prevent Lyme disease is to prevent tick bites and remove ticks quickly and effectively if bitten. Using an insect repellent with DEET is effective at repelling ticks, and wearing long pants tucked into socks will help protect the legs from tick bites. Hikers should wear light-colored clothing so ticks can be easily seen. If a tick is seen on the body, it should be removed with fine tweezers; never attempt to burn or suffocate a tick. In addition, drying clothing on high heat will kill any ticks hiding in clothing. Rinsing clothing in cool water is ineffective.

53. Number 2 is correct.

Rationale: The client will likely require more insulin during his illness because the body produces more glucose while fighting infection. The client's blood sugar should be closely monitored.

54. Number 4 is correct.

Rationale: Naegele's Rule is used as follows to calculate the date of confinement:

October 10, 2015	Find the first day of the last menstrual period.
October 10, 2015 + 1 year = October 10, 2016	Add 1 year.

October 10, 2016 − 3 months = July 10, 2016	Subtract 3 months.
July 10, 2016 + 7 days **= July 17, 2016**	Add 7 days.

55.   Number 1 is correct.

Solution:

1 lb = 0.45 kg 0.45 kg × 86 lbs = 38.7 kg (round up to 39 kg)	Convert the child's weight in pounds to kilograms.
20 mg (per kilo) × 39 kg = 780 mg/day **in total** to be administered	Find how many milligrams **total** per day must be administered for the child's weight, if 20 mg/kg per day is required.
780 mg/3 doses **= 260 mg q8hr**	Find how many milligrams PER DOSE must be administered by dividing the total amount of milligrams by 3.

56.   Number 2 is correct.

Rationale: The incident report should include only factual information, nothing that adds to the story, makes assumptions, or speculates as to what occurred. If the nurse did not witness the other scenarios, he should not allege or assume they occurred.

57.   **Answer:**

Step 1: stop the infusion and disconnect Ringer's lactate

Step 2: scrub the catheter hub

Step 3: attach the flush syringe and flush catheter with normal saline

Step 4: withdraw a blood sample and discard

Step 5: withdraw the blood sample for the lab

58.   Number 3 is correct.

Rationale: A dual diagnosis refers to a co-occurring diagnosis of a mental disorder and a substance abuse disorder, such as bipolar disorder and alcoholism. Clients with dual diagnoses are at greater risk for homelessness, hospitalization, HIV, and hepatitis. Hypertension is not a mental disorder or substance abuse problem; patients who have hypertension and a mental disorder like major depressive disorder are not considered to have a dual diagnosis if they do not also have a substance abuse disorder. Both schizophrenia and depression are mental disorders, but a patient diagnosed with both who does not also have a substance abuse disorder does not have a dual diagnosis. The same can be said for patients with both depression and obsessive-compulsive disorder.

59.   Number 3 is correct.

Rationale: Clients near the end of life may lose interest in eating, and the nurse should respect the client's desire to make decisions about his treatment and care. In these cases, feeding tubes should be avoided, as should encouraging the client to eat any meals.

60.   Number 3 is correct.

Rationale: An autologous blood donation refers to a blood donation given by an individual for his own use. An allogenic blood donation is when a donor gives blood to be stored in a blood bank for use by an unknown recipient. Xenogeneic blood donations are blood donations between two different species. A directed donation occurs when the donor gives blood to be used by a specific person, such as a friend or family member.

61. Number 2 is correct.

Rationale: Plumbism, also known as lead poisoning, may occur if a child is exposed to lead paint. Living in a home built before 1976 may put children at risk, because paint manufactured before this date may contain lead. Signs and symptoms of lead poisoning in children include weight loss, developmental delay, learning disability, vomiting, and hearing loss. The most important factor in lead poisoning is exposure to lead dust and paint, not nutrition or tap water consumption. Phototherapy is prescribed to newborns with high levels of bilirubin, which can cause jaundice. Jaundice is not a known cause of lead poisoning.

62. Numbers 2 and 4 are correct.

Rationale: The client's exposure to prolonged sunlight while taking isotretinoin or sulfamethoxazole would concern the nurse because both cause increased photosensitivity. Photosensitivity is not a known side effect of tetrahydrozoline or levonorgestrel.

63. Number 2 is correct.

Rationale: Common physical characteristics seen in children with Down syndrome include small, low-set ears; hyperflexibility; enlarged tongue; flat facial features; and a single deep crease in the palm. Upward slanting eyes, not downward slanting eyes, are characteristic of children with Down syndrome.

64. Number 1 is correct.

Rationale: *Gravida* indicates the total number of pregnancies, regardless if the pregnancies were carried to term. The current pregnancy is included in determining *gravida*. *Parity* refers to the number of births after 20 weeks of gestation (including viable births, nonviable births, and stillbirths). Multiples such as twins or triplets are counted as one birth.

65. Number 4 is correct.

Rationale: Glossopharyngeal neuralgia is a condition caused by damage to cranial nerve IX (the glossopharyngeal nerve). Signs and symptoms may include episodes of pain in the throat, ears, tongue, and tonsils that can be triggered by swallowing or talking. Episodes of vertigo may be associated with vestibular neuritis, damage to cranial nerve VIII. Difficulty in moving the tongue is linked to damage to cranial nerve XII (hypoglossal nerve). Double vision is noted in abducens nerve palsy, damage to cranial nerve VI.

66. Answer: one tablet.

Solution:

1 gr = 60 mg	Convert grains to milligrams.
60 mg × 5 = 300 mg	Multiply the quantity in milligrams by 5 (since 5 grains were ordered) to find the amount ordered in milligrams.
= **one tablet**	The quantity in milligrams is equal to one tablet: 300 mg.

67. Number 3 is correct.

Rationale: A child is not usually able to point to a certain object when asked until 24 months of age. Imitating certain gestures, independently holding a bottle, and responding to his name are milestones a child usually reaches around 12 months of age.

68. **Answer:**

1. stay with the client until the panic attack is over
2. reduce external stimuli in the immediate area

3. instruct the client to take slow, deep breaths
4. incorporate physical activity into the client's daily routine
5. work with the client to develop coping mechanisms

69. Number 4 is correct.

Rationale: During a hearing test, the nurse should stand 1 – 2 feet away from the student, ask the student to cover one ear, whisper a phrase while facing the student, and ask the student to repeat the phrase. Then the nurse should repeat the test with the student covering the other ear.

70. Numbers 1, 2, 3, and 4 are correct.

Rationale: Social withdrawal, agitation, auditory hallucinations, and disorganized speech are all signs and symptoms of schizophrenia. Others include abnormal motor behavior, delusions, catatonia, inability to sleep, and feelings of apathy. Lack of attention to personal hygiene is not a symptom of schizophrenia.

71. Number 2 is correct.

Rationale: Placing the baby on his back to sleep is recommended by the American Academy of Pediatrics, because stomach or side sleeping carries a higher risk of SIDS. Other risk factors include low birth weight, young maternal age, maternal smoking during pregnancy, co-sleeping with parents or siblings, anemia, and male gender.

72. Number 2 is correct.

Rationale: Clients with cholecystitis have an inflamed gallbladder and should avoid high-fat foods. A low-potassium and low-phosphorus diet is associated with the renal diet followed by clients with kidney disease. Increased vitamin B 12 may be recommended for someone with pernicious anemia.

73. Number 4 is correct.

Rationale: Raynaud's disease is a disorder in which the blood vessels in the fingers and toes contract when the client is cold or stressed, causing temporary discoloration and pain. It is most common in young adult females.

74. Number 3 is correct.

Rationale: During the primary stage of syphilis, a chancre sore may be seen at the site of infection. A rash, swollen lymph nodes, fatigue, weight loss, and achy joints may be noted during the secondary stage. During the latent stage of syphilis, most clients do not experience any signs or symptoms. The damage that occurs in the final stage, tertiary syphilis, is irreversible and can include tissue tumors, blindness, heart disease, and death.

75. Number 4 is correct.

Rationale: Mean arterial pressure (MAP) is the average arterial pressure during one cardiac cycle. It is calculated using a formula:

MAP = (2 × diastolic pressure) + systolic pressure/3	Use the formula for MAP.
(2 × 84) + 132 = 300	Calculate and solve.
300/3 **= 100 mmHg**	

76. Number 1 is correct.

Rationale: Tetracycline is an antibiotic prescribed for many bacterial infections. Patients should be instructed that this medication should be avoided in pregnancy, can cause photosensitivity, and cannot be taken with dairy products or other sources of calcium. Aluminum, iron, and zinc deactivate the medication, and tetracycline should not be taken with sources of these minerals, such as antacids.

77. Number 2 is correct.

Rationale: Purpura are reddish-purple non-blanching skin discolorations (sized 0.3cm – 1cm) caused by bleeding under the skin. Ecchymosis is a hematoma larger than 1 cm in size. Petechia is a small hematoma less than 3mm. A bruise is bleeding under the skin caused by trauma.

78. Number 2 is correct.

Rationale: The nursing priority is to administer oxygen in accordance with the airway, breathing, and circulation priority model. Once the client is receiving supplemental oxygen, the nurse can assess and further intervene.

79. Number 2 is correct.

Rationale: A client in restraints should be checked at least every 30 minutes for circulatory compromise. The restraints should be released every 2 hours to check skin integrity and range of motion.

80. Answer: 31 drops/min

Solution:

total volume of solution/time in minutes	Use the formula.
1,500 mL/720 min = 2.08 mL/min	Substitute and solve.
2.08 mL/min × drop factor	
2.08 mL/min × 15 drops/1 mL = 31.2 drops/min	
31 drops/min	Round to the nearest whole number.

81. Number 1 is correct.

Rationale: The nurse's first action should be to activate the emergency disaster response plan. The other actions are important, but should take place after the emergency disaster plan is officially activated and underway.

82. Number 4 is correct.

Rationale: Autonomy refers to the client's right to make her own health care decisions. Fidelity is an ethics term that refers to loyalty and trust; confidentiality is based on a client's right to privacy and protection of health information. Justice is an ethical term in regards to fairness.

83. Number 4 is correct.

Rationale: Rubella is an airborne illness spread by coughing or sneezing, not skin-to-skin contact. The incubation period for rubella is 3 – 7 days, and signs and symptoms include high fever, runny nose, and cough.

84. Number 4 is correct.

Rationale: Agoraphobia is the fear of open spaces; these clients tend to stay indoors in a familiar space. Sociophobia refers to the fear of people or social situations. Anthropophobia is a related disorder that refers to the fear of being in the company of other people. The fear of strangers or foreigners is known as xenophobia.

85. Number 2 is correct.

Rationale: Flumazenil is given as an antagonist to benzodiazepines. Lorazepam and alprazolam are both benzodiazepines and would exacerbate the problem. Naloxone is given for opiate overdoses.

86. Number 4 is correct.

Rationale: The patient has recently attempted suicide and is at a high risk of harming herself. She should not be left alone or assigned a roommate until she is no longer a risk to herself or others. A staff member should stay with the client at all times to keep the client safe.

87. Number 2 is correct.

Rationale: A bandage saturated with blood could contain infectious blood-borne pathogens and should be disposed of as medical waste in a biohazard bag. It should never be disposed of in the regular trash, even if it is double bagged. To ensure safe disposal, only sharps (such as used syringes) should be thrown away in the sharps container.

88. Number 2 is correct.

Rationale: The most therapeutic response is to address the client's concerns and answer honestly. Since the boy has just begun puberty, it is probable that he will grow taller than girls his age within a few years. Girls tend to hit height growth spurts before boys, and this is normal and expected development. The other responses invalidate the boy's feelings and do not explain anything about puberty.

89. Number 2 is correct.

Rationale: In case of a fire, the nurse should attempt to open the window to breathe in fresh air and be seen by emergency personnel. Hiding in the closet or under the bed is dangerous because emergency responders may be unable to find those in need of help. The door to the room should be shut to attempt to contain the fire in the hall.

90. Numbers 1, 3, and 5 are correct.

Rationale: A client with fluid volume excess may show decreased urinary output, jugular vein distention, and tachycardia. Other signs and symptoms include hypertension, bounding pulse, edema, and dyspnea.

91. Number 2 is correct.

Rationale: In the team model of nursing care delivery, an RN leads a team to provide care for a client. The functional model of care refers to a delivery model in which each member of the staff is assigned a particular task or assignment to complete. In the total patient care model, one nurse assumes responsibility for all of the care for a particular client during the shift. The modular delivery model is when client assignments are based on location on the unit.

92. Number 4 is correct.

Rationale: Client-related factors include mechanical ventilation use, a complex medication regimen, and isolation precaution requirements. Nurse-to-client ratio is a staff-related factor.

93. Number 4 is correct.

Rationale: Serotonin syndrome occurs if an excess amount of serotonin enters the central nervous system or peripheral nervous system. The classic clinical triad of abnormalities seen in serotonin syndrome includes cognitive, autonomic, and somatic effects.

94. Number 2 is correct.

Rationale: Thrush is an oral fungal infection caused by candida yeast. It can be treated with an antifungal medication such as fluconazole (Diflucan). Fluconazole is not an antiviral, analgesic, or antibiotic.

95. Number 3 is correct.

Rationale: Normal findings in a newborn include a respiratory rate between 30 and 50 breaths/minute and a heart rate between 120 and 160 beats/minute. RR 46 breaths/minute and HR 153 beats/minute would fall within normal limits.

96. Number 3 is correct.

Rationale: The BUN-to-creatinine ratio is used as a tool in determining kidney function: The ratio indicates if the levels are proportionate to each other. It is calculated by dividing BUN by creatinine.

18/0.7 = 25.7:1, which rounds to 26:1

97. Number 2 is correct.

Rationale: Clients at a higher risk for aspiration include those who have a nasogastric tube, those on mechanical ventilation, and those with a condition that leads to difficulty swallowing, such as dysphagia. Total parenteral nutrition has no effect on aspiration risk.

98. Number 4 is correct.

Rationale: Capsaicin, derived from chili peppers, is a topical pain relief ointment used for strains/sprains, arthritis, and muscle aches. Aloe gel is often used for burns and psoriasis. Zinc oxide and hydrocortisone are anti-itch ointments.

99. Number 3 is correct.

Rationale: As people age, they have greater difficulty distinguishing between blue and green, due to yellowing of the eye lens. They have less difficulty differentiating among the other colors mentioned.

100. Number 3 is correct.

Rationale: During the first 24 hours post-op following an ileostomy, expected drainage is between 1,500mL and 2,000 mL.

101. Number 2 is correct.

Rationale: Risk factors for colon cancer include being African American, being over 50, and having a past medical history of diabetes. Other risk factors include a personal or family history of colon cancer; a high-fat, low-fiber diet; a history of inflammatory intestinal disease; obesity; smoking; and a sedentary lifestyle.

102. Number 4 is correct.

Rationale: Normal urine specific gravity values fall between 1.000 and 1.030. An increased value over 1.035 indicates dehydration, which may be seen in a client who has been experiencing pronounced vomiting and diarrhea.

103. Number 1 is correct.

Rationale: Cushing's disease is a disorder in which there is an increased secretion of adrenocorticotropic hormone, which leads to immunosuppression. An immunosuppressed client should be placed in a private room if possible. Pityriasis rosea is a bothersome, but usually harmless, skin rash. It is not contagious. Patients with diabetes mellitus normally need not be isolated. Heterochromia iridium, or multicolored irises, is almost always harmless and requires no treatment.

104. Number 1 is correct.

Rationale: Clients with celiac disease must follow a strict gluten-free diet. Chicken, carrots, potatoes, and cheese are gluten free and acceptable food choices for this client. Wheat bread, regular spaghetti, and flour tortillas all contain gluten. Any croutons in the Caesar salad would have gluten, too, if they are made from regular bread.

105. Number 4 is correct.

Rationale: Achondroplasia is a type of dwarfism marked by shortened proximal limbs, short fingers and toes, a large head, and a small midface with a flattened nasal bridge. Physical characteristics such as alopecia, failure to thrive, a small face, and a recessed jaw are seen in children with progeria. Enlarged hands and feet, skull expansion at fontanelle, and an enlarged tongue are characteristics found in people with acromegaly. Children with Down syndrome may present with poor muscle tone, slanted eyes, and a single palmar crease.

106. Numbers 1, 4, and 5 are correct.

Rationale: Clients with osteoarthritis should try to maintain a healthy weight; this has been shown to decrease joint pain and reduces stiffness. Using heat will help to ease stiffness, and moderate exercise three times a week is recommended. High-impact exercise should be avoided as it risks harming bone and tissue. Acetaminophen, not aspirin, is the first-choice drug to reduce osteoarthritis-related pain.

107. Number 2 is correct.

Rationale: Hepatitis B is transmitted via infectious blood, dirty needles, and sexual contact, and from mother to newborn. Hepatitis C is most commonly spread by infectious blood and needles. Contaminated food and water can transmit hepatitis A, while hepatitis E is transmitted only by contaminated water.

108. Numbers 1, 2, 3, 4, and 5 are correct.

Rationale: Meningitis is an illness that causes inflammation of the meninges. It can be caused by a bacterial, viral, or fungal infection; certain parasites; or a noninfectious origin such as cancer, certain drugs, or connective tissue disorders.

109. Number 2 is correct.

Rationale: The nurse would be alarmed if a 12-month-old presented with BP 65/55, RR 50, HR 130, as these are values within normal limits for a child aged newborn – 3 months. Normal vital signs for a 12-month-old are as follows: BP 80 – 100/ 55 – 65; RR 25 – 40, and HR 80 – 120. The other vital signs shown are in the normal limits for the age ranges listed.

110. Number 2 is correct.

Rationale: Erikson believed school-age children deal with the psychological crisis industry versus inferiority. Ego integrity versus despair is expected in mature adults over age 65. Trust versus mistrust is associated with infants, and ego identity versus role confusion is associated with adolescents.

111. Number 4 is correct.

Rationale: A non-rebreather mask delivers the highest percentage of oxygen compared to a venturi mask, nasal cannula, or simple face mask. If the client does not improve with the non-rebreather mask, the physician is likely to intubate the client and place him on mechanical ventilation.

112. Number 4 is correct.

Rationale: The RN cannot delegate an admission assessment to an LPN. Initial, comprehensive, and baseline assessments, such as a new client admitted to the floor, are the responsibility of an RN. An LPN may perform a focused assessment on a stable client.

113. Number 4 is correct.

Rationale: An order with a trailing zero, or a zero that follows a decimal point, needs to be clarified by the physician. Here, the lorazepam (Ativan) 1.0 mg could be mistaken for 10 mg.

114. Number 2 is correct.

Rationale: An African American woman over the age of 65 is at highest risk for a CVA. Other risk factors include smoking, family history of stroke or heart attack, sedentary lifestyle, high cholesterol, and a history of atrial fibrillation.

115. Numbers 2, 3, and 4 are correct.

Rationale: Signs and symptoms of a transplanted kidney rejection include increased blood pressure, weight gain, and pain at transplant site. Other indications are decreased urinary output, elevation in creatinine level, fever, and sudden edema.

116. Number 3 is correct.

Rationale: Scarlet fever is an infectious disease usually found in young children; it is distinguished by high fever, sore throat, and a characteristic rash. A possible complication is rheumatic fever. It can be treated with antibiotics. It is caused by an erythrogenic toxin. There is no vaccine for scarlet fever.

117. Number 1 is correct.

Rationale: Addison's disease is caused by the adrenal glands producing insufficient amounts of certain hormones. It requires lifelong medication therapy, and can lead to a life-threatening condition called Addisonian crisis. People with Addison's disease should not use salt substitutes. Clients with Addison's crave sodium in their diets and should be allowed salt. Salt substitutes are dangerous because they contain potassium; people with Addison's disease should limit dietary potassium.

118. Number 4 is correct.

Rationale: Because of a blunted immune response, elderly clients may not show many of the typical early signs and symptoms of pneumonia like chest pain, fever, and dyspnea. Instead, elderly clients may seem confused or have a change in mental status.

119. Number 1 is correct.

Rationale: Cases of genital herpes are not required to be reported to the CDC. Cases of chlamydia, hepatitis B, and gonorrhea must be reported, as well as chancroid, HIV, and syphilis.

120. Number 4 is correct.

Rationale: Long-term use of corticosteroids has been associated with osteoporosis. It is also associated with hypertension, hyperglycemia, edema, weight gain, cataracts, and increased risk of infection.

121. Number 3 is correct.

Rationale: The MMR vaccine is administered subcutaneously. It can be administered over the triceps using a 23- to 35-gauge, 5/8-inch needle. The skin should be pinched and the needle inserted at a 45-degree angle to avoid injecting into the muscle.

122. Number 2 is correct.

Rationale: Orthostatic hypotension is a condition in which one experiences low blood pressure when sitting or standing suddenly after lying down. The nurse should suggest the client wear support stockings, which will encourage venous return and prevent blood from pooling in the legs.

123. Numbers 2, 3, and 5 are correct.

Rationale: A cataract refers to the clouding of the eye lens. Signs and symptoms may include cloudy vision, double vision, diminished night vision, and halos seen around lights. Nausea and vomiting and severe eye pain are more typically associated with glaucoma.

124. Number 2 is correct.

Rationale: If possible, the nurse should utilize the hospital interpreter services. Using a certified interpreter is the most reliable method of communicating with a client who speaks another language. In addition, interpreters affiliated with a hospital specialize in medical and health terminology.

125. Number 1 is correct.

Rationale: Primary disabilities for children diagnosed with fetal alcohol syndrome are functional disabilities stemming from central nervous system (CNS) damage in utero. Poor motor skills, learning impairments, poor impulse control, hyperactivity, and memory problems are all examples of primary disabilities. Secondary disabilities of fetal alcohol syndrome emerge over time and are secondary to CNS damage. Examples include promiscuous behavior, future drug and alcohol dependency, and clinical depression.

126. Number 4 is correct.

Rationale: Pregnant women need 400 – 800 mcg of folic acid per day. Folic acid is a B vitamin linked to helping to prevent neural tube defects. Foods high in folic acid include strawberries and other citrus fruits, whole grains, legumes, leafy greens such as spinach and lettuce, and avocado.

127. Number 1 is correct.

Rationale: An overdose of acetaminophen can lead to hepatotoxicity, causing acute liver injury, permanent liver damage, or death. The nurse's priority would be obtaining lab tests used to determine liver function. Liver function can be determined by analyzing the liver enzymes aspartate transaminase and alanine transaminase.

128. Number 4 is correct.

Rationale: Type IV hypersensitivity reactions are cell mediated and are delayed reactions. Examples of type IV hypersensitivity reactions include allergic contact dermatitis, Crohn's disease, and graft versus host disease. Others include type I diabetes mellitus, multiple sclerosis, and celiac disease. A penicillin allergy is a type I hypersensitivity reaction.

129. Number 3 is correct.

Rationale: Azoospermia (sperm count of zero) usually occurs 3 – 4 months after a vasectomy. Until a semen analysis is performed to confirm a sperm count of zero, a backup method of birth control should be used.

130. Number 4 is correct.

Rationale: Benztropine (Cogentin) is an anticholinergic sometimes prescribed to reduce extrapyramidal side effects caused by first generation antipsychotics such as Haldol. Flumazenil is used to treat benzodiazepine overdose. Donepezil is an acetylcholinesterase inhibitor commonly prescribed for clients diagnosed with Alzheimer's disease. Naloxone is an opioid antagonist.

131. Number 1 is correct.

Rationale: The nurse should fully assess the client before determining what action or intervention to take.

132. Number 1 is correct.

Rationale: The goal of primary prevention is to prevent illness and disease before they occur, such as immunizing against disease. Secondary preventions reduce the impact and harm from an injury or disease that has already occurred. Mammogram screenings, testing and treating babies born to mothers with syphilis, and developing exercise programs to prevent MI are all examples of secondary prevention. A support group for depression is a tertiary prevention; it attempts to reduce the harmful impact of an ongoing illness or disease.

133. Numbers 1, 3, and 5 are correct.

Rationale: Anthrax can be transmitted to humans through cutaneous, inhalation, and gastrointestinal routes. Cutaneous anthrax occurs when anthrax spores enter the skin through an open sore or cut. Inhalational anthrax occurs when anthrax spores are inhaled into the lungs. Gastrointestinal anthrax is transmitted by consuming contaminated meat or drinking water contaminated by anthrax bacteria.

134. Number 3 is correct.

Rationale: Toddlers aged 2 1/2 – 3 years old typically engage in *parallel play*: They will play alongside others, but not necessarily play together. Playing alone with no interaction with others is seen in children under age 2. Playing in single-sex groups is typical of children aged 4 – 6, while playing in a mixed group of boys and girls is common with children aged 3 – 4.

135. Number 1 is correct.

Rationale: The classic Cushing's triad includes increased blood pressure, irregular respirations, and decreased heart rate. This triad indicates an emergency situation of increasing intracranial pressure, usually leading to brain herniation or death if not immediately treated. Cardiac arrhythmia is not part of the Cushing reflex triad.

136. Answer:

1. sinoatrial node
2. atrioventricular node
3. bundle of His
4. bundle branches
5. Purkinje fibers

137. Number 1 is correct.

Rationale: Intrapersonal communication is the communication process within an individual's internal thoughts or language. Horizontal communication is communication among individuals or groups on the same level in a hierarchy (often in reference to a workplace). Interpersonal communication is verbal and nonverbal information exchange (face-to-face communication) between two or more people. Vertical communication is communication among individuals or groups on different levels in a hierarchy (such as between subordinates and superiors).

138. Number 1 is correct.

Rationale: Many clients recognize their daily medications, and the nurse should be concerned if the client states the medication is different from what she usually takes. The nurse should not administer the medication until he verifies the order. There may indeed have been a medication error, so the nurse should not tell the client the medication is correct. The nurse should not report that there has been a medication error before verifying with the MAR and pharmacy, because there may not be an error at all. While it may be helpful to explain to the client that medications can vary in appearance even if they are the same substance, in this situation the nurse should verify the medication before making any assumptions.

139. Number 3 is correct.

Rationale: An open- ended question requires the client to respond in a descriptive method; it necessitates more than a one-word answer. The nurse wants to foster a therapeutic relationship by asking the client to describe his anxiety levels on the weekend. Close-ended questions can usually be answered with a one-word response such as *yes* or *no*.

140. Number 2 is correct.

Rationale: Bioterrorism agents classified as Category A include anthrax, botulism toxin, plague, and smallpox. Typhoid, malaria, and Ebola are not Category A bioterrorism agents.

141. Number 3 is correct.

Rationale: Clients participating in research studies have the right to quit at any time and should be informed they are free to leave the study whenever they choose.

142. Number 3 is correct.

Rationale: A 3-in-1 TPN solution includes dextrose, amino acids, and lipids. TPN also may be prepared as a 2-in-1 solution, which only includes dextrose and amino acids, with lipids administered separately.

143. Number 3 is correct.

Rationale: Someone with current symptoms of a common cold or the flu cannot donate blood. A potential donor must be free of cold or flu symptoms on the day of donation. Those with hyperthyroidism, new mothers, and people who are at least 3 years recovered from tuberculosis after completing treatment are eligible to donate blood.

144. Number 1 is correct.

Rationale: DMD is carried by an X-linked recessive gene. It is transmitted by the mother: If the mother is a carrier, one of her X chromosomes has the mutation. Therefore, there is a 50% chance a female child will be a DMD carrier (females have two X chromosomes). There is a 50% chance a male child will inherit the disease and have DMD (males only have one X chromosome).

145. Number 3 is correct.

Rationale: On a neutropenic diet, clients should avoid unpasteurized dairy products, raw or undercooked meats, uncooked eggs, and uncooked, raw vegetables. Fresh, uncooked fruits are only acceptable if they can be peeled, such as bananas or oranges.

146. Number 1 is correct.

Rationale: The anticipated action of vasopressin administered during a cardiac arrest is to raise blood pressure. This is an antidiuretic drug, which works by reabsorbing water in the renal tubules.

147. Number 4 is correct.

Rationale: Modifiable risk factors are lifestyle changes a person can make in order to reduce their risk of developing a certain disease. A high-stress lifestyle, smoking, and obesity are all modifiable risk factors for CAD. Risk factors such as age, gender, race, and family history are nonmodifiable.

148. Number 1 is correct.

Rationale: BMI is a health screening tool calculated by considering an individual's height and weight. A BMI over 30 is considered obese. If BMI falls between 25 and 29.9, the individual is considered overweight. A BMI between 18.5 and 24.9 is considered a normal/healthy weight, and BMI under 18.5 is considered underweight.

149. Number 3 is correct.

Rationale: Due to many factors, older adults are at risk for malnutrition. Complications caused by malnutrition include an increased risk of falls due to weakness, poor wound healing, and an increased risk for infections. Malnutrition does not contribute to chronic heart failure; however, chronic heart failure does put a client at risk for malnutrition.

150. Number 4 is correct.

Rationale: Fungal infections such as Fusarium require treatment with antifungal medications such as Vfend. Combivir is an antiretroviral drug used to treat HIV-1 infections. It is not a cure but does help delay the process of the disease when taken in combination with other drugs. Famvir is an antiviral prescribed for the herpes zoster (shingles) virus. Cipro is a quinolone antibiotic.

FOUR: Practice Test Four

1. A nurse starts an IV medication for a client. It is ordered as IV push, and she pushes the medication slowly over two minutes. The client then becomes restless, complains of chest pain, has difficulty breathing, and becomes cyanotic. The nurse recognizes this is most likely caused by

    1. an allergic reaction to the drug.

    2. pneumothorax.

    3. septic shock.

    4. pulmonary embolism.

2. An 80-year-old man with a decubitus ulcer has just been admitted to the floor. Upon assessment of the wound, the nurse notes that an area of skin under the wound extends and creates another opening in the skin 4 centimeters away. She would chart this as

    1. tunneling.

    2. dehiscence.

    3. undermining.

    4. evisceration.

3. What airborne precautions should the nurse anticipate when a client with measles is admitted to the hospital? **Select all that apply.**

    1. wear a surgical face mask upon entering client's room

    2. require client to wear a face mask in the hallway during transport

    3. require client to be placed in a negative pressure airflow room

    4. wear a fit-tested N-95 respirator at all times when in client's room

    5. have the client enter through the facility's dedicated isolation entrance

4. The nurse is working on a discharge teaching plan for a client prescribed phenelzine (Nardil), a monoamine oxidase inhibitor (MAOI drug). The nurse knows teaching was successful if the client states,

 1. "I will not be able to have wine and aged cheese anymore."
 2. "I should avoid all dairy products from now on."
 3. "Taking this medication with vitamin K–containing foods is dangerous."
 4. "I will need to decrease my dietary fiber now."

5. A client is being treated with internal radiation (brachytherapy). The nurse explains to the client that

 1. visitors should wear gown, gloves, and mask when coming in the room.
 2. visitors are not allowed until the client is no longer receiving radiation therapy.
 3. visitors must stay at least 6 feet away from the client.
 4. visitors should not bring any cards or gifts into the room because they can become radioactive.

6. A 19-year-old male is rushed to the emergency room with a GI bleed after a car accident. The priority intervention is

 1. asking the client what he remembers about the accident.
 2. obtaining a full set of vitals.
 3. completing a full abdominal assessment.
 4. administering ordered pain medication STAT.

7. A woman with hypothyroidism has been taking levothyroxine (Synthroid) for 5 years. She has just been prescribed warfarin (Coumadin). The nurse immediately calls the health care provider to review these orders and anticipates the physician will

 1. order lab work.
 2. increase the dose of warfarin.
 3. discontinue the levothyroxine.
 4. decrease the dose of warfarin.

8. A woman has undergone a mastectomy of her right breast and has been brought to the recovery unit. The nurse explains that the client should

 1. keep her right arm elevated on a pillow.
 2. keep her right arm elevated above her head.
 3. keep her right arm level with the heart.
 4. keep her right arm slightly lower than her heart.

9. The nurse manager has noticed that one of the nurses has been late three times this month. What should the nurse manager do first?

   1. call a staff meeting to review attendance policy and consequences for tardiness
   2. make a note in the nurse's file documenting her tardiness
   3. call the nurse into a private meeting
   4. report the nurse to human resources

10. A client on the post-op floor underwent surgery 4 days ago. The night nurse reports to the nurse coming on to dayshift that the client complained all night of pain, even though she received every dose of prescribed pain medication. The client currently rates the pain at a 10 out of 10. The day shift nurse should first

    1. call the physician and ask her to prescribe a different medication.
    2. work with the client on alternative pain relief measures such as guided imagery.
    3. administer the next dose of pain medication, but observe the client swallow it to ensure she is really taking the medication.
    4. complete a full head-to-toe assessment on the client.

11. An operating room nurse just received a client scheduled for a laparoscopic cholecystectomy, but discovers the consent form has not been signed. What is the most appropriate action?

    1. bring the client a new consent form and have him sign it right away
    2. call the surgeon and ask how she would like to proceed
    3. inform the nursing manager there is no signed consent form
    4. ask the unit manager if the surgery can be rescheduled for later in the day

12. A woman is receiving outpatient treatment at a mental health center. She starts crying and tells the nurse her husband has filed for divorce. The **best** response from the nurse is

    1. "I am so sorry. I am divorced too, but it worked out for the best."
    2. "About half of marriages end in divorce these days."
    3. "You have to let him go and move on with your life."
    4. "Tell me what happened."

13. A 56-year-old male with a long history of alcohol abuse is brought to the detox center per terms of his probation. He had his last drink 6 hours ago and seems confused and agitated. The nurse expects the physician to order

    1. naloxone hydrochloride (Narcan).
    2. chlordiazepoxide hydrochloride (Librium).
    3. disulfiram (Antabuse).
    4. propofol (Diprivan).

14. A home health nurse visits a 7-year-old boy on neutropenic precautions. His mother cares for him during the day. Which of the following statements by the mother indicates a need for further teaching?

    1. "I will call the doctor if my son has a temperature above 38°C."
    2. "My son should protect his skin by showering every other day instead of daily."
    3. "His aunt cannot visit until 3 weeks have passed since her flu shot."
    4. "I will need to throw out the flowers he got as a get-well gift."

15. A nursing instructor demonstrates to several students how to wrap an amputated limb in a bandage using a figure eight technique. Which of the following correctly states the benefits of this technique? **Select all that apply.**

    1. prevents blood clots from forming
    2. reduces post-operative swelling
    3. minimizes pain and discomfort
    4. prevents exposure to air

16. A client with chronic kidney disease has just been admitted to the floor. The admitting nurse reviews a list of OTC medications the client takes at home and is concerned when he sees

    1. Mylanta antacid.
    2. iron supplements.
    3. daily baby aspirin.
    4. fish oil supplements.

17. A new graduate nurse has an argument with a coworker regarding how the medication cart should be organized. The nurse asks his coworker to step into the break room to discuss their disagreement. This is an example of what type of conflict management?

    1. competing
    2. confronting
    3. accommodating
    4. avoiding

18. The nurse is caring for a 10-year-old boy with hemophilia. The nurse suspects the child has developed hemarthrosis when she observes

    1. jaundice.
    2. increased heart rate.
    3. popping sounds in the joints.
    4. redness or swelling over the joints.

19. A 49-year-old female suffered a stroke that resulted in dysphagia. The dietician orders a diet of dysphagia-pureed foods. Which of the following foods would be an appropriate choice?

    1. beef stew
    2. hard-boiled egg
    3. custard
    4. sliced peaches

20. A labor and delivery nurse is assessing a newborn baby boy. Which finding would indicate possible microcephaly?

    1. depressed fontanelles during feeding
    2. hypoactivity
    3. head circumference in lowest tenth percentile
    4. absent fontanelles

21. A nurse is leading a parenting class for new parents. She explains that most babies say their first word by age

    1. 6 months.
    2. 12 months.
    3. 10 months.
    4. 18 months.

22. The physician orders 1.25 L of normal saline (NS) to infuse over 10 hours. The nurse should set the IV pump at what flow rate (mL/hr)?

    1. 55 mL/hr
    2. 125 mL/hr
    3. 175 mL/hr
    4. 200 mL/hr

23. A manic client is admitted to an inpatient psychiatric center. He is hyperactive, talking quickly, acting aggressively, and pacing. The nursing staff should

    1. outline realistic expectations for the client's behavior.
    2. ignore the client's behavior.
    3. allow the client to eat lunch with other clients to observe the interaction.
    4. assign an RN to stay with the client at all times.

24. Which of the following signs would indicate imminent death in a hospice patient?

    1. tightly clenched muscles
    2. steady, deep respirations
    3. slow pulse rate
    4. fixed, dilated pupils

25. A pediatric nurse volunteers at a health screening fair. The nurse examines a patient. Which of the following findings may be indicative of type 1 diabetes and require further investigation?

    1. stomach bloating, swollen lymph nodes, increased thirst

    2. sudden weight loss, blurry vision, muscle weakness

    3. sudden weight gain, ringing in the ears, difficulty sleeping

    4. feeling hungry all of the time, increased thirst, waking up at night to urinate

26. A student nurse overhears her instructor using the term *pink puffer*. The student knows this term refers to a client with which condition?

    1. chronic bronchitis

    2. chronic obstructive pulmonary disease (COPD)

    3. emphysema

    4. allergic asthma

27. As serum calcium levels rise, which hormone is excreted?

    1. prolactin

    2. melatonin

    3. aldosterone

    4. parathyroid

28. A medication error has occurred, and the client has received double the ordered dosage of magnesium sulfate. The nurse anticipates the physician will order what medication STAT?

    1. chlordiazepoxide (Librium)

    2. vitamin K

    3. naloxone (Narcan)

    4. calcium gluconate

29. A client diagnosed with lung cancer asks the nurse what the term *M0* refers to. The nurse says that M0 means

    1. no distant metastasis present.

    2. distant metastasis present.

    3. distant metastasis cannot be evaluated.

    4. metastasis present only in immediate lymph nodes.

30. A client comes into the emergency room after a chemical splashed into her eye at work. The **priority** nursing intervention is to

    1. cover the eye with a sterile cloth.

    2. determine what chemical splashed into the eye.

    3. irrigate the eye with normal saline solution.

    4. test vision in the affected eye.

31. A nurse is working with an immobile client and doing passive range-of-motion (ROM) exercises on his legs. The client states the exercise is too painful and does not want to continue. The nurse should

    1. ask the client to first rate the pain level on a scale of 0 – 10.

    2. ask the provider to order PRN pain medication to be given before exercise.

    3. continue the exercise and encourage the client to work through any pain.

    4. stop the exercise if the client complains of pain.

32. A child was exposed to the hepatitis A virus, became ill, and made a full recovery 2 years ago. The child is now immune to the hepatitis A virus and will likely be protected for the rest of her life. This type of immunity is referred to as

    1. active artificial immunity.

    2. naturally acquired active immunity.

    3. artificially acquired passive immunity.

    4. naturally acquired passive immunity.

33. The nurse cares for two children brought into an emergency shelter. Law enforcement suspects the children have been neglected. The nurse should assess

    1. visual acuity using the Snellen chart.

    2. blood pressure and pulse rate.

    3. height and weight.

    4. bruises on the knees and elbows.

34. The floor nurse sees a new order in a client's chart for levothyroxine (Synthroid) 125 mcg PO every day. The pharmacy sends up Synthroid 0.1 mg tablets. How many tablets should the nurse administer? Calculate and fill in the blank.

_____

35. The nurse is working with a nursing student to administer an enema solution to a client. The client states she feels painful cramping. The nurse should intervene by

    1. squeezing the enema bag so the flow rate is faster.

    2. explaining to the client that this is a normal feeling and continuing with the enema.

    3. clamping the tube for 1 minute and then starting the enema at a slower rate.

    4. discontinuing the enema until the provider can order a PRN pain medication.

36. During the planning stage of the nursing process, the nurse should

    1. collect pertinent data about the client.

    2. consider goals and select the best nursing interventions.

    3. evaluate success of the interventions.

    4. create a nursing diagnosis based upon the assessment.

37. A client has been diagnosed with pernicious anemia. What breakfast should the nurse suggest to increase dietary B12?

1. banana nut muffin, bowl of grits, green tea
2. bran waffles, grapefruit, iced coffee
3. whole grain oatmeal with strawberry slices, orange juice
4. scrambled eggs, beef sausage patty, milk

38. A client must take oral potassium supplements every day. The nurse explains to the client that the potassium supplements

1. need to be stored in the refrigerator.
2. should only be taken in the evening before bed.
3. should be diluted in a glass of cold water or juice.
4. need to be taken on an empty stomach.

39. A 15-year-old male is brought into the emergency room after being hit by a car while riding his bicycle. The team quickly assesses him for injury and notes on the neurologic exam the client responds to external stimuli by arching back his head, extending and internally rotating the arms and legs, extending the elbows, pronating the wrists, and clenching his teeth. The team suspects injury to

1. the frontal lobe.
2. the spinal column.
3. the midbrain.
4. the cerebral hemisphere.

40. A 52-year-old female with mitral valve stenosis is admitted to the floor. She asks the nurse why she got this condition because it does not run in her family. The nurse explains most cases of mitral stenosis are due to a history of

1. right-sided heart failure.
2. hypercholesterolemia.
3. rheumatic fever.
4. viral meningitis.

41. Which of the following are risk factors for developing glaucoma? **Select all that apply.**

1. asthma
2. pernicious anemia
3. diabetes mellitus
4. obesity
5. hypertension

42. A client's lab results have just come in. The nurse reviews the electrolytes and contacts the health care provider regarding which result?

1. chloride 167 mEq/L

2. calcium 9.3 mg/dL

3. phosphate 3.8 mg/dL

4. sodium 141 mEq/L

43. A client in the recovery ICU is on mechanical ventilation. The nurse notices the client has frothy secretions around his mouth, and the nurse hears adventitious breath sounds with the stethoscope. The nurse should

1. increase the oxygen level on the ventilator.

2. suction the endotracheal tube.

3. lower the head of the bed.

4. call the rapid response team.

44. A nurse prepares to administer a transfusion of RBCs and takes the client's vital signs. The client's temperature is 102.7°F, but other vitals are within normal limits. The nurse should

1. transfuse the RBC as ordered.

2. administer an antipyretic and transfuse the RBCs.

3. transfuse the RBCs but monitor the temperature hourly.

4. not transfuse the RBCs and instead contact the physician.

45. A new graduate nurse is assigned to a 30-year-old female requiring NG tube feeding. The preceptor reminds the graduate nurse to check placement of the NG tube before administering the feeding. The **best** way to do this is by

1. verifying placement with an X-ray before each feeding.

2. aspirating gastric contents and testing the contents on a pH paper.

3. auscultating bowel sounds after administering a 30 cc air bolus.

4. auscultating bowel sounds after administering the first 10 cc of tube feeding.

46. The nurse is caring for a client with staphylococcus epidermidis. The client is on a vancomycin IV. What nursing consideration should the nurse be aware of regarding this medication?

1. The client should only order from the low-residue-diet menu.

2. The nurse should assist the client to ambulate.

3. The nurse will need to draw blood before administration to determine trough levels.

4. The client should be monitored for cardiac arrhythmias.

47. A 42-year-old female has thrombocytopenia with a platelet count of 75,000. The nurse should

   1. monitor for bleeding.

   2. place the client on neutropenic precautions.

   3. limit visiting hours.

   4. encourage a diet high in iron.

48. An 8-year-old boy is diagnosed with a Wilm's tumor. The nurse would expect what finding on assessment?

   1. occult blood in the stool

   2. yellowing of the sclera

   3. vision loss

   4. enlarged abdomen

49. The nursing assistant is taking vitals for a client on mechanical ventilation. Which of the following findings should the nursing assistant report to the nurse immediately?

   1. respiratory rate 26 breaths/minute

   2. heart rate 82 beats/minute

   3. blood pressure 152/86 mmHg

   4. temperature 102.1°F

50. A 32-year-old male client has just undergone a liver biopsy and is released to the post-op floor for observation. The nurse should have the client lie in what position?

   1. semi-Fowler's

   2. on his right side

   3. supine

   4. on his left side

51. The nurse is caring for a client who received tissue plasminogen activator 2 hours ago. The nurse would be **most** concerned by which of the following in the client?

   1. blood pressure of 134/91

   2. bright red blood streaks in the stool

   3. temperature of 40.1°C

   4. ankle edema

52. A school nurse is suspicious that a child is being physically abused at home. The nurse's responsibility is to

   1. ask the child if the suspicions of abuse are accurate and true.

   2. speak with the caregivers to share the abuse suspicions.

   3. accurately and fully document this in the child's chart.

   4. report the situation to the local authorities.

53. A med-surg nurse is floating to the post-op floor for a few days. The float nurse sees one of the regular post-op nurses taking medication out of the med cart and ingesting several pills. The float nurse should immediately

   1. inform the state board of nursing.

   2. inform the nursing supervisor who works on the post-op floor.

   3. report the nurse to human resources.

   4. confront the post-op nurse about stealing and abusing medications.

54. A nurse is asked to prepare a client for placement of a central venous catheter that will be inserted into the right jugular vein. The nurse asks the client to

   1. lie in a supine position with the head turned to the right.

   2. sit in a high-Fowler's position with the head turned to the left.

   3. lie in the Trendelenburg position with the head turned to the left.

   4. lie in a supine position with the head positioned straight.

55. A 46-year-old male has been placed under therapeutic hypothermic care after a myocardial infarction (MI). The nurse correctly explains to the family,

   1. "Therapeutic hypothermia increases the production of neurotransmitters in the brain."

   2. "Therapeutic hypothermia will repair damaged cardiac tissue."

   3. "Therapeutic hypothermia will help protect the brain from injury by slowing metabolism."

   4. "Therapeutic hypothermia will slow the heart rate to reduce likelihood of another MI."

56. A labor and delivery nurse is caring for a newborn baby whose mother was a regular cocaine user during the entire pregnancy (prenatal cocaine exposure). The nurse expects the newborn to

   1. present with irritability, trouble sleeping, and a shrill cry.

   2. present with lethargy, poor muscle tone, and inability to cry.

   3. require pharmaceutical support for cocaine withdrawal.

   4. benefit from a regular breastfeeding schedule.

57. An ICU nurse monitors a client recovering from a head injury. The client's intracranial pressure (ICP) has been between 15 and 19 mmHg throughout the shift. However, after the nurse suctions the client's endotracheal tube, the ICP jumps to 28 mmHg. It decreases a few minutes later to 20 mmHg. The **best** intervention by the nurse is to

   1. increase the rate of the sedative IV drip.

   2. chart the findings and continue to monitor the client.

   3. reposition the client.

   4. contact the physician.

58. The director of nursing is working on an occupational health and safety manual for the staff. She wants to include a section describing how factors in the environment can increase safety and reduce risk and injury. The term for this study is

   1. occupational therapy.
   2. accident analysis.
   3. ergonomics.
   4. body mechanics.

59. A critically injured woman is rushed to the ER. She needs an immediate blood transfusion, and there is no time to cross-match blood type. The nurse anticipates the physician will call for

   1. 1 unit of AB positive blood.
   2. 1 unit of O positive blood.
   3. 1 unit of AB negative blood.
   4. 1 unit of O negative blood.

60. The nurse is caring for a 28-year-old female with a long history of heroin addiction. The client tells the nurse that she started off using a small amount recreationally, but as time went on, she needed more and more heroin to feel a high. The nurse recognizes this as

   1. addiction.
   2. dependence.
   3. tolerance.
   4. withdrawal.

61. A client newly diagnosed with type 1 diabetes mellitus asks the nurse why it is important to rotate insulin injection sites. The nurse explains this is done to avoid

   1. tissue scarring.
   2. insulin resistance.
   3. localized edema.
   4. lipodystrophy.

62. A 3-year-old child had a PPD skin test 2 days ago. When the mother brings the child back to the clinic to have the nurse check the results, the nurse notes a 10 mm area of induration. This is considered

   1. an inconclusive skin test.
   2. a positive skin test.
   3. a negative skin test.
   4. too early to determine the results.

63. The nurse expects a child with a deficiency in factor VIII to be diagnosed with

1. hemophilia A.

2. pernicious anemia.

3. sickle cell disease.

4. Tay-Sachs disease.

64. A client is prescribed heparin 2,000 units SC q8 hours. The pharmacy sends heparin 5,000 units/mL. How many mL should the nurse administer every 24 hours?

1. 0.4 mL/ day

2. 0.8 mL/ day

3. 1.2 mL/ day

4. 1.4 mL/day

65. A nurse creates a care plan for a client diagnosed with a cerebellar brain tumor. The correct nursing diagnosis for this client is "Client at risk for injury related to

1. impaired balance."

2. decreased visual acuity."

3. decreased level of consciousness."

4. impaired ability to make decisions."

66. The nurse is teaching a group of premenopausal women how to conduct self-breast exams. The nurse should instruct the women to perform self-breast exams

1. on the first day of the menstrual cycle.

2. one week after the menstrual cycle.

3. immediately after the menstrual cycle.

4. on the first day of every month.

67. The nurse knows the **best** intervention for preventing a postoperative infection is

1. wearing gown, gloves, and mask in the client's room.

2. administering a prophylactic antibiotic.

3. placing the client in a private room.

4. following hand hygiene protocols.

68. A 16-year-old girl presents with peptic ulcers, constipation, low self-esteem, irregular menstrual cycle, and dental erosion. Her weight has fluctuated between 96 and 128 pounds over the past year. The nurse suspects the girl is suffering from

1. binge eating disorder.

2. bulimia nervosa.

3. pernicious anemia.

4. anorexia nervosa.

69. A 5-year-old boy ingested aspirin tablets, thinking they were candies. The nurse is **most** concerned about

    1. metabolic acidosis.

    2. metabolic alkalosis.

    3. respiratory alkalosis.

    4. respiratory acidosis.

70. A client in cardiac arrest shows to be in torsades de pointes, and magnesium sulfate is ordered STAT. The **priority** nursing intervention is

    1. monitor client for bradycardia and respiratory depression.

    2. prepare client for synchronized cardioversion.

    3. monitor client for tachycardia and hyperventilation.

    4. prepare client for Swan catheter.

71. A labor and delivery nurse is caring for a client in active labor. The fetal monitor shows late decelerations. The nurse should first

    1. place the client in high-Fowler's position in preparation to push.

    2. place the client in left lateral recumbent position.

    3. increase the rate of IV Pitocin.

    4. call the physician and report fetal distress.

72. A 4-year-old girl has been transferred to a step-down recovery room after a tonsillectomy yesterday. The nurse should place the child in what position while she sleeps?

    1. semi-Fowler's position

    2. supine position

    3. prone position

    4. side-lying position

73. A public health nurse works with a specific population. Many of the clients use herbal remedies at home. The nurse would express concern if which of the following clients reported using herbal remedies?

    1. 13-year-old girl with a toothache

    2. 42-year-old man with xerostomia

    3. 59-year-old woman with nasopharyngitis

    4. 20-year-old woman with psoriasis

74. A client with Graves' disease is brought to the ER with a suspected thyroid storm. The nurse expects to see what signs and symptoms?

    1. seizures, jaundice, irregular heartbeat, vomiting
    2. bradycardia, septic shock, polyuria
    3. increased cranial pressure, thready pulse, rash across chest
    4. poor muscle tone, dyspnea, cyanosis

75. Which of the following is a metabolic, life-threatening adverse reaction to general anesthesia?

    1. hypothermia
    2. hyperthermia
    3. hypoglycemia
    4. hyperglycemia

76. A teenage girl is brought to the outpatient psychiatric clinic for treatment of anxiety and depression. How should the nurse **best** evaluate the client's risk for suicide?

    1. ask the client if she has had any suicidal thoughts or plans
    2. ask the girl's parents what changes in behavior they have noticed
    3. ask the client if she has been taking her antidepressant medication as prescribed
    4. do not mention the subject of suicide until the client brings it up herself

77. A client diagnosed with Alzheimer's disease initiates the same conversation repeatedly, becomes aggressive when stressed, needs reminders to perform ADLs, and is easily lost in his neighborhood. This client is likely in what stage of Alzheimer's disease?

    1. pre-Alzheimer's
    2. early/mild
    3. moderate
    4. late to severe

78. An ICU nurse is caring for a client receiving total parenteral nutrition (TPN) via IV. The client's infusion ended 2 hours ago and the pharmacy has not yet sent another bag. The client is diaphoretic and tachycardic, and states he feels weak, dizzy, and fatigued. The nurse suspects

    1. dehydration.
    2. fluid volume overload.
    3. hyperglycemia.
    4. hypoglycemia.

79. A 22-year-old woman has just been diagnosed with myasthenia gravis. She asks the nurse what causes this disease. The **most** accurate response from the nurse is

   1. "This is a disease caused by a chromosomal defect in utero. It is a structural abnormality in the chromosome that causes nerve cells in your body to become inflamed and not function properly."

   2. "This is an autoimmune disease in which antibodies attack the muscles and muscle atrophy occurs. The muscles will become weak and begin to waste."

   3. "This is an autoimmune disease in which antibodies destroy acetylcholine at the neuromuscular junction. This prevents your muscles from contracting normally."

   4. "This is a hereditary condition caused by a recessive gene. It causes nervous tissue to be broken down, and damage occurs to the brain and spinal cord."

80. A client is scheduled for a colposcopy. The nurse assists the client into which position?

   1. Sim's position

   2. supine position, with the head of the bed elevated 15 degrees

   3. left-side-lying position, knees to chest

   4. lithotomy position

81. A client comes into the dermatology office and shows the nurse a rash she is very concerned about. The nurse examines areas of skin on the elbows and scalp that are inflamed and covered with silvery-white scales. The nurse determines this is **most** likely

   1. scabies.

   2. plaque psoriasis.

   3. urticaria.

   4. contact dermatitis.

82. After a traumatic accident, the client must have his left arm amputated in an emergency procedure. When the client wakes from anesthesia and sees his arm has been amputated, he becomes extremely distressed. He cries uncontrollably and yells about how angry he is at the doctor. The **best** therapeutic action from the nurse is to

   1. close the door to the client's room and return to check on him periodically.

   2. sit quietly with the client until he calms down.

   3. explain to the client that he should not be angry because there was no other choice.

   4. call the hospital chaplain to come speak with the client.

83. A 9-year-old child weighing 40 kilograms has an order for piperacillin (Pipracil) via IV infusion. The recommended daily dose for this medication is 240 – 300 mg/kg/day IV div. q8h. What is the maximum daily dose of piperacillin this client can receive per day? Calculate and fill in the blank.

_____

84. A client with a past history of substance abuse and opioid addiction comes to the hospital after falling off a ladder. Upon assessment, the client reports his pain is a 9 out of 10 on the pain scale. The nurse should

    1. chart "The client states his pain is 9/10."

    2. chart "The client has a past history of addiction and is claiming he has severe pain."

    3. ask the client if his pain level is really as high as he states.

    4. report to the physician the client is likely seeking drugs.

85. A 22-year-old pregnant client is diagnosed with autoimmune hemolytic anemia. The nurse anticipates immediate treatment with

    1. IgA.

    2. IgG.

    3. IgE.

    4. IgD.

86. A client's serum sodium level is 113 mEq/L. The nurse would expect which findings upon assessment?

    1. headache, confusion, muscle weakness, fatigue

    2. hypertension, muscle cramps, respiratory depression

    3. cardiac arrhythmia, tetany, tachycardia

    4. confusion, nystagmus, tetany, hallucinations

87. A client with chronic kidney disease (CKD) is being evaluated by the transplant team. The client's glomerular filtration rate (GFR) is 14 mL/min. This places the client in which stage of CKD?

    1. stage 1

    2. stage 5

    3. stage 4

    4. stage 2

88. A woman comes to a community health clinic and expresses concern she may have been exposed to HIV. The community nurse draws blood for an ELISA test, which comes back as positive. The nurse should

    1. ask the client to come into the clinic to tell her in person she is HIV positive.

    2. request the client come in and follow up with a Western blot test.

    3. explain to the client this shows she has been exposed to HIV, but does not have HIV.

    4. call and tell client that she is HIV positive.

89. Ideally, the first dose of what vaccine is given at birth?

    1. IPV

    2. Hib

    3. DTaP

    4. hepatitis B

90. A client confides in the nurse that a close friend recently died from pancreatic cancer. The client asks what the risk factors are for pancreatic cancer. The nurse should respond with

    1. "Being a female of Asian descent is linked to an increased risk of pancreatic cancer."

    2. "Drinking two or fewer alcoholic beverages per week is linked to an increased risk of pancreatic cancer."

    3. "Past history of acute pancreatitis before age 20 is linked to an increased risk of pancreatic cancer."

    4. "Cigarette smoking is linked to an increased risk for pancreatic cancer."

91. A nurse graduated from nursing school 3 years ago. He worked at one hospital on the telemetry unit for 6 months. He then transferred to the cardiac care unit (CCU) at a teaching hospital, and has been working there for 2.5 years. According to the novice-expert model of nursing, he is considered

    1. novice.

    2. expert.

    3. competent.

    4. advanced beginner.

92. According to Maslow's hierarchy of needs, "lack of prejudice" falls under which level of human need fulfillment?

    1. love and belonging

    2. self-actualization

    3. safety

    4. esteem

93. A triage nurse is reviewing messages from four clients. The nurse's **priority** is which client?

    1. 69-year-old male with cloudy urine and fever of 100.3°F

    2. 42-year-old female with pain in jaw and back that has become more intense in past 15 minutes

    3. 56-year-old female with hot flashes and inability to sleep the past four nights

    4. 10-year-old boy with a closed fracture of the tibia, who rates his pain level as 7 out of 10

94. A client prescribed furosemide (Lasix) should choose which meal for lunch?

    1. chicken breast, white rice, apple

    2. turkey sandwich on wheat bread, celery sticks, grapefruit

    3. egg salad, cooked carrots, strawberries

    4. baked salmon, spinach salad, banana

95. A client who has been taking Coumadin (warfarin) was stabbed in the upper arm. His prothrombin time is over twice the normal amount. The nurse anticipates an order for

    1. fresh frozen plasma

    2. whole blood

    3. platelets

    4. packed red blood cells

96. A client requires IV insulin. The pharmacy sends up a bag labeled 1,000 units of insulin in a 250 mL bag of 0.9% NaCl. The pump is set to infuse at 5 mL/hr. How much insulin does the client receive per hour?

    1. 20 units/hour

    2. 50 units/hour

    3. 25 units/hour

    4. 15 units/hour

97. After a train accident, the nurse is assigned to triage the injured. Based upon the triage protocol, which individual should be seen last?

    1. 66-year-old male with no visible injuries, but who is experiencing tachycardia and seems confused

    2. 16-year-old female with fixed, dilated pupils who is unresponsive and has clear fluid draining from right ear

    3. 25-year-old female with an abrasion to left eye and a swollen ankle, who is unable to put weight on right leg

    4. 80-year-old male with chest pains and shortness of breath

98. An RN delegates patient assignments to an LPN and nursing assistant. Later, the RN overhears a nursing assistant arguing with a patient regarding a late breakfast tray. The nursing assistant begins to raise his voice as the disagreement continues. The **best** action from the RN is to

    1. call the nursing assistant out of the room and speak with him about the incident.

    2. apologize to the patient and assign another nursing assistant to that room.

    3. report the nursing assistant to the nursing manager for poor patient care.

    4. write an incident report and give a copy to the nursing assistant and nurse manager.

99. An 8-year-old girl is scheduled for a tonsillectomy. The child arrives at the surgery center with her legal guardian. The nurse should

   1. inform the legal guardian the surgeon will be in soon with the consent form to sign.

   2. ask the legal guardian if one of the parents can come in to sign the consent.

   3. check the client's chart to see who signed consent forms in the past.

   4. tell the surgeon that no parent is present to sign the consent.

100. The **priority** nursing intervention for a client with sickle cell crisis is to

   1. administer pain medication.

   2. administer packed RBC.

   3. administer oxygen.

   4. administer IV fluids.

101. Which of the following statements regarding proper use of a cane is correct?

   1. When standing, the cane should reach a height even with the natural waist.

   2. When walking downstairs, the cane should be placed down on the step first, followed by the injured leg, and then the good leg.

   3. The elbow should be straight when holding the cane.

   4. The cane should be held in the hand of the same side that needs support.

102. The charge nurse notices another nurse on the floor reading the chart of a client who is not under her care. When confronted, the nurse says, "This client is my neighbor, and I'm just concerned about him." Which is the correct response by the charge nurse?

   1. "As long as you don't share any information, it's okay."

   2. "Why don't you just let his nurse update you on his status?"

   3. "You should not be reading the client's chart if you are not involved in his care."

   4. "Go with the doctor when he rounds on this client so you will be able to answer the family's questions."

103. The nurse is precepting a student nurse in the ICU. Which statement regarding student nurses is correct? **Select all that apply.**

   1. The student nurse can administer client medications on his own.

   2. The student nurse may assist other nurses in turning and repositioning their clients.

   3. The student nurse may read his assigned client's chart and access lab results to determine interventions.

   4. The student nurse should take all opportunities to provide direct client care under the preceptor's oversight.

   5. The student nurse may report details of the assigned client's case to others in the post-clinical conference as long as client privacy is maintained.

104. The nurse is caring for a 42-year-old client who has a *do not resuscitate* (DNR) order on the chart. The client tells the nurse, "I've changed my mind about the DNR. I would like to cancel that and be given whatever care is needed to keep me alive." Which response by the nurse is correct?

    1. "I will notify your health care provider right away."

    2. "I'm glad to hear this. You shouldn't be a DNR at your age."

    3. "Let me call your family and tell them you have changed your mind."

    4. "You cannot change a DNR once it's on your chart. It is a legal document."

105. The nurse is developing a care plan for a client with hepatitis A. The nurse knows that the **primary** routes of transmission of this hepatitis virus are which of the following? **Select all that apply.**

    1. sputum

    2. blood

    3. feces

    4. contaminated food

106. The nurse is preparing to test a client who has the herpes virus. Which of the following tests should the nurse perform?

    1. Rinne test

    2. stress test

    3. Tzanck test

    4. patch test

107. The nurse is preparing to administer a unit of red blood cells (RBCs) to an anemic client. From starting the infusion (puncturing the blood pack) to completion, infusion of the pack should occur within which time period?

    1. 8 hours

    2. 6 hours

    3. 4 hours

    4. 2 hours

108. The nurse is caring for a client who suffers from post-traumatic stress disorder (PTSD) following the loss of her husband and children in an automobile accident while they were on a family vacation. Which interventions by the nurse are appropriate for this client? **Select all that apply.**

    1. assist the client to develop adequate coping techniques

    2. encourage the client to try different relaxation techniques

    3. listen to the client in a supportive and nonjudgmental manner

    4. allow the client a safe and secure environment to express her feelings

    5. encourage the client to avoid going out in public until she has worked through all the stages of grief

109. The nurse is working with a client in the psychiatric unit. The client has memory gaps, which she fills in with detailed fantasies that she believes to be true. The nurse understands that the client is exhibiting which type of abnormal thought process?

_____

110. The nurse is caring for a client with bipolar disorder. The client has been manipulating some of the staff and other clients in order to get her way. Which actions by the nurse are appropriate in managing this client? **Select all that apply.**

  1. giving support when the client exhibits positive behaviors

  2. setting clear limits and communicating expected behaviors

  3. role playing with the client to demonstrate appropriate behaviors

  4. treating the client more like a friend in order to show respect for her as a person

  5. giving the client small gifts, such as extra dessert, in order to encourage appropriate behavior

In questions 111 – 114, identify each intramuscular injection site on the diagram using the corresponding letter.

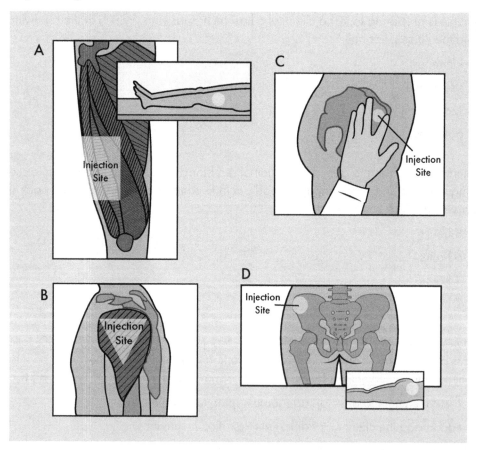

111. deltoid muscle

112. ventrogluteal muscle

113. dorsogluteal muscle

114. vastus lateralis muscle

115. The nurse is caring for an obese client who had a diagnostic laparotomy with midline incision one week ago. The client just called the nurse to report a "popping" sensation in the abdomen. Upon assessment, the nurse notes loops of bowel protruding through the incision. Which is the **priority** nursing action for this client?

    1. monitor vital signs

    2. stay with the client

    3. call for help and have the surgeon notified

    4. place the client in low Fowler's with the knees bent

116. A client has orders for zoledronic acid (Reclast). Which lab value finding would prompt the nurse to notify the prescriber?

    1. ferritin level of 78 ng/mL

    2. magnesium level of 2.3 mEq/dL

    3. creatinine clearance of 29 mL/min

    4. platelet count of 135,000 cells/mcL

117. A client with a T5 spinal cord injury suddenly begins sweating profusely in the face and neck. Vital signs reveal sudden bradycardia and significant increase in blood pressure. Which is the **priority** nursing action?

    1. administer nitrate or nifedipine

    2. check the client for fecal impaction

    3. check the client for bladder distention

    4. place the bed in the high Fowler's position

118. The nurse is caring for a client with stage 3 moderate chronic kidney disease. Which laboratory value would be expected for this client?

    1. GFR of 92 mL/min

    2. GFR of 63 mL/min

    3. GFR of 39 mL/min

    4. GFR of 16mL/min

119. The nurse is auscultating a client's breath sounds. Low-pitched grating and rubbing are noted on inhalation and exhalation. What will the nurse chart under assessment findings?

    1. ronchi

    2. stridor

    3. friction rub

    4. fine crackles

120. Which assessment finding would the nurse expect in a client with long-term venous insufficiency with the presence of a venous ulcer?

   1. decreased or absent pedal pulses with cool or cold foot
   2. the presence of stasis ulcers over the medial malleolus
   3. skin atrophy and pallor with elevation of the affected leg
   4. decreased circumference in the affected leg due to venous constriction

121. The nurse is caring for a client whose native language is Korean; he speaks only a few words of English. The health care provider has determined that the client needs to undergo a coronary artery bypass graft. Which is the appropriate action by the nurse?

   1. ask the client's spouse to give consent for the procedure before explaining it to the client
   2. ask the client's spouse to translate for the health care provider and explain the procedure to the client
   3. communicate with the client by showing pictures of the intended surgery while a family member translates
   4. request a licensed translator to interpret for the health care provider and client during the conversation

122. The nurse is admitting a new client to the medical unit. When asked about advance directives, the client says, "I'm not really sure what that is, but I trust my doctor to do whatever he thinks I need." Which is the correct action by the nurse?

   1. tell the client not to worry about it, because the client can always add the advance directives later
   2. tell the client that she can pay her lawyer to draw one up and have a copy sent to the hospital
   3. explain what advance directives are and how they benefit the client, and offer to give the client a copy so she can read it and ask questions
   4. omit further discussion about advance directives, and chart that the client does not have one and refuses further information

123. A nurse on the orthopedics floor is asked by another nurse to witness her waste 1 mg of morphine. The nurse draws the full 2 mg dose of morphine into the syringe and tells the first nurse, "This client does not get enough pain relief with 1 mg of morphine, so I just go ahead and give 2 mg to keep him comfortable because the doctor won't change the dose." Which is the correct action by the first nurse?

   1. tell the other nurse to call the doctor back and request an increase in the dosage
   2. refuse to sign off on the waste and report the incident to the charge nurse or unit manager
   3. sign off the waste, and suggest that the nurse give it over two separate doses 30 minutes apart
   4. sign off the waste, but tell the nurse to give it slowly to be sure that the client can tolerate the dose

124. The nurse has just administered an IM injection to a client. In which of the following ways should the nurse dispose of the needle?

   1. re-cap the needle and discard it in the nearest puncture-resistant container
   2. break the needle and discard it in the nearest puncture-resistant container
   3. discard the needle in a puncture-resistant container in the central medication area
   4. discard the needle in a puncture-resistant container in the client's room

125. A nurse is preparing to lift a client up in bed. Which of the following should the nurse do to help avoid injuring his back?

   1. keep his feet together
   2. instruct the client to not help
   3. tighten his stomach and leg muscles
   4. elevate the head of the bed to about 30 degrees, if the client can tolerate it

126. An elderly adult has been admitted with a diagnosis of hypertension with a history of dementia. Which of the following nursing diagnoses has the **highest priority** for this client?

   1. ineffective coping
   2. activity intolerance
   3. ineffective tissue perfusion
   4. risk for injury

127. The nurse is caring for a client who has verbalized the desire to commit suicide. He has a detailed, concrete plan in place. The nurse places the client on suicide precautions, which include assigning the client a 24-hour sitter. The client becomes angry and refuses the sitter. Which action by the nurse is the **most** appropriate?

   1. place the client in soft wrist restraints
   2. have security sit outside the client's door
   3. assign a sitter despite the client's refusal
   4. allow the client to leave against medical advice (AMA)
   5. tell the client that a friend can come sit with him instead

128. The clinic nurse is seeing a client who suffers from caregiver strain due to caring for her elderly parents who have dementia and live with her. Which action by the nurse during the assessment is **most** important?

   1. ask the client about her support systems
   2. ask the client what she does for relaxation
   3. ask if her parents' insurance covers adult day care for them
   4. offer to give her a list of nursing homes to care for her parents

129. The nurse plans on administering a medication using the Z-track intramuscular technique. The nurse knows the following steps are required during the procedure. **Select all that apply.**

   1. Draw 0.2 – 0.5 cc of air after aspirating the prescribed medication.
   2. Use the vastus lateralis muscle.
   3. Replace the needle used for medication withdrawal with a new one prior to injection.
   4. Insert the needle at 45-degree angle.

130. The nurse is preparing to administer regular and NPH insulin to the client. He knows to do which of the following steps?

   1. insert air first into the regular insulin
   2. insert air first into the NPH insulin
   3. draw up regular insulin first
   4. draw up NPH insulin first

131. The nurse is preparing to administer the first dose of intravenous immunoglobulin (IVIG) to a 50-year-old female adult client admitted to the hospital with Guillain-Barre syndrome. Which nursing intervention is appropriate regarding administration?

   1. administer IVIG transfusion at a constant rate
   2. monitor vital signs within 15 minutes prior to administration and within 30 minutes after starting the infusion
   3. administer IVIG at room temperature
   4. should chills occur during the infusion, continue the infusion and provide the client with a blanket

132. The unit nurse is teaching a nursing student about increased intracranial pressure (ICP). The nurse knows the teaching was effective if the student nurse makes which statement?

   1. "Altered level of consciousness is a late sign of increased ICP."
   2. "Elevated temperature is the earliest indication of increased ICP."
   3. "Late signs of increased ICP include narrowed pulse pressure and a lowered heart rate."
   4. "Late signs of increased ICP include increased systolic blood pressure and a widened pulse pressure."

133. The nurse reviews the chart of a client diagnosed with nephrotic syndrome and expects to note which finding associated with this diagnosis?

   1. lipiduria
   2. hypolipidemia
   3. hyperalbuminemia
   4. decreased coagulation

134. The nurse is caring for a client with a permanent tracheostomy who is able to eat. Which is the correct action by the nurse in managing this tube?

1. if the tube must be capped, place the cap before deflating the cuff
2. inflate the cuff and remove the inner cannula before capping the tube
3. inflate the cuff (if the tube is not capped) for meals and 1 hour afterward to prevent aspiration
4. deflate the cuff (if the tube is not capped) for meals and 1 hour afterward to prevent aspiration

135. The nurse is supervising a student nurse on the oncology unit who is providing care for a client with neutropenic precautions. Which action by the student nurse requires intervention by the supervising nurse?

1. Vital signs, including temperature, are monitored every 4 hours.
2. The student nurse inspects the client's mouth at least every 8 hours.
3. The student nurse delivers a potted plant to the room sent by the client's family.
4. The student nurse washes her hands before performing client care or touching client belongings.

136. The nurse is caring for a client who is 12 weeks pregnant and presented with the following symptoms: mild uterine cramping with spotting of blood. The cervical os is closed upon examination. How should the nurse chart the findings?

1. missed miscarriage
2. complete miscarriage
3. inevitable miscarriage
4. threatened miscarriage

137. The nurse is caring for a client who lives below the poverty level. While providing discharge teaching, the nurse notes that the client has received a prescription for warfarin (Coumadin) and will need to return to the clinic for regular lab work. Which of the following is **most** appropriate for the nurse to ask the client?

1. "Which pharmacy do you use for your medications?"
2. "Do you know when your next appointment is for lab work?"
3. "Do you have a car or someone to take you to get your lab work done?"
4. "Can you tell me the side effects that you should report to your physician?"

138. The nurse is delegating tasks to an experienced, unlicensed assistive personnel (UAP). Which of the following clients should the nurse delegate to the UAP?

1. a client with multiple pressure ulcers requiring daily dressing changes
2. a client with a permanent tracheostomy requiring daily tracheostomy care
3. a client recovering from pneumonia with orders to ambulate in the hall BID
4. a client who just received pain medication and needs to have her pain level assessed in 30 minutes

139. The nurse has received report on the day's assigned clients. Which of the following clients should the nurse see **first**?

   1. a client complaining of nausea and vomiting after eating breakfast
   2. a client complaining of itching and burning at the IV site while receiving normal saline
   3. a client who is post-op day 1 from a hernia repair with a pain level of 6 on a scale of 1 – 10
   4. a client who has been given the first dose of an antibiotic and complains of tingling in and around the mouth

140. The nurse is working on a postsurgical floor with an LPN. A new client has just arrived. Which task is appropriate for the nurse to delegate to the LPN?

   1. taking the client's vital signs
   2. flushing the client's PICC line with heparin
   3. administering morphine 2 mg IV push for pain
   4. starting total parenteral nutrition (TPN) to the client's PICC line

141. The nursing assistant finds a client on the floor. Once the client is safe, which of the following should the nurse do next?

   1. document the event in the client's medical record only
   2. document the event in the client's medical record and file an incident report
   3. document the event in the client's medical record and have the nursing assistant file an incident report
   4. have the nursing assistant file an incident report

142. The nurse is administering afternoon medications, which include an antihypertensive med and aspirin for pain relief. Which of the following should the nurse do first before administering the medications?

   1. match the client's date of birth and name on his wristband with the same information on the medication order
   2. ask the client his name and date of birth
   3. ask the client to confirm the medication ordered and compare this with the medication order
   4. match the client's name and room number with the medication order

143. The physician orders an MRI of the spine with infusion for an adult female. Which of the following findings in the client's history should the nurse report to the physician?

   1. allergy to shellfish
   2. congestive heart failure (CHF)
   3. chronic cystitis
   4. metformin administered daily

144. The nurse is preparing a client with acquired immunodeficiency syndrome (AIDS) for discharge home. Which of the following statements by the client indicates a need for further teaching by the nurse?

   1. "I do not need to limit my time in public places."
   2. "I may share food from serving dishes with others at a restaurant."
   3. "I may use public restrooms."
   4. "I may donate blood."

145. The nurse is visiting a client at home who is using a transdermal fentanyl patch. The nurse knows the client requires additional education based on which of the following statements?

   1. "I apply the patch when I have breakthrough pain."
   2. "I store my patches in a private location away from my grandchildren's reach."
   3. "I remove my old patch before applying a new one."
   4. "I enjoy orange juice for breakfast."

146. The nurse is observing a student nurse administer an otic medication to an adult client. The nurse knows the student nurse requires additional teaching when which of the following actions is observed?

   1. positions client in prone position
   2. follows the six rights of medication administration
   3. applies nonsterile gloves
   4. pulls the pinna back and up

147. The nurse is assessing the reflexes of a full-term newborn infant. Which of the following is true regarding newborn reflexes?

   1. The Babinski reflex disappears after 1 year of age.
   2. Complete fencing response disappears by 2 months.
   3. The stepping or "walking" reflex is present until 3 – 4 months.
   4. The Moro reflex is present at birth and disappears by 6 months.

148. The nurse is caring for a client with compartment syndrome. The client's husband asks what causes the condition. Which of the following will the nurse share with the client's husband? **Select all that apply.**

   1. It can be present in severe burns.
   2. Most cases are caused by fractures.
   3. It can be caused by severe infiltration of IV fluids.
   4. It occurs with failure to ambulate after surgical procedures.
   5. Untreated high blood sugars are a contributing factor in some cases.

149. A client is prescribed heparin 5,000 units subcutaneously every 12 hours for deep vein thrombosis prophylaxis. The pharmacy dispenses a vial containing 10,000 units/1 ml. How many milliliter(s) of heparin should the nurse administer?

_____

150. The nurse is caring for a client who has just returned from surgery for an ascending colostomy. The nurse plans to include reinforcement teaching for the client and spouse. Which statements should the nurse include in the teaching? **Select all that apply.**

   1. The colostomy will begin functioning within 24 hours.

   2. A large amount of bleeding may be present at the stoma site.

   3. The first stools will be liquid and will gradually become more formed.

   4. A healthy stoma is reddish-pink and moist and protrudes about 2 cm from the abdominal wall.

PRACTICE TEST FOUR ANSWER KEY

1. Number 4 is correct.

    Rationale: Pulmonary embolism is a possible risk of IV therapy. It is caused by air accidentally being pushed into a vein via an IV. If the air embolism travels to the lung, a dangerous pulmonary embolism can occur. Other signs and symptoms can include hypotension, confusion, stroke, and heart failure. The nurse would be alerted to the most likely cause based on her recent intervention. Septic shock and pneumothorax both have additional symptoms that develop over a longer period of time. While an allergic reaction to the medication given is possible, chest pain would be unlikely.

2. Number 1 is correct.

    Rationale: Tunneling occurs when a wound spreads and travels to another break or opening in the skin. Undermining is less extensive than tunneling and would not create as large an area to the decubitis ulcer. Dehiscence is the separation and disruption of previously joined wound edges. In evisceration, wound edges separate and the intestines protrude.

3. Numbers 2, 3, 4, and 5 are correct.

    Rationale: A client with measles should be placed under airborne precautions. The client should wear a mask when in the hallway and should enter through a separate entrance of the hospital to avoid the waiting/reception area. Any staff entering the client's room should wear a fit-tested N-95 respirator mask—put on prior to entering the room and removed upon exiting the room. In addition, any client under airborne precautions (tuberculosis, measles, varicella, and disseminated herpes zoster) should ideally be placed in an airborne infection isolation room.

4. Number 1 is correct.

    Rationale: Clients who take MAOI drugs should avoid foods with tyramine, which could trigger a hypertensive crisis. Tyramine can be found in aged cheeses, fermented meats, alcoholic beverages, pickled foods, chocolate, fava beans, and sauerkraut. These clients may still eat some dairy products. Foods with vitamin K might be avoided by clients prescribed blood thinners. Dietary fiber is important for healthy digestion and including it in the diet should be encouraged.

5. Number 3 is correct.

    Rationale: Clients undergoing brachytherapy emit a small amount of radiation. Brachytherapy is an internal radiation treatment that is inserted directly into a tumor and therefore limits exposure to healthy surrounding tissues. Visitors should stay at least 6 feet away and should avoid direct contact with the client, but they need not wear personal protective equipment. Short periods of time with the client are unlikely to be harmful because the sources of radiation used have a short half-life. Items the client uses in the room and the client's body fluids are not radioactive, and once the implant is removed, the client no longer emits radiation.

6. Number 2 is correct.

    Rationale: The nursing priority is to obtain and determine baseline vitals, as well as to assess for abnormalities in blood pressure, respiration, and pulse rate, which may be signs of the body compensating for blood loss. The nurse can then prioritize care by talking with the client while taking vitals and ask about accident recall, assess the abdomen, and provide pain medication after assessing pain.

7. Number 1 is correct.

    Rationale: Levothyroxine enhances the effects of warfarin, which could place patients at a higher risk for bleeding. A nurse should anticipate that the physician would evaluate the clotting time of the client more frequently and adjust the medication accordingly.

8. Number 1 is correct.

Rationale: Clients who have undergone a mastectomy should keep the affected arm slightly elevated in order to promote drainage and not impede circulation. A pillow generally allows the hand to remain higher than the elbow, which assists with lymphatic fluid drainage. The arm position in correlation with the heart is not important.

9. Number 3 is correct.

Rationale: The nurse manager should first speak with the nurse privately to hear her explanation regarding her recent tardiness, and to review the consequences of this behavior in accordance with the agency attendance policy. Then the nurse manager should make a note in the employee's file stating what was discussed during the meeting. If the behavior does not improve, the nurse manager should follow the chain of command.

10. Number 4 is correct.

Rationale: The nurse should fully assess the client to determine the source and cause of the pain before attempting any interventions. Based on the findings of the assessment, he would then provide pain medication and contact the physician. The nurse could work with the client at a later time when the patient is comfortable to review guided imagery technique.

11. Number 3 is correct.

Rationale: It is the surgeon's responsibility to have the consent form signed, and it must be signed before she performs this procedure (protocol differs for emergency situations). If the form has not been signed, the nurse should go up the chain of command and report this to the nurse manager. The nurse manager would work with the surgeon and facility policy to determine the next course of action.

12. Number 4 is correct.

Rationale: The nurse should practice therapeutic communication by exploring the situation, allowing the client to verbalize her thoughts and feelings openly. The first three choices are not open-ended questions; some are judgmental and do not allow the client to express her feelings.

13. Number 2 is correct.

Rationale: Librium is commonly used with clients experiencing acute alcohol withdrawal to manage anxiety and withdrawal symptoms. Naloxone hydrochloride is given to reverse the effects of opioids. Disulfiram would be provided post acutely to help with ongoing alcohol abuse. Propofol is a sedative that is used during surgical anesthesia.

14. Number 2 is correct.

Rationale: Patients on neutropenic precautions have a low white blood cell count and require preventative measures to avoid potential infections. A daily bath or shower, along with wearing fresh, clean clothing, is recommended for neutropenic clients. Patients should avoid crowds or people exhibiting signs of illness. Tasks such as gardening or playing in the dirt should be avoided. The patient should not clean up after pets, but petting his dog or cat and then performing hand hygiene is appropriate.

15. Number 2 and 3 are correct.

Rationale: The figure eight technique for bandaging helps to reduce edema by promoting venous return; it also minimizes discomfort. The bandage should be worn at all times, but should be removed completely and rewrapped several times each day. Proper bandaging ensures that the residual limb is shaped and molded. Activity is important in the postoperative period for prevention of blood clots and exposure to air is not harmful.

16. Number 1 is correct.

Rationale: Patients with chronic kidney disease (CKD) can experience a buildup of magnesium. Magnesium is excreted by the kidneys, and decreased kidney function may lead to a dangerous level of magnesium in the body. Magnesium-based antacids, like Mylanta, should be avoided by CKD patients. Iron may be prescribed for anemia. Baby aspirin may be appropriate for other health conditions. Taking fish oil does not have any contraindications in patients with CKD.

17. Number 2 is correct.

Rationale: Confronting is a type of conflict management in which the issue is immediately addressed and resolved. Competing conflict management is when one's own needs are advocated over another's. In accommodating, another party's needs are prioritized. Avoidance involves failing to discuss the topic in question and letting concerns go unaddressed.

18. Number 4 is correct.

Rationale: Hemarthrosis is a condition of bleeding in the joint spaces. It is a complication of hemophilia. Signs and symptoms may include redness or warmth in the joints, joint swelling or pain, and limited movement. Jaundice and increased heart rate are not symptoms of hemophilia. Popping sounds in the joints are not signs of hemarthrosis.

19. Number 3 is correct.

Rationale: Clients who follow a dysphagia-pureed diet have difficulty swallowing and need foods that have been pureed or blended until smooth. Custard would be an acceptable choice. The other food choices would be too difficult to swallow and would put the client at risk for choking.

20. Number 3 is correct.

Rationale: A baby with microcephaly typically has a head circumference in the lowest tenth percentile. Other signs and symptoms may include facial distortions, dwarfism, and seizures. Hyperactivity, not hypoactivity, is a symptom of microcephaly. Depressed fontanelles could indicate a nutritional problem or dehydration in the infant. Absent fontanelles might be a sign of other medical conditions, such as craniosynostosis.

21. Number 2 is correct.

Rationale: At 6 months, most babies make new sounds. They might recognize their name. By 9 months, they string sounds together that do not represent words. Most babies began to speak their first word by 12 months of age, for example, "mama" and "dada." By 18 months of age, babies should be able to say several single words.

22. Number 2 is correct.

Solution:

1.25 L NS × 1,000 = 1,250 mL	Convert the amount of saline in liters to milliliters.
1,250 mL/10 hrs = **125 mL/hr**	To find the flow rate in milliliters per hour, divide the volume in milliliters by the time in hours.

23. Number 1 is correct.

Rationale: Since the client is showing hyperactive and manic behavior, he should be placed in a quiet environment and behavioral limits should be set. Ignoring the client is not therapeutic. If the client is agitated and aggressive, regular meals with other clients might place them in danger. Unless the client is threatening to harm himself, one-on-one observation is not the first step to take. If the aggressive behavior escalates, additional measures for client safety would be considered.

24. Number 4 is correct.

Rationale: Signs of imminent death include fixed and dilated pupils, weak and rapid pulse, shallow respirations, and atonic muscles. Clenched muscles could be a sign that the patient is in pain and might need additional assessment. Steady, deep respirations and a slower pulse rate are a sign of a stable patient.

25. Number 4 is correct.

Rationale: Signs of Type 1 diabetes include polyphagia (increased hunger), polydipsia (increased thirst), and polyuria (increased urine output). While some of the answers in responses 1, 2, and 3 are correct, they are not all indicative of the specific signs of type 1 diabetes. Swollen lymph nodes, muscle weakness, bloating, ringing in the ears, and difficulty sleeping are associated with other medical diagnoses.

26. Number 3 is correct.

Rationale: *Pink puffer* is used to describe a client with emphysema based on the symptoms, which include increased CO_2 retention, minimal cyanosis, pursed-lip breathing, dyspnea anxiety, and a barrel chest. *Blue bloater* is used to describe a client with chronic bronchitis, based on the symptoms of dusky color due to cyanosis, recurrent cough with sputum, hypoxia, increased respiratory rate, and respiratory acidosis. Asthma and COPD do not carry the same symptoms.

27. Number 4 is correct.

Rationale: Parathyroid hormone aids in the regulation of calcium and phosphorus levels in the body. The other hormones do not have a critical relation to calcium excretion.

28. Number 4 is correct.

Rationale: Calcium gluconate is given as an antidote to counteract magnesium sulfate toxicity. Magnesium sulfate toxicity is dangerous because it can cause respiratory depression and hypotension. Chlordiazepoxide (Librium) is used to assist patients in alcohol withdrawal. Naloxone (Narcan) is used in case of an opioid overdose. Vitamin K would be given to increase clotting.

29. Number 1 is correct.

Rationale: M0 refers to no distant metastasis being present; the cancer has not spread to the lymph nodes or other parts of the body. M1-4 indicates ascending degrees of metastatic involvement, including distant nodes. MX means metastasis cannot be evaluated.

30. Number 3 is correct.

Rationale: The priority nursing intervention is to flush the eye with normal saline for at least 10 minutes. After or during the irrigation, the nurse would address the chemical that was splashed into the eye and would potentially cover the eye with a sterile cloth. After treatment, vision testing would be appropriate.

31. Number 4 is correct.

Rationale: If a client experiences pain during passive ROM exercises, the nurse should stop and not force the joint movement; the client could become injured. The nurse would then assess the client's pain level and document. The physician could then make a decision on the future plan of care and whether modifications, medications, or a referral to physical therapy is appropriate.

32. Number 2 is correct.

Rationale: Naturally acquired active immunity occurs when a person is exposed to a pathogen and develops an immune response. This immune response will lead to immunological memory, thus protecting the person from illness if exposed to the same pathogen again in the future. Naturally acquired passive immunity occurs when antibodies are passed from an immune mother to her baby through breast milk or the placenta. Artificially acquired immunity is immunity acquired from vaccine sources.

33. Number 3 is correct.

Rationale: Neglected children may have atypical growth patterns or delays in physical development. By assessing height and weight, the nurse can determine if the children are growing as expected, or if there is a potential clue to abuse or neglect. Bruises on knees and elbows are common injuries in children and not necessarily signs of neglect. Blood pressure and pulse would not be good indicators of neglect if there are no acute injuries. A Snellen chart is used to determine visual acuity and would not be an indicator of neglect.

34. Answer: 1.25 tablets

Solution:

125 mcg/1000 = 0.125 mg levothyroxine (Synthroid)	Convert micrograms to milligrams.
0.125 mg/0.1 mg × 1 tablet **= 1.25 tablets**	Calculate and solve.

35. Number 3 is correct.

Rationale: Abdominal cramping and discomfort are possible if the enema flow rate is too rapid. The nurse should briefly stop the flow and restart at a slower rate. Squeezing the enema bag to increase the flow rate exacerbates client discomfort and could result in reflux or vomiting. A PRN pain medication should not be necessary at the proper flow rate.

36. Number 2 is correct.

Rationale: During the planning stage, the nurse should develop a care plan of interventions based on the identified goals. The steps of the nursing process are assessing (answer 1), analyzing, planning, implementing (answer 4), and evaluating (answer 3).

37. Number 4 is correct.

Rationale: Foods high in B12 include eggs, lamb, beef, shellfish, some cheeses, seafood, and milk. While the other foods need not be avoided, diet should focus on consuming B12–rich foods.

38. Number 3 is correct.

Rationale: Oral potassium supplements can cause GI distress; they should be dissolved in a full glass of water or juice and taken close to mealtime, though the time of day does not matter. Taking them without food can cause additional GI distress. Potassium can be stored at room temperature.

39. Number 3 is correct.

Rationale: Decerebrate posturing includes arching back the head, extending and internally rotating the arms and legs, extending the elbows, pronating the wrists, and clenching the teeth. Decerebrate posturing is indicative of an injury to the midbrain. Frontal lobe injuries usually affect emotions, while cerebral hemisphere injuries can affect problem-solving, memory, and coordination. Injuries to the spinal cord may result in paralysis.

40. Number 3 is correct.

Rationale: The most common cause of mitral valve stenosis is rheumatic heart disease caused by a past history of rheumatic fever. Infective endocarditis is another, less common, cause of mitral valve stenosis. Right-sided heart failure, hypercholesterolemia, and viral meningitis do not cause mitral valve stenosis.

41. Numbers 3, 4, and 5 are correct.

Rationale: Diabetes mellitus, obesity, and hypertension are all risk factors for developing glaucoma. Other risk factors include cardiovascular disease, uveitis, long-term use of steroids, family history, and being of East Asian or African descent. Asthma and pernicious anemia are not associated with risk factors for glaucoma.

42. Number 1 is correct.

Rationale: The normal electrolyte level of chloride is between 97 and 107 mEq/L. Hyperchloremia may be caused by kidney disease, diarrhea, and diuretic use. The other levels listed are within normal ranges.

43. Number 2 is correct.

Rationale: A client on mechanical ventilation may experience secretions that require suctioning. The nurse should watch for signs that the client needs to be suctioned, such as visible secretions, adventitious breath sounds, and restlessness. Increasing oxygen and lowering the head of the bed are not therapeutic interventions for the symptoms that the patient is experiencing. The rapid response team is not indicated unless the patient is in distress.

44. Number 4 is correct.

Rationale: An elevated temperature may indicate an underlying infection or illness, and the nurse should speak with the health care provider before continuing with the RBC transfusion.

45. Number 2 is correct.

Rationale: The best practice to verifying NG tube placement is by aspirating gastric contents and checking the pH. If the pH is above 5.5, the placement is assumed to be correct and the nurse can continue with the feeding. While an X-ray is an accurate determination of testing NG tube placement, checking before each feeding is not feasible for practice. An air bolus can be used, but is not as effective as pH paper. Auscultation of bowel sounds is not effective as the client will have bowel sounds despite placement of the tube.

46. Number 3 is correct.

Rationale: The nurse will need to draw blood to monitor peak and trough levels of vancomycin in order to reduce the chance of side effects caused by toxicity. A low-residue diet and assistance with ambulation are unrelated to the vancomycin administration. Cardiac arrhythmia can be caused by antibiotics, but is not a common reaction.

47. Number 1 is correct.

Rationale: A client with low platelet counts (thrombocytopenia) is at risk for bleeding, and the nurse should monitor for bruising, nosebleeds, blood in the urine or stool, and petechia. Neutropenic precautions would be utilized if the client had a low white blood cell count. Visiting hours do not need to be restricted. While adequate iron should be encouraged, it is not the best nursing intervention.

48. Number 4 is correct.

Rationale: Wilm's tumor is a malignant tumor of the kidney in children. Signs and symptoms include large abdominal mass, blood in the urine, hypertension, fatigue, and nausea/vomiting. The other symptoms indicated are not known symptoms of a Wilm's tumor.

49. Number 4 is correct.

Rationale: Clients on mechanical ventilation are susceptible to infection because bacteria and viruses can enter the endotracheal tube and infect the lower respiratory system. An increased temperature could indicate a possible infection and should be reported immediately. The other vital signs are findings that would be considered within normal limits.

50. Number 2 is correct.

Rationale: The client will need to lie on his right side for several hours after the liver biopsy to reduce the chance of bleeding. The other positions increase the risk for bleeding.

51. Number 2 is correct.

Rationale: Tissue plasma activator (tPA) is used to dissolve clots in certain clients who have experienced a stroke or myocardial infarction. Blood in the stool or any other sign of bleeding (LOC changes, hypotension, and tachycardia) may indicate a hemorrhage and is an emergency situation. The other choices do not indicate an emergency situation that would be caused by the administration of tPA.

52. Number 4 is correct.

Rationale: As a mandated reporter, the nurse has a legal responsibility to report any suspicions of child abuse to the authorities. The nurse would then document his actions in the child's chart. Legal authorities and social services would intervene to assess the child and interview the caregiver.

53. Number 2 is correct.

Rationale: The float nurse should adhere to the chain of command and immediately report the nurse to the nursing supervisor. The nursing supervisor will then work with human resources to take steps to discipline the nurse according to hospital policy and the state board of nursing.

54. Number 3 is correct.

Rationale: The client should be placed in the Trendelenburg position with the head turned left. This position will reduce the risk of an air embolism and allow the physician best access to the vein. High-Fowler's places the patient at 90 degrees, Trendelenburg places the patient with the head lower than the body, and supine places the patient flat on the bed. These positions do not optimize central venous placement.

55. Number 3 is correct.

Rationale: Therapeutic hypothermia is used after an MI as a method to reduce injury to the brain. Hypothermia slows the brain's oxygen demand by lowering metabolism, and it reduces the production of free radicals and neurotransmitters.

56. Number 1 is correct.

Rationale: A newborn exposed to cocaine in utero may be irritable, have difficulty sleeping/feeding, have a shrill cry, and be underweight. Most infants exposed to cocaine in utero respond well to additional soothing and swaddling in the first week after birth and do not need pharmacological support. Since cocaine can be found in breast milk, the medical team will need to determine the risk versus benefit of breastfeeding.

57. Number 2 is correct.

Rationale: Intracranial pressure can increase with suctioning or repositioning the client, and a temporary jump in ICP is expected in these situations. If the ICP returns to normal, no further intervention is needed, and the nurse should chart the findings and continue to monitor the client.

58. Number 3 is correct.

Rationale: Ergonomics refers to how factors in the working environment can reduce the risk of musculoskeletal injuries and to improve workers' safety and comfort. Occupational therapy is a discipline that involves working with people with impairments to help them maintain or recover meaningful activities. Accident analysis looks at how an accident or injury took place. Body mechanics refers to how people carry out tasks such as sitting, lifting, and carrying,

59. Number 4 is correct.

Rationale: In an emergency situation, where there is no time to cross-match blood type, a client can be given a blood type O negative transfusion. O negative is considered a universal blood type and can be received by anyone. It is optimal for emergency situations. The other blood types could cause an ABO incompatibility reaction.

60. Number 3 is correct.

Rationale: Tolerance refers to the need for more of the drug over time to reach the same effect; this term best describes the client's experience. Addiction refers to the physiological and physical craving of a drug or substance. Dependence is when the body depends on the drug after repeated use, and if the drug is removed (withdrawal), physical side effects can occur.

61. Number 4 is correct.

Rationale: Insulin lipodystrophy can occur if insulin is injected repeatedly into the same area of skin. This leads to formations of fat deposit that can cause unpredictable absorption of insulin at the site. While localized edema can occur at the injection site, this is not harmful and will quickly resolve. Tissue scarring will not occur in fatty tissue. Insulin resistance is a precursor to the development of type 2 diabetes.

62. Number 2 is correct.

Rationale: In most healthy people with normal immune systems, an induration of 15 mm or greater is considered a positive reading. However, a 10 mm area of induration is considered positive for children under 4 years of age, IV drug users, travelers recently arrived from high-risk areas, and those exposed to mycobacterium at work. A negative skin test would have not induration or would have a small area (less than 5 mm in individuals who do not have a compromised immune system). TB tests must be read between 48 and 72 hours after taken for accurate results.

63. Number 1 is correct.

Rationale: A deficiency in clotting factor VIII would lead to a diagnosis of hemophilia A, a disorder that causes increased bleeding due to a lack of an essential blood clotting protein. It is more commonly seen in males and is caused by an X-linked recessive trait. Pernicious anemia usually occurs later in life and is a type of anemia that can be corrected with B12. Sickle cell and Tay-Sachs are also inherited diseases, but manifest with different symptoms from hemophilia.

64. Number 3 is correct.

Solution:

2,000 units × 1 mL/5,000 units = 0.4 mL	Find the milliliters of heparin 5,000 units/mL the client will require per dose.
0.4ml × 3 doses/day **= 1.2 mL/ day**	Multiply the volume of the dose by 3 to find the amount administered in 24 hours. (Administering a dose every 8 hours equals three doses in a 24-hour period.)

65. Number 1 is correct.

Rationale: A tumor in the cerebellum may affect the client's coordination, balance, and motor control. An occipital lobe tumor might cause vision disturbances. A temporal lobe tumor might cause problems with decreased levels of consciousness or impaired decision-making.

66. Number 3 is correct.

Rationale: Premenopausal women should conduct self-breast exams immediately after their menstrual cycle ends because this is the time the breasts are least tender. If a woman is prone to fibrocystic breast changes, they will be less pronounced immediately after menses.

67. Number 4 is correct.

Rationale: Hand washing is the most effective intervention for breaking the chain of infection. While barriers such as a gown, gloves, and mask might help in preventing transmission, hand washing is the first and most effective step to medical asepsis. Unless the patient is compromised or undergoing certain procedures, antibiotics are generally not indicated and may cause long-term resistance to antibiotics. A private room is not always feasible and hand washing is still indicated.

68. Number 2 is correct.

Rationale: Signs and symptoms of bulimia nervosa include peptic ulcers, constipation, low self-esteem, irregular menstrual cycle, and dental erosion. Gastric reflux, electrolyte imbalance, swollen salivary glands, and depression may also be seen. A client with bulimia nervosa may have a normal weight, but can also be underweight or overweight depending on diet, exercise, and binge habits.

69. Number 1 is correct.

Rationale: Salicylate (aspirin) toxicity can lead to metabolic acidosis in children and adults. Signs and symptoms of metabolic acidosis include hypoxia, Kussmaul respirations, nausea/vomiting, cardiac arrhythmia, and seizures. An overdose of aspirin would not likely cause the other conditions listed.

70. Number 1 is correct.

Rationale: Magnesium sulfate is a CNS depressant and can cause marked bradycardia and respiratory depression. The nursing priority is to monitor the client's vital signs for CNS depression after this drug is administered. Tachycardia and hyperventilation are not side effects of magnesium sulfate. A Swan catheter and synchronized cardioversion are not indicated.

71. Number 2 is correct.

Rationale: The nurse's priority is to increase oxygen to the fetus. The fastest way for the nurse to accomplish this is by turning the mother on her left side. The nurse should then stop the Pitocin drip and administer oxygen. A high-Fowler's position could impede the blood supply to the fetus. Increasing IV Pitocin would cause stronger contractions that would also put the fetus at risk for compromised blood flow. The nurse should contact the physician after intervening with the mother and fetus.

72. Number 4 is correct.

Rationale: The child should be placed in a side-lying position while sleeping so oral secretions can drain without presenting the risk of airway obstruction. The child may choke on secretions from drainage if placed in the other positions.

73. Number 1 is correct.

Rationale: The nurse would express concern if a child with a toothache was using herbal remedies. A toothache can indicate a problem and should be evaluated by a dentist for more comprehensive treatment. There is no objection to adults using herbal remedies for xerostomia (dry mouth), nasopharyngitis (common cold), or psoriasis.

74. Number 1 is correct.

Rationale: A thyroid storm is a life-threatening complication of hyperthyroidism seen in clients with Graves' disease. Signs and symptoms may include seizures, jaundice, irregular heartbeat, and vomiting.

Agitation, dehydration, and heart failure may also be seen. The other answer groups are not specific to Graves' disease.

75. Number 2 is correct.

Rationale: Malignant hyperthermia, not hypothermia, is a dangerous adverse reaction to certain drugs used in general anesthesia. Hypoglycemia and hyperglycemia could possibly be a concern if the patient has a diagnosis such as diabetes, but both would be addressed preoperatively.

76. Number 1 is correct.

Rationale: The nurse should ask the client directly if she has experienced any thoughts of suicide or self-harm, and if she has ever made a suicide plan. While the nurse can ask questions 2 and 3, they are not the best way to determine if the client is suicidal. Because of the client's history, suicidal intent should be determined.

77. Number 3 is correct.

Rationale: Alzheimer's disease is a form of dementia that develops over time and gradually worsens. A client who initiates the same conversation repeatedly, displays aggression when stressed, and becomes easily lost in familiar places is showing signs consistent with the moderate stage of Alzheimer's disease. A client with pre-Alzheimer's would not have changes in function. Early and mild Alzheimer's is characterized by memory lapses but no changes in medical function that reflect dementia. Late to severe Alzheimer's is reflected by medical deficiencies such as incontinence, abnormal reflexes, and rigidity.

78. Number 4 is correct.

Rationale: Total parenteral nutrition (TPN) is high in dextrose, and if it is suddenly stopped, the client can become hypoglycemic. The patient could also be dehydrated, but the priority would be blood glucose control.

79. Number 3 is correct.

Rationale: Myasthenia gravis is an autoimmune disease in which antibodies destroy acetylcholine at the neuromuscular junction, causing muscles to be unable to contract normally. The muscles become weak and fatigued. While muscle wasting can occur in severe instances, it is not indicative of the condition. The brain and spinal cord are not damaged from myasthenia gravis.

80. Number 4 is correct.

Rationale: A colposcopy is a painless gynecological procedure, usually done after an abnormal pap smear. The client is placed in a lithotomy position, and a colposcope is used to view the cervix with a bright light. The other positions do not offer the best position to facilitate the medical procedure.

81. Number 2 is correct.

Rationale: Plaque psoriasis is a noncontagious skin disorder in which plaquey areas of inflammation and silvery-white patches of skin develop on the knees, elbows, scalp, and back. Scabies present as a pimple-like rash. Urticaria is also known as hives and presents as red skin with areas of red itchy welts. Contact dermatitis causes skin to be red and inflamed without silvery-white scales.

82. Number 2 is correct.

Rationale: The client is working through feelings of shock, anger, and sadness. The most therapeutic response from the nurse is to sit quietly with the client until he calms down. The nurse should not leave the client alone. The nurse can ask if the client would like to see a chaplain or a counselor but should not assume his wishes, as he did not ask to speak with the chaplain. The nurse should wait for the client to express his own feelings and not tell the client how to feel about the situation.

83. Answer: 12,000 mg/day

Solution:

240 – 300 mg/kg/day	Review the recommended daily dose of piperacillin (Pipracil).
300 mg × 40 kg = 12,000 mg/day	Find the maximum therapeutic daily dose for a 40 kg individual.
12,000 mg/day	Maximum dose for 40 kg child.

84. Number 1 is correct.

Rationale: Pain is subjective and is always what the client states. Therefore, the nurse should chart "The client states his pain is 9/10." If the client mentions that he has a history of addiction, the information can be charted. With prior opioid addiction, clients may experience pain more intensely. Pain management should not be withheld and levels should not be questioned.

85. Number 2 is correct.

Rationale: The client will likely require treatment with immunoglobulin G (IgG) because it is the only immunoglobulin treatment able to cross the placental barrier.

86. Number 1 is correct.

Rationale: Normal sodium levels in an adult are between 135 and 145 mEq/L. Signs and symptoms of hyponatremia may include headache, confusion, muscle weakness, and fatigue. Seizures, loss of appetite, and irritability may also occur. The other symptom groups do not all fit with symptoms of hyponatremia.

87. Number 2 is correct.

Rationale: Calculating glomerular filtration rate is the best way to determine kidney function. It is calculated with a formula that considers a client's age, gender, race, and serum creatinine level. A GFR < 15 mL/min indicates stage 5, end-stage CKD. These clients require dialysis or kidney transplant for survival. A GFR of 15 to 29 indicates stage 4 kidney disease, and preparation for dialysis or transplant is usually indicated. Stages 1 – 3 of kidney disease are less severe and can often be managed with medication and lifestyle changes.

88. Number 2 is correct.

Rationale: The ELISA test is often the first test used for HIV screening. It can detect antibodies to HIV, and DNA/RNA of HIV in the blood. If the ELISA test is positive, further testing must be done, such as the Western blot test. Although false positives are rare, one positive ELISA test is not diagnostic of HIV. Because of possible HIPAA violation and the severity of the diagnosis, discussing HIV test results over the phone should not be done.

89. Number 4 is correct.

Rationale: Hepatitis B is the only vaccine the Centers for Disease Control and Prevention (CBC) typically recommends be administered at birth. The second dose is usually administered 1 – 2 months after the first dose. IPV, Hib, and DTaP series start at 2 months of age.

90. Number 4 is correct.

Rationale: Smokers are two to three times more likely than nonsmokers to develop pancreatic cancer, and smoking is considered a major risk factor for developing the disease. Other risk factors include African American race, obesity, familial history, PMH of certain cancers (breast, lung, bladder, etc.), chronic pancreatitis, liver cirrhosis, and diabetes. Alcohol abuse is linked to an increased risk of pancreatic cancer; however two or fewer alcoholic beverages a week is considered social alcohol consumption.

91. Number 3 is correct.

Rationale: A nurse who has been working in the same, or similar, position for 2 – 3 years is considered a competent nurse. Competent nurses are expected to use their experience to analyze problems that arise, and have developed solid critical thinking skills. However, a nurse at the competent level does not yet have the intuition and life or situational experience an expert nurse can rely on. The novice-expert model is based on Dr. Patricia Benner's work, which describes a novice as a beginner with no experience, an advanced beginner as a nurse who can demonstrate marginally acceptable performance, and an expert nurse as one who has a background to practice independently.

92. Number 2 is correct.

Rationale: In Maslow's hierarchy of needs, the highest level of fulfillment is self-actualization, which includes morality, creativity, problem-solving, spontaneity, acceptance of facts, and lack of prejudice. Esteem follows as the next need and presents as the human desire to be accepted and valued by others. Love and belonging and safety follow esteem on the hierarchy of needs pyramid.

93. Number 2 is correct.

Rationale: The nurse should prioritize by first assessing for risks to airway, breathing, or circulation. The woman reporting jaw and back pain may be experiencing a myocardial infarction, which is a priority situation. While all of the other situations should be addressed, they should be triaged appropriately as they are not emergencies.

94. Number 4 is correct.

Rationale: A client taking furosemide (Lasix) is at risk for hypokalemia, because this medication is a (potassium wasting) loop diuretic. Salmon, spinach, and bananas are all foods high in potassium. While the other foods are not harmful, they are not the most beneficial for replacing potassium in the body.

95. Number 1 is correct.

Rationale: Prothrombin time is a measure of the clotting tendency of the blood. Since warfarin is an anticoagulant, this client is at an increased risk for hemorrhage. Clients who are taking warfarin and are in an emergency situation where they are actively bleeding can be given fresh frozen plasma to quickly reverse the effects of warfarin and reach homeostasis. Red blood cell transfusions are utilized to treat hemorrhage. Platelets are used to prevent hemorrhage in patients with thrombocytopenia or platelet function defects.

96. Number 1 is correct.

Solution:

1,000 units / 250 mL = 4 units/mL	Find the number of units of insulin per milliliter.
4 units/mL × 5 mL/hr **= 20 units/hr**	Multiply the number of units per milliliter by the milliliters per hour to find the number of units administered per hour.

97. Number 2 is correct.

Rationale: The 16-year-old female is not likely to survive her injuries. Fixed, dilated pupils, unresponsiveness, and probable severe head trauma are indicators of a very poor prognosis. Clients who are not expected to survive, even with treatment and intervention, are not the triage priority. Triage should prioritize critical clients who have a chance of survival if treated quickly, and then should see clients with less serious injuries.

98. Number 1 is correct.

Rationale: The RN needs to speak with the nursing assistant privately and directly regarding the incident as soon as possible. The nurse needs to assess the situation before determining the best action to take.

Answers 2, 3, and 4 might be appropriate at a later time, but the nurse should directly address the situation as it is occurring.

99. Number 1 is correct.

Rationale: If a minor child is in the care of a legal guardian, the guardian has the right to sign medical consent forms. There is no need to require a parent to sign the consent instead or to check the chart for that information. A legal guardian retains the rights to make decisions for the minor child's medical care.

100. Number 4 is correct.

Rationale: All of the interventions listed are important during a sickle cell crisis; however, administering IV fluids is the priority. Hydration can stop the sickling process of the blood cells by causing hemodilution.

101. Number 2 is correct.

Rationale: A cane can offer stability and balance to clients who have minor injuries, pain, or weakness. The proper order for coming down the stairs is to place the cane down on the step first, then step with the injured leg, and then step down with the good leg. The cane should reach a height even with the wrist, and the elbow should be slightly bent when holding the cane. Additionally, the cane should be held opposite of the side that requires support.

102. Number 3 is correct.

Rationale: This nurse is guilty of a HIPAA violation regarding client privacy. Even though the nurse and client are neighbors, no one other than those providing direct care to the client should be viewing the client's medical record, including lab results or progress notes. A nurse should only access the records of her specific clients. Even if the information is not shared with anyone else, viewing nonclient records still violates HIPAA. Asking the client's nurse for information is also inappropriate. The nurse should not round on other clients with the physician. HIPAA violations are grounds for dismissal and disciplinary action by the state's board of nursing. Nurses must exercise due diligence in protecting the privacy of all clients.

103. Numbers 2, 3, 4, and 5 are correct.

Rationale: Nurses often help turn and reposition other nurses' clients, so this is an appropriate action for a student nurse. Student nurses should read the chart for their assigned client and be familiar with the medical history, current diagnosis, diagnostic tests, and medications. This allows the student nurse to see how care is provided for various conditions and allows opportunities to ask questions of the licensed nurse. The student nurse should work closely with the preceptor and perform as much hands-on care as he is qualified to do under state nursing law and facility policy. If the student nurse is not qualified to provide the care, he still has the opportunity to observe and ask questions in preparation of advancing his skills. Post-clinical conferences allow groups of student nurses to share interesting procedures or observations that facilitate learning among the group. HIPAA rules still apply; the student nurses are reminded not to share client names or any identifying data when sharing with the group.

A student nurse may not administer medications on his own. Instead, the precepting nurse should accompany the student nurse in medication administration, once the student nurse has passed the medication exam and is allowed by the instructor to administer medications. Before giving any medication, the student nurse should be able to explain to the preceptor what the medication is for, contraindications, and side effects. The precepting nurse is still responsible for the student nurse's actions and can be held liable for medication errors by the student nurse.

104. Number 1 is correct.

Rationale: Clients have the right to change DNR orders or advance directives whenever they choose. It is important to notify the health care provider immediately so that the DNR order may be rescinded. Response 2 is inappropriate because the nurse is expressing her opinion about what the client should do. Response 3 is inappropriate because the client is of legal age and has rights protected under HIPAA to make her own decisions regarding care. Response 4 is incorrect because although a DNR is a legal document, the client retains the right at any time to change her mind regarding treatment.

105. Numbers 3 and 4 are correct.

Rationale: Hepatitis A is transmitted when an uninfected person ingests food or water that is contaminated with the feces of an infected person. Hepatitis C is transmitted through blood. Hepatitis B is transmitted through various body fluids, including sputum.

106. Number 3 is correct.

Rationale: The Tzanck test will determine the presence of cells from the herpes virus. The stress test assesses cardiac response to increased workload. The Rinne test compares bone conduction to air conduction in the ears. The patch test identifies the cause of allergic contact sensitization.

107. Number 3 is correct.

Rationale: Transfusion rates for a unit of RBCs should occur within 4 hours. The 2-hour infusion would be appropriate for a client experiencing an emergency situation. The 6-hour and 8-hour infusion rates are too long.

108. Numbers 1, 2, 3, and 4 are correct.

Rationale: There are several nursing interventions to help the client suffering from PTSD. Most clients will require a combination of different techniques to maximize coping skills. Every client is different, and some clients will try many techniques before finding what works best for them. The nurse should help the client develop adequate coping techniques and practice using a variety of techniques. The client should also be encouraged to try relaxation techniques. Listening to the client in a supportive and nonjudgmental manner paves the way for therapeutic communication and offers a safe environment for the client. A client who does not feel as if the environment is safe and secure is less likely to express her feelings and may delay her progress. There is no need for the client to wait until she has worked through all the stages of grief before going out in public; doing so may delay healing and keeps the client from attending to the necessary duties of everyday life, such as working, shopping for food, and keeping physician appointments.

109. (Correct response: Confabulation)

Rationale: Clients experiencing confabulation may fill in memory gaps with elaborate, detailed fantasies which they believe to be true. They are not intentionally trying to deceive others; their fantasies are often based on old memories.

110. Numbers 1, 2, and 3 are correct.

Rationale: The nurse can best manage the behavior of the client by showing support when the client exhibits positive behaviors. The nurse should set clear, enforceable limits and communicate expectations to the client. The client should also be informed of consequences of not complying. Role playing demonstrates appropriate behaviors to the client and allows her to practice best responses before a situation arises. Treating the client more like a friend is inappropriate; the nurse should maintain a professional relationship with the client and not try to be her friend. This only confuses the client; it also makes the situation worse for other staff members and can lead to infighting among staff. Giving small gifts to encourage desired behavior is a form of bribery. The nurse should not try to bribe or manipulate the client, nor should the nurse accept gifts from the client. Consistent treatment by all staff members gives the client a stable and safe environment in which to work on her behavior.

111. Answer: B

112. Answer: C

113. Answer: D

114. Answer: A

115. Number 3 is correct.

Rationale: This client is experiencing wound evisceration, which is an emergency. The first priority is to call for help and have the surgeon notified. While waiting on another nurse to bring needed supplies, the nurse stays with the client and positions him in a low Fowler's with the knees bent to prevent tension on the incision. Monitor vital signs as soon as equipment is available. The wound should be covered with a sterile normal saline dressing and kept moist. After the surgeon arrives, the client is prepared for surgery if ordered.

116. Number 3 is correct.

Rationale: Reclast is contraindicated in clients with a creatinine clearance less than 35 mL/min. The other lab values are within normal range and do not affect administration of this medication.

117. Number 4 is correct.

Rationale: This client is experiencing autonomic dysreflexia, which requires immediate treatment to prevent hypertensive stroke. Placing the client in the high Fowler's position reduces blood pressure by promoting gravitational pooling of blood in the lower extremities. The nurse should notify the health care provider immediately and assess for the cause. Bladder distention and fecal impaction are common causes; if the client has a urinary catheter in place, the nurse should check for kinks in the tubing. If indicated, preparation to catheterize the client should begin immediately. Nitrate or nifedipine are the most common drugs used for treatment.

118. Number 3 is correct.

Rationale: The client with a glomerular filtration rate (GFR) of 92 mL/min has a normal value but may have physical findings or genetic traits that indicate stage 1 kidney disease. A GFR of 63 mL/min indicates stage 2, or mild chronic kidney disease (CKD). A GFR of 39 mL/min is consistent with stage 3, or moderate CKD. A GFR of 16mL/min indicates stage 5, end-stage kidney disease.

119. Number 3 is correct.

Rationale: Low-pitched grating and rubbing is indicative of friction rub. Rhonchi are either low-pitched, continuous rattling sounds (sonorous) or high-pitched and continuous (sibilant) sounds. Stridor occurs on inspiration and is loud, high-pitched crowing that can be heard without a stethoscope. Fine crackles are brief and high pitched.

120. Number 2 is correct.

Rationale: Stasis ulcers often form as a result of edema or minor injury to the leg. They occur more often medially than laterally over the malleolus of the affected limb. Decreased or absent pulses with cool or cold feet is a finding of arterial ulcers. Skin atrophy and pallor with elevation are another indication of arterial ulcers. Edema is often present due to valvular damage from the backup of blood and venous hypertension.

121. Number 4 is correct.

Rationale: All hospitals should have access to licensed translators, via telephone or in person, for most languages. Language barriers do not preclude the client from being told exactly what procedure is being suggested by the health care provider. A licensed translator understands the nuances of slang or colloquial language, and is experienced in explaining medical procedures in everyday language that the client can understand. Even if the family member appears to be fluent in English, the information conveyed to the client may be selectively edited in order to influence the client's decision. Informed consent may not be given unless all the client's questions and concerns have been answered, including risks and possible surgical outcomes. The spouse does not need to give consent for the client unless the client is incapable of doing so. While showing pictures to the client may help him understand the procedure, a licensed translator provides explanations without bias or trying to influence the client's decision. Without the use of a licensed translator, the health care provider is at legal risk of performing surgery without fully informed consent.

122. Number 3 is correct.

Rationale: The Patient Self-Determination Act of 1990 requires that all clients of health care facilities be informed of their right to refuse care or specify their wishes should they become unable to speak for themselves. Giving the client a copy to read allows the nurse to answer questions and explain that the client may choose which interventions she does or does not want. For example, a client may refuse to be on a ventilator but will accept tube feedings for nutrition. If the client fills out the advance directives, it should be witnessed by two nonfamily members or other neutral parties and placed on the client's chart. While the directives can be added later, the nurse should not tell the client not to worry about it. The directives may be forgotten, and should an emergency arise, the client will not have as much autonomy in her care. Advance directives do not need to go through a lawyer in most cases, and waiting to have them drawn up and sent causes unnecessary delays for the client. The nurse should never simply drop the discussion and chart that the client refused them. The nurse is duty bound to make the client fully aware of all of her rights. It is important to avoid any actions that may endanger a client or lead to potential legal action.

123. Number 2 is correct.

Rationale: The nurse should refuse to sign off on the waste and immediately report the incident. The nurse is bound by duty, law, and ethics to refuse to cover up for another nurse's illegal actions. The second nurse is practicing medicine without a license, as it is beyond the scope of practice for the nurse to change a medication dose. The first nurse is also guilty and can be found liable if any harm comes to the patient. While suggesting the second nurse notify the physician for a dosage change is a reasonable action, the first nurse has been informed that the client has already received a greater-than-ordered dose and must report this information. Options 3 and 4 do not negate the fact that the second nurse is breaking the law and putting the client at risk.

124. Number 4 is correct.

Rationale: Needles should be placed in the nearest puncture-resistant container intact. Needles should not be re-capped or broken.

125. Number 3 is correct.

Rationale: Engaging the core (stomach) and leg muscles provides the safest traction for moving a client in bed. Feet should be shoulder width apart. The client should be instructed to help as much as possible. The head of the bed should be flat, if the client can tolerate it.

126. Number 4 is correct.

Rationale: Older adults with dementia are at risk for injury due to increased risk for falls. They may not recognize their limitations given the ineffective tissue perfusion that occurs with hypertension. Ineffective coping, activity intolerance, and ineffective tissue perfusion would not be the highest priority.

127. Number 3 is correct.

Rationale: The nurse should assign a sitter, because keeping the client safe after he has verbalized a suicide plan is more important than the client's right to refuse care. Placing the client in restraints does not guarantee his safety and may escalate the situation. If the client manages to get out of the restraints, he might hang himself with them. Having security sit outside the door does not provide direct observation of the client and uses up a limited resource of the facility. Allowing the client to leave AMA leaves the nurse and the facility vulnerable to legal action if the client commits suicide after leaving. Having a friend come sit does not guarantee safety; the friend may provide him with the means to commit suicide, such as bringing drugs for him to overdose on.

128. Number 1 is correct.

The most important information for the nurse to find out is what support systems the client has available. The nurse must remember that this information is key in order to know how to approach the client and how to plan care. If the client has few or no support systems, the priority is to help her find resources to help her. Asking the client what she does for relaxation is little help if she has no support system. Asking about her parents' insurance coverage for adult day care may be an option to explore down the road, but it takes a back seat to determining the client's support systems. Offering a list of nursing homes is not appropriate at this time and does not offer timely help with her situation. Once the nurse understands the client's support systems, she can make appropriate decisions on where to proceed next.

129. Numbers 1 and 3 are correct.

Rationale: Withdrawing air after aspirating the prescribed medication creates an air-lock to seal in the medication once injected. The needle used for medication is replaced with a new one prior to injection so no drug is on the outside of the needle shaft. The ventrogluteal muscle is used for Z-track injection. The needle is inserted at a 90-degree angle.

130. Numbers 2 and 3 are correct answers.

Rationale: Air is inserted first into the cloudy insulin (NPH) followed by insertion of air into the regular insulin. Regular (clear) insulin is drawn up first followed by cloudy insulin (NPH).

131. Number 3 is correct.

Rationale: IVIG is stored under refrigeration yet should be administered at room temperature, typically within 30 minutes of removal from cold storage. The IVIG infusion rate is slow at first and increased gradually every 15 to 30 minutes as tolerated by the client until the maximum infusion rate may be administered. Vital signs should be monitored 15 minutes prior to administration, 15 minutes after initiation of infusion, and at every rate change. Chills, considered an adverse reaction to IVIG, warrant stopping the infusion.

132. Number 4 is correct.

Rationale: Increased ICP includes increased systolic blood pressure and widened pulse pressure, along with a decreased heart rate. Altered level of consciousness is the earliest and most sensitive manifestation of increased ICP. The client may have an elevated temperature, but this is not the earliest sign. Narrowed pulse pressure is not present with increased ICP.

133. Number 1 is correct.

Rationale: Lipiduria is a key feature of nephrotic syndrome. Other key findings include hyperlipidemia, hypoalbuminemia, and increased coagulation.

134. Number 3 is correct.

Rationale: Inflating the cuff (if the tube is not capped) during meals and for 1 hour afterward prevents aspiration. The client should sit up for all meals. When capping the tube, the cuff is first deflated and the inner cannula removed prior to capping in order to avoid blocking the airway. The cuff is not inflated prior to capping. The cuff must be inflated for meals.

135. Number 3 is correct.

Rationale: Clients on neutropenic precautions are at high risk of infection. Fresh flowers and potted plants should not be placed in the client's room. It is important to monitor vital signs, including temperature every 4 hours as increased temperature may indicate infection. Inspecting the client's mouth on a regular basis and providing oral care helps limit bacteria and allows visualization for oral changes. Strict adherence to standard precautions including hand hygiene is important with all clients, but especially those who are immunocompromised.

136. Number 4 is correct.

Rationale: Threatened miscarriage presents with mild uterine cramping, spotting of blood, and a closed cervical os. A missed miscarriage refers to a pregnancy in which the fetus has died but the products of conception may be retained in utero for several weeks. The cervical os remains closed, and there may or may not be bleeding or cramping. With an inevitable or incomplete miscarriage, a moderate to heavy amount of bleeding is present with an open cervical os.

137. Number 4 is correct.

Rationale: Warfarin is a high-alert drug and clients should know which side effects to report to their physician. Bloody, black, or tarry stools; pink urine; or excessive bleeding should be reported immediately. Which pharmacy the client uses is not as important as knowing which side effects to report. Knowing the next lab appointment is important but not as important as knowing the side effects of warfarin. Clients must undergo regular laboratory testing to ensure that the warfarin is at a therapeutic level. Clients living at poverty level often lack reliable transportation to return to clinics for follow-up lab work. The nurse should ensure that the client has transportation for lab work to prevent the risk of bleeding. If the client expresses doubt about being able to return for labs, the nurse should notify the health care provider and ask for a social worker consult. The social worker may know of free transportation for low-income individuals or be able to provide a bus or cab voucher. Nurses collaborate with other disciplines to ensure the best care for the client. The nurse is often the only one that the client confides in regarding obstacles to care.

138. Number 3 is correct.

Rationale: Assisting a client to ambulate in the hall is within the scope of practice for a UAP. The nurse cannot delegate dressing changes, such as the first two clients need. Only the licensed nurse may assess clients, including assessing pain levels. When delegating tasks, the nurse is responsible for delegating the appropriate task to qualified personnel. Clients who are not stable, who have dressing changes, who need further assessments performed, or whose outcomes are unpredictable should not be delegated to UAPs. The nurse is ultimately responsible for the task being carried out properly.

139. Number 4 is correct.

Rationale: The client experiencing tingling in and around the mouth may be having an allergic reaction to the antibiotic. The nurse should immediately assess the client's airway and breathing, as the client is at risk for the tongue swelling and blocking the airway. The other clients may be seen after assessing the client for an allergic reaction. While it is important to address the other clients' needs quickly, the nurse always addresses potentially life-threatening situations first.

140. Number 1 is correct.

Rationale: Taking vital signs is within the scope of practice for LPNs. Flushing central lines and hanging TPN to a PICC line is beyond the scope of practice for an LPN. Administering IV medications should only be done by the registered nurse, as LPNs are not licensed to do so.

141. Number 3 is correct.

Rationale: Documentation of the event in the client's medical record is required. The one who discovers the event (the nursing assistant) should complete the incident report.

142. Number 1 is correct.

Rationale: The 2016 Hospital National Patient Safety Goals by the Joint Commission on Accreditation of Hospitals states that at least two ways to identify patients are needed to promote patient safety. Asking the client to state his name and date of birth is only one form of identification. Asking the client to confirm the medication ordered and comparing this with the medication order are not two viable means of identifiers. The room number is not used as a client identifier.

143. Number 4 is correct.

Rationale: Metformin within 48 hours of a contrast study can result in lactic acidosis. The physician will need to withhold Metformin on the day of contrast administration and for an additional 48 hours; instead, use another hypoglycemic agent during this period. Allergy to shellfish is not a contraindication to the use of a contrast dye nor is CHF or chronic cystitis.

144. Number 4 is correct.

Rationale: The human immunodeficiency virus (HIV), which causes AIDS, is concentrated mostly in blood and semen. The client should not donate blood. Someone with HIV does not need to limit time in public places. As HIV is not transmitted by sharing food, there are no restrictions on this activity. Use of public restrooms by persons with HIV is an acceptable practice.

145. Number 1 is correct.

Rationale: A transdermal patch of fentanyl is to be worn continuously to provide round-the-clock pain relief. A potent opioid analgesic, fentanyl needs to be stored in a safe location where others may not access the drug. Orange juice may be ingested while on fentanyl; however, grapefruit juice should be avoided as it increases the effect of the drug.

146. Number 1 is correct.

Rationale: Positioning the client in a prone position is unnecessary. Instead, position the client with the affected ear uppermost or tilt the client's head to the side if he is sitting or lying on the unaffected site. The six rights of medication administration should be followed (right client, medication, dose, route, time, documentation). Nonsterile gloves should be applied after hand washing. The pinna is pulled back and up to straighten the ear canal to facilitate the medication reaching the proper location.

147. Number 1 is correct.

Rationale: The Babinski reflex disappears after 1 year of age. The complete fencing response disappears by 3 – 4 months. The stepping or "walking" reflex is present until 3 – 4 weeks. The complete Moro reflex response remains intact until 8 weeks.

148. Numbers 1, 2, and 3 are correct.

Rationale: Severe burns can lead to compartment syndrome because edema increases pressure in the compartments, which house muscles, nerves, and blood vessels. Fractures are present in 75% of all cases of compartment syndrome. Severe infiltration of IV fluids also increases compartment pressure due to edema surrounding the area of infiltration. Failure to ambulate after surgery is not a cause of compartment syndrome. Blood sugar levels do not affect compartments.

149. Answer: The nurse should administer 0.5 mL of heparin.

Rationale:

10,000 units/1 mL = 5,000 units/X	Set up a proportion (dose on hand/quantity on hand = dose desired/X)
10,000 units × X = 5,000 units × 1 mL	Calculate.
X = 5,000 units × 1 mL/10,000 units	Solve for X.
X = 0.5 mL	

150. Numbers 3 and 4 are correct.

Rationale: The first stools are liquid and gradually become more formed. The healthy stoma is reddish-pink and moist and protrudes about 2 cm from the abdominal wall. Only a small amount of bleeding should be present at the stoma site. The colostomy will begin functioning in 2 to 3 days.

Question Bank

SAFE AND EFFECTIVE CARE ENVIRONMENT—MANAGEMENT OF CARE

1. The nurse is caring for a middle-aged woman who walks 3 miles every morning. The nurse notes that during her morning walk, the client called her son and stated that she thought she was having a heart attack. Which symptom, identified by the client, is the **most** common and consistent with a myocardial infarction (MI)?

    1. palpitations
    2. lower extremity edema
    3. uncomfortable feeling of pressure in the chest
    4. nausea

2. The nurse assists the client to the operating room table and supervises the operating room technician preparing the sterile field. Which action, completed by the surgical technician, indicates to the nurse that a sterile field has been contaminated? **Select all that apply.**

    1. A sterile object is held below the table surface and returned to the sterile field.
    2. The outer inch of the sterile towel hangs over the side of the table.
    3. A partially emptied container of sterile betadine is replaced within the sterile field.
    4. Sterile packages are opened with the first edge away from the technician.

3. The nurse is responsible for his own actions while on duty caring for clients. What is the name of this ethical principle? **Fill in the blank.**

    _____

4. The nurse is caring for a client on the orthopedic unit who had a total knee replacement on the left side. The nurse knows the client will be ready for discharge when she is able to do which of the following activities?

   1. ambulate 100 feet with crutches or walker
   2. get up and down a flight of stairs
   3. flex the surgical knee 30 degrees
   4. fix a snack

5. A client undergoes total shoulder replacement on the left shoulder. Which statements by the client indicates he requires further teaching? **Select all that apply.**

   1. "I look forward to soaking in my hot tub when I get home from surgery."
   2. "The surgery will eliminate my pain within 24 hours."
   3. "I will receive therapy for several weeks after my surgery."
   4. "Walking is an exercise I'll be able to do after surgery."

6. Which diagnostic tool is most commonly used to determine the location of the myocardial damage?

   1. electrocardiogram (ECG)
   2. echocardiogram
   3. cardiac enzymes
   4. cardiac catheterization

7. The charge nurse is teaching unit nurses about droplet precautions. Which statement by one of the nurses indicates further teaching is needed by the charge nurse?

   1. "Mumps is a viral infection that requires droplet precautions."
   2. "Pharyngeal diphtheria is a viral infection that requires droplet precautions."
   3. "Pertussis is a bacterial respiratory infection that requires droplet precautions."
   4. "Mycoplasma pneumonia is a bacterial respiratory infection that requires droplet precautions."

8. The nurse is working with an unlicensed assistive personnel (UAP) in the medical-surgical unit. Which client should be assigned to the UAP?

   1. a client with cervical cancer who has an internal radiation implant
   2. a client who is receiving blood as treatment for hypovolemic shock
   3. a client who had an abdominal wound dehiscence 24 hours earlier and requires dressing changes
   4. a client who is post-op day 2 following a laparoscopic hernia repair and gets up to the chair for meals

9. A client is being treated for pulmonary hypertension. The nurse knows that the involvement of nursing, pharmacy, cardiology, physical therapy, and nutritional services is an example of which of the following approaches?

   1. continuity of care
   2. case management
   3. quality improvement
   4. interdisciplinary

10. An 84-year-old adult male requires nonurgent surgery. The client is considered to have diminished decision-making capacity due to a diagnosis of Alzheimer's. The nurse questions his ability to provide informed consent for the procedure. The **best** action for the nurse to take in this situation is which of the following?

    1. as this is nonurgent surgery with few risks, allow the client to sign the consent form
    2. contact administrative personnel for a determination consistent with hospital policy
    3. have the client's 54-year-old second cousin sign the consent form
    4. request the physician sign the consent form

11. A nurse assigned to a client with congestive heart failure (CHF) is providing shift report. Which nursing interventions would be appropriate to include? **Select all that apply.**

    1. The nurse should reduce fluid intake to less than 1,000 ml per shift.
    2. The nurse should keep the client in a supine position as much as possible.
    3. The nurse should encourage alternating activity with rest periods.
    4. The nurse should assess the ankles, legs, and feet for pitting edema.

12. A nurse is caring for a client in the immediate post–cardiac catheterization period. Which intervention should the nurse include in the client's care?

    1. monitor vital signs every 30 minutes for the first 2 hours
    2. assess the insertion site
    3. maintain the client in a prone position
    4. keep the client NPO for 2 hours

13. The nurse is preparing to interpret an electrocardiogram rhythm strip. Identify the order for interpreting the strip. Use all the options.

    1. measure the P-R interval
    2. determine the heart rate and rhythm
    3. analyze the P waves
    4. measure the QRS duration

14. A client is admitted with inflammatory bowel syndrome (Crohn's disease). Which nursing measures would be included in the client's care plan? **Select all that apply.**

    1. high-fat diet
    2. lactulose therapy
    3. daily weight
    4. corticosteroids

15. The nurse is caring for an elderly client who is 1 day post–hip replacement surgery. Which nursing interventions should be included on the care plan? **Select all that apply.**

    1. apply compression stockings
    2. ambulate with walker
    3. encourage coughing and deep breathing every 2 hours
    4. limit fluid intake

16. The school nurse is monitoring the diet of a child with cystic fibrosis. Which type of diet would the family be advised to follow?

    1. low calorie, high fiber
    2. low fiber, low fat
    3. low sodium, gluten free
    4. high fat, high calorie

17. A charge nurse is preparing client care assignments for the upcoming shift. A client who underwent a laminectomy is scheduled to return from the recovery care unit. Which staff member should receive this client?

    1. graduate nurse with 3 months of experience
    2. RN with 1 year of experience
    3. certified nursing assistant with 5 years of experience
    4. charge nurse with 2 years of experience

18. A toddler in gastric distress is admitted to the pediatric intensive care unit. The toddler becomes anxious and tries to remove the IV. The mother offers to help calm the child. Which action by the nurse is **most** appropriate?

    1. paint a smiley face on the dressing covering the IV site
    2. give the child a puzzle to complete
    3. ask the mother to read the child's favorite book
    4. administer a sedative to the child

19. Which assignment made by a charge nurse should be questioned?

    1. a student nurse assigned to a newly admitted child with acute leukemia who is receiving a blood transfusion

    2. an RN assigned to a teenaged child diagnosed recently with bacterial meningitis

    3. a CNA assigned to a stable male client who is 3 days post-stroke

    4. an LPN assigned to a newly admitted child with acute leukemia who is receiving IV fluids

20. A 4-month-old infant is admitted to the pediatric unit for a 10-day course of antibiotics. The parents are only able to visit on weekends. Which action indicates the nurse understands the emotional needs of the infant?

    1. The nurse care plan calls for soothing music to be played several times per day.

    2. The nurse self-assigns care for the infant each shift worked.

    3. The nurse assigns a male nurse to care for the infant as much as possible.

    4. The nurse places the infant in a room close to the nursing station.

21. The school nurse is assessing the readiness of a 16-year-old athlete who is diabetic. As the teenager becomes more physically active during the day, which management strategies should the nurse advise? **Select all that apply.**

    1. monitor blood glucose level before exercise

    2. always carry some form of high-protein, high-fat snack

    3. let the coach know the athlete is a diabetic

    4. inject insulin at least 30 minutes prior to athletic event

22. The nurse is caring for a client with an infected leg wound. The client develops a fever of 102°F. Which action by the nurse is the **priority** for this client?

    1. obtain a wound culture

    2. administer acetaminophen

    3. administer IV antibiotic as scheduled

    4. perform the scheduled dressing change

23. The nurse is performing a dressing change on a client with a stage 3 sacral wound. Once the old dressing is removed, the nurse would perform which step next?

    1. wash hands

    2. chart the findings

    3. assess the wound

    4. prepare the sterile field

24. A newly graduated nurse has completed hospital orientation and has just started working with her own clients. Which of the following assignments is **most** appropriate for this nurse?

    1. a nonverbal client hospitalized for seizures

    2. a client undergoing peritoneal dialysis at the bedside

    3. a client who had a negative heart catheterization the day before

    4. an elderly client who just returned from surgery for a below-the-knee amputation

25. The nurse is working with a newly hired unlicensed assistive personnel (UAP). Several activities of daily living need to be completed for the nurse's clients. Which task should the nurse delegate to the UAP?

    1. performing oral care on a client with a bleeding disorder

    2. turning a client with a tibial fracture with external fixation

    3. assisting a client admitted with COPD exacerbation to the chair

    4. reinforcing teaching on use of the inhaler for a client with asthma

26. The RN is assigning a client to the LPN. The RN understands that the **best** assignment for the LPN is which client?

    1. a client receiving blood for a GI bleed

    2. a client with a PICC line requiring TPN

    3. a client who will receive enemas in preparation for a colonoscopy

    4. a client who needs preoperative teaching for bowel resection surgery

27. A local volunteer singing group performs in the activity room of a long-term care facility. The group's leader asks the nurse if they may take a photo of themselves with several of the clients. The nurse gives permission to the leader, who then posts the photo on Facebook. Upon notification of this situation, the facility administration immediately terminates the nurse. What Health Insurance Portability and Accountability Act (HIPAA) violation did the nurse commit?

    1. breach of confidentiality

    2. failure to seek administrative approval

    3. unethical conduct

    4. unprofessional conduct

28. A nurse manager and a case manager are talking to a group of new nurses about the differences of case management and care coordination. The nurse manager understands which to be true regarding the differences?

    1. With care coordination, the stakeholder can be an insurance company or a hospital.

    2. The main goal of case management is to promote a better quality of life for the client.

    3. Case management is based on a holistic approach and an understanding of client-family dynamics.

    4. In care coordination, the client defines the scope of work based on a plan that is created with input from the client.

29. The newly graduated nurse is caring for an elderly client on the medical-surgical floor. The nurse recalls learning about client advocacy. Which actions by the nurse indicate an understanding of client advocacy? **Select all that apply.**

   1. The nurse speaks to the daughters regarding care-making decisions, since the client is elderly and may not understand.
   2. The nurse tells the family that they should really consider making the client an organ donor in case something happens.
   3. The nurse makes sure the client understands treatment options, including possible outcomes if the client refuses treatment.
   4. The nurse obtains an interpreter for the client if her native language is not English and she only understands her native language.
   5. The nurse asks the client for a copy of advance directives or a living will, or provides information if the client does not have one.

30. A nurse manager is educating a group of nursing students about the Patient's Bill of Rights. The nurse knows that the student nurses have an understanding of the bill when one of the nurses makes which statement?

   1. "Clients have the right to view their medical records but may not copy any of the information contained in the records."
   2. "Clients may be declined care at an emergency department or need preauthorization for care if they do not have premium-level insurance."
   3. "Clients have the right to a quick and objective review of any claim that they levy against a health care facility, physician, or health care plan."
   4. "It is the admitting nurse's job to verify the client's past medical history, medications, and treatments, even if the client refuses to cooperate in giving the information."

31. Nurses are expected to understand the principles of triage when caring for multiple clients. The ICU charge nurse is reviewing assignments. Based on the principles of triage, to which client would the charge nurse give **priority** for treatment? **Select all that apply.**

   1. a client on a ventilator who has an alarm sounding
   2. a client who has just returned from an open appendectomy
   3. a client ready to transfer to the floor after the nurse calls report
   4. a client who has been talking with family and is now unresponsive
   5. a client receiving a new antibiotic who complains of tingling in the mouth
   6. a client who has not eaten yet and is a type 2 diabetic with a morning blood sugar of 90

32. A nurse on a busy surgical floor is working with an unlicensed assistive personnel (UAP). The nurse understands that which task cannot be delegated to the UAP?

   1. assisting a stable client to set up her meal tray for easy access
   2. assisting a client with an arm cast onto the bedpan
   3. calling report on a client who is being transferred to the observation floor
   4. helping a client ambulate in the hall who is post-op day 2 from a cardiac catheterization with stent placement

33. The nurse in the senior dementia unit noticed an increase in client falls over the last six months. She worked with other unit nurses and the nurse manager to develop a new fall risk assessment tool and updated the unit policies regarding falls. Which activity did the nurse engage in?

    1. delegation

    2. peer review

    3. consultation

    4. client referral

    5. quality improvement

34. The ED nurse is attending orientation for nurses new to working in the ED. As part of the training, the ED nurse would expect to report which conditions to the proper authorities? **Select all that apply.**

    1. West Nile virus

    2. herpes simplex

    3. gunshot wounds

    4. elder abuse or neglect

    5. bites from an unknown dog

35. The RN is precepting a nursing student in the surgical ICU. The client is diabetic and asks the student nurse about insulin. Which response by the RN is **best**?

    1. ask the family to step out of the room to ensure client privacy

    2. tell the client that he should ask the health care provider when she rounds

    3. inform the client that the student nurse cannot answer questions regarding medication

    4. allow the nursing student to answer the client's question while the RN is present and can provide additional information if needed

36. The nurse is caring for a client who is a Jehovah's Witness and is scheduled for hip replacement surgery. The client refuses to sign consent for blood due to religious reasons. The client's daughter has the power of attorney in case the client is unable to state his wishes regarding health care. The daughter tells the nurse, "I'm afraid if something goes wrong, dad might need blood. I want to sign a blood consent form since I'm his power of attorney." The daughter is not a Jehovah's Witness. Which action by the nurse is the **best** in this situation?

    1. notify the charge nurse so that she can ask the night shift nurse to handle the situation

    2. go and get a blood consent form for the daughter to sign, noting that she has power of attorney over the client

    3. notify the surgeon that the client's daughter has power of attorney and will be signing a blood consent form so that an order may be obtained for a type and cross

    4. remind the daughter that the client clearly does not wish to receive blood, and that a power of attorney cannot override client wishes that have been clearly stated when he was able to give or refuse consent

37. The nurse manager has approval to add one LPN to the RNs in the medical-surgical unit. Which nursing actions does the nurse manager expect the LPN to be able to perform according to **most** state board of nursing practice acts? **Select all that apply.**

    1. draw blood from a PICC line

    2. access a port with a Huber needle

    3. perform hemodynamic monitoring

    4. transcribe written physician orders

    5. perform finger-prick blood glucose testing

38. The nurse is caring for a client when the attending physician comes in to round on the client. At the nurses' station, the nurse smells alcohol on the physician's breath when he hands her the chart with new orders. Which action by the nurse is appropriate?

    1. notify the nurse manager and or/charge nurse

    2. confront the physician about the smell of alcohol

    3. tell the client and request a consult with another physician

    4. enter the new orders as written, since there was only a morning lab draw ordered

39. A newly graduated nurse has been assigned a client who has a chest tube following a thoracotomy. The new nurse is not experienced with chest tube management. Which action by the nurse is **most** appropriate regarding this assignment?

    1. ask for a different group of clients

    2. ask to be floated to another area in the facility

    3. refuse the assignment, since she is not familiar with chest tubes

    4. accept the assignment and ask for another nurse to help her with the chest tube

40. A nurse is precepting a nursing student in the pediatrics unit. The student nurse is preparing to administer an injection to a 14-month-old infant. Which statement by the student nurse indicates a need for further teaching by the licensed nurse?

    1. "I will use a needle that is 7/8 inch to 1 inch long."

    2. "I will give this injection at a 90-degree angle of insertion."

    3. "I will give this injection in the vastus lateralis with a 27-gauge needle."

    4. "I can give this injection with a 25-gauge needle in the dorsogluteal area."

41. The nurse is admitting a new client complaining of severe abdominal pain. When asked about valuables, the client says he has $1,500 cash in his wallet. He is from out of state and does not have anyone who can take his wallet into safekeeping for him. Which statement by the nurse **best** addresses this situation?

    1. "I can keep it locked up in the charge nurse's office for you."

    2. "It should be fine. Just hide it in a drawer when you go down for a CT scan."

    3. "I can call security to bring a form to fill out, and they will lock it up for you."

    4. "You will have to call someone to come get it. We can't let you keep it in your room."

42. The nurse is caring for a client with dyspnea. Which interventions can the nurse delegate to an unlicensed assistive personnel (UAP)? **Select all that apply.**

    1. assessing lung sounds

    2. checking a pulse oximetry

    3. administering oxygen via nasal cannula

    4. encouraging the client to cough and deep breathe

    5. showing the client how to use an incentive spirometer

43. The ED nurse is working in triage on a summer weekend. The following clients present at the same time. Which client does the nurse anticipate being seen **first**?

    1. a 58-year-old man with abdominal pain and nausea

    2. an infant with fever, a shrill cry, diarrhea, and nuchal rigidity

    3. a 38-year-old jogger who twisted her ankle, has a good pedal pulse, and has no deformity

    4. a 46-year-old client who was working outside and has tachypnea, diaphoresis, and fatigue

    5. an ambulatory child who fell off a bicycle and hit his head on grass while wearing a helmet

44. The charge nurse in the medical unit is preparing a bed assignment for a stable client diagnosed with necrotizing fasciitis. The client has a history of diabetes and hepatitis. There are four beds available. The nurse knows that the **best** roommate for this client is which of the following?

    1. a client with gout in the large toe

    2. a client with fever, vomiting, and diarrhea

    3. a client with MRSA

    4. a client with severe dementia with a tendency to wander

45. The nurse is caring for a client who is post-op day 1 for a coronary artery bypass graft (CABG). The nurse knows that continuity of care for this client is ensured by doing which of the following? **Select all that apply.**

    1. using standardized handoff reports

    2. knowing how to perform a chart check

    3. following up on outstanding lab reports and incomplete orders

    4. knowing the proper procedures to transfer clients to another floor

    5. telling the next shift that they will need to draw blood that was due on the current shift

46. The nurse reports to work and finds that a client from the previous day has been assigned to another nurse. The nurse had a great rapport with the client and wonders how he did during the night. She decides to look at the client's chart to read the progress notes. Which statement is correct regarding the nurse's actions?

    1. She should go to the client's room and see how he is doing.
    2. She has legal access to the client's chart since she was involved in his care.
    3. The nurse is violating HIPAA regulations and should not be accessing the client's chart.
    4. She should wait and ask the other nurse how the client is doing and not view the client's chart.

47. A nurse is talking to a nursing student about quality improvement and nurse-sensitive indicators. The nurse knows that the nursing student understands quality improvement when she identifies which to be nurse-sensitive indicators? **Select all that apply.**

    1. fall injury rates
    2. restraint utilization rates
    3. staying within the unit budget
    4. upgrading computer charting programs
    5. pressure ulcer prevalence and incidence
    6. client satisfaction with pain management

48. The nurse is charting on his client, who had an open appendectomy the previous day. Which are appropriate nursing documentation entries? **Select all that apply.**

    1. The client appeared anxious when several family members came to visit.
    2. The client appeared angry when the health care provider changed her medications.
    3. The client tolerated 80% of the lunch tray with no complaints of nausea or stomach cramping.
    4. The abdominal dressing is clean, dry, and intact with a 3-cm area of light staining noted in the center.
    5. The client ambulated 200 feet in the hall with a cane. No dyspnea or syncope noticed. Tolerated well.

49. The ED nurse has triaged a client who was in a severe motor vehicle accident. He is unconscious with fractures to the left femur and left humerus and ulna. CT also reveals a large amount of internal hemorrhaging. No identification was found on the client at the scene. What is the correct action by the nurse?

    1. prepare the client for emergency surgery
    2. try to obtain informed consent from a family member
    3. wait until the client is conscious, and then obtain the consent
    4. ask police to run the tag number so the client can be identified
    5. inform the health care provider that consent cannot be obtained at this time

50. The nurse notices an increase in the prevalence of deep vein thrombosis among clients in a surgical unit. The nurse collects data, develops a preventative program with peers, and works with her manager to implement a new policy and procedure. Which of the following **best** describes the nurse's actions?

    1. collaboration
    2. consultation
    3. informatics
    4. performance improvement

51. The nurse is caring for an elderly client with osteoporosis who has fractured her mid-shaft clavicle. Which nursing intervention would be included on the plan of care?

    1. immobilize the affected shoulder with a sling
    2. encourage weight-bearing exercise
    3. increase fluids to 1,500 cc/day
    4. prepare for surgical repair

52. The nurse is caring for a client admitted for right-sided renal artery stenosis. Where should the nurse anticipate auscultating for a renal bruit?

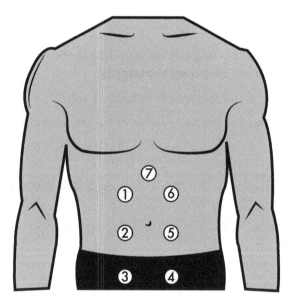

    1. right renal artery
    2. right iliac artery
    3. left renal artery
    4. left iliac artery

53. The school nurse is monitoring the diet of a child with celiac disease. What lunch menu item would the nurse recommend to the family?

   1. ham and cheese sandwich

   2. chef salad with oil and vinegar dressing

   3. chili with corn bread

   4. vegetarian pizza with lactose-free cheese

54. The role of the nurse as patient advocate is accurately identified in which of these statements?

   1. Nurses evaluate only the negative outcomes of patient advocacy.

   2. Nurses provide only physical and emotional support.

   3. Advocacy practices are limited to within health care settings.

   4. Nurses work with patients, their families, other health care team members and third-party persons.

55. Which statement concerning informed consent is false?

   1. Persons 17 years of age and younger may not give informed consent.

   2. A married minor may not give informed consent.

   3. A pregnant minor may give informed consent.

   4. An adult 18 years of age and older may give informed consent.

56. Identify the position in this diagram.

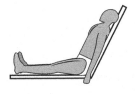

_____

57. Identify the position in this diagram.

_____

58. Identify the position in this diagram.

_____

59. Identify the position in this diagram.

_____

60. Identify the position in this diagram.

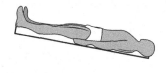

_____

61. Identify the position in this diagram.

_____

62. The nurse is talking with a client about primary and secondary prevention of cancer. Which statements are examples of primary prevention? **Select all that apply.**

1. removing colon polyps to prevent colon cancer

2. limiting alcohol to no more than 1 ounce per day

3. colonoscopy at age 50 years and then every 10 years

4. yearly mammogram for all women older than 40 years

5. getting vaccinated against human papilloma virus (HPV)

6. eating a low-fat diet high in fiber, including fruits and vegetables

63. The nurse is reviewing the facility's emergency preparedness plan. Which statement is true regarding emergency preparedness?

1. Nurses play supporting roles during and after a disaster or emergency.

2. The critical incident stress debriefing team analyzes what went wrong and what went right with the plan.

3. The administrative review meets with team members shortly after the event to promote effective coping strategies to staff.

4. Without stress management and intervention during and after an event, staff members are at risk of developing post-traumatic stress disorder (PTSD).

64. The nurse is educating a client on meningitis. Which statements would the nurse include in the teaching? **Select all that apply.**

1. The CDC recommends an initial vaccine at age 6 or upon entering first grade.

2. Immunocompromised clients and older adults are at increased risk of meningitis.

3. Viral meningitis is the most common type; typically, no organisms are isolated from CSF cultures.

4. Young preschool-age children have the highest rates of infection from life-threatening meningococcal infection.

5. A booster vaccine is given at age 11 or 12 to children living in crowded spaces, such as group homes or summer camps.

65. A nurse is preparing a sterile field for a client who is having a central venous catheter placed for IV therapy. Which action reflects a break in the sterile field?

1. The nurse uses sterile gloves to place objects on the sterile field.

2. The nurse stays near the sterile field at all times without turning away from it.

3. The nurse removes a sterile syringe from the sterile field using clean gloves but does not touch the sterile field itself.

4. The nurse opens a syringe, carefully peeling the wrapper away from the syringe without touching it so that it can be removed by a clinician wearing sterile gloves.

66. The nurse is caring for a client with limited mobility and right-sided paralysis. The nurse needs to pull the client up in the bed. Which statement reflects correct performance of this action?

    1. The nurse stands behind the head of the bed, places her hands under the client's axillae, and pulls him up.

    2. The nurse rolls the client to his left side, stands behind the head of the bed, and pulls the client up with the draw sheet.

    3. The nurse places the bed in the Trendelenburg position and alternates pulling on each side of the draw sheet, maneuvering the client up in the bed.

    4. The nurse calls for another nurse, places the client supine with arms folded across his chest, and each nurse pulls client up using both sides of the draw sheet at the same time.

67. The nurse sees a small fire in a trash can at the nurses' station. She retrieves the fire extinguisher. Which is the correct method to put out the fire?

    1. pull the pin, squeeze the handles, aim at the top of the fire, and sweep downward to contain the flames

    2. squeeze the handles firmly, aim hose at the top of the fire, and then spray downward in a sweeping motion until flames are extinguished

    3. pull the pin, aim hose at the outside of the trash can, and coat it thoroughly to contain the fire before spraying flames inside trash can

    4. pull the pin, aim the hose at the fire's base, squeeze the handles, and sweep from side to side slowly to ensure even coverage and extinguish flames

68. The nurse is preparing to administer Protonix 40 mg PO to a client. The medication dispenser system is out of the tablets, but the nurse realizes that he can override and pull out IV Protonix instead. The client has a patent IV, and the nurse decides this will save time instead of calling the pharmacy for the missing medication. Which of the six rights of medication administration has the nurse violated?

    1. right dose

    2. right time

    3. right route

    4. right patient

    5. right medication

    6. right documentation

69. The nurse is caring for a client with influenza. Which precautions would the nurse expect to be in place for this client?

    1. contact

    2. droplet

    3. airborne

    4. protective environment

70. A nurse is preparing to administer IV Rocephin for infection to a client. The client has a central venous line infusing blood but no other IV access. The blood still has 30 minutes left to infuse. The Rocephin is due now. How should the nurse proceed?

   1. hold the Rocephin since it will be too late to give it after the blood completes infusing
   2. draw up the Rocephin in a syringe after reconstitution and inject it into the blood bag so it can infuse with the blood
   3. stop the blood, flush the line with 0.9% NS, administer the Rocephin, and then flush the line with the NS before restarting blood
   4. allow the blood to finish infusing before giving Rocephin; the Rocephin will be administered during an acceptable time frame for "on time" administration

71. The nurse is setting up a room for an admission. Which equipment would the nurse remove from service and then notify maintenance? **Select all that apply.**

   1. a bed that is missing a rail but is still usable
   2. an IV pump with a current safety inspection sticker
   3. a rolling recliner with all wheels in the fully locked position
   4. a new extension cord for a radio that a previous client left behind
   5. a feeding pump with a frayed electrical cord and a current safety inspection sticker

72. The nurse is caring for a client who is paralyzed on the left side due to a stroke. The unlicensed assistive personnel (UAP) is assisting the nurse with a bed bath. Which action by the UAP requires intervention by the nurse?

   1. The UAP places dirty linen on the floor during the bed change.
   2. The UAP first washes his hands and dons gloves before beginning the bath.
   3. The UAP drapes the client for privacy and warmth during the course of the bath.
   4. The UAP asks the client if she needs to use the bedpan before beginning the bath.

73. The nurse is preparing to perform suctioning on a client with a tracheostomy who is not on a mechanical ventilator. Which of the following actions by the nurse are appropriate? **Select all that apply.**

   1. The nurse instills normal saline into the airway before suctioning.
   2. The nurse applies intermittent suction for 15 seconds while pulling the catheter straight out.
   3. The nurse hyperoxygenates the client with the manual resuscitation bag before suctioning.
   4. The nurse quickly inserts the catheter during inspiration until resistance is met or the client coughs.
   5. The nurse quickly inserts the catheter during expiration until resistance is met or the client coughs.
   6. The nurse applies intermittent suction for 10 seconds while rotating the catheter back and forth between the dominant thumb and forefinger.

74. The nurse has given a client an injection and then notes that the sharps container is full. Which is the correct action by the nurse?

 1. exchange the full container for a new one

 2. place the syringe on top of the container so it will not roll off

 3. force the syringe into the top of the container as well as it will fit

 4. put the syringe into her pocket and dispose of it in another room

75. The nurse is caring for a client with a left pneumothorax and a water-seal chest tube. Which of the following indicates a need for further action by the nurse? **Select all that apply.**

 1. The client is resting in a semi-Fowler's position.

 2. The client is resting in a Trendelenburg's position.

 3. The suction control chamber has constant gentle bubbling.

 4. Constant bubbling is present in the water seal after clamping off suction.

 5. Tidaling is present in the water seal chamber and corresponds to respiration.

76. The nurse is caring for a client who just returned from a supratentorial craniotomy, during which a large tumor was removed. Which of the following interventions by the nurse are appropriate for this client? **Select all that apply.**

 1. elevate the head of the bed 30 degrees

 2. elevate the head of the bed 90 degrees

 3. monitor neurological status every 2 hours

 4. monitor for signs of increased intracranial pressure

 5. apply antiembolism stockings to the client once he is alert

 6. turn the client every 2 hours from the operative side to the nonoperative side

77. The nurse is caring for a client with an internal cervical radiation implant. When performing morning care, the nurse notes the implant lying on the bed. Which nursing action should be done **first**?

 1. notify the health care provider

 2. apply gloves and attempt to reinsert the implant

 3. retrieve the implant with long-handled forceps and place into a lead container

 4. don a lead apron and retrieve the implant with long-handled forceps and place into a lead container

78. The nurse is supervising the unlicensed assistive personnel (UAP) while providing care for a client with an internal radioactive implant. Which action by the UAP requires immediate intervention by the nurse?

 1. The UAP assists the client in setting up the meal tray.

 2. The UAP wears a dosimeter badge while performing client care.

 3. The UAP closes the door to the room upon entering and exiting.

 4. The UAP places soiled linen in a laundry cart and takes it to the soiled utility area.

79. The nurse is preparing to administer metoprolol (Lopressor) to a new client. Which of the following actions by the nurse are correct? **Select all that apply.**

    1. hold for a heart rate greater than 80 bpm

    2. check the client's blood pressure and apical pulse

    3. check the client's allergies before giving any medications

    4. verify the client's identity using two patient identifiers

    5. tell the client not to take the medication with grapefruit juice

80. The nurse is caring for a client with Guillain-Barre syndrome. Due to paralysis, the client is unable to press the call button with his finger. The nurse must make accommodations for this client to be able to call for help. Which action by the nurse is correct?

    1. leave the client's door open and instruct him to yell loudly for help

    2. ask a family member to stay around the clock so she can call for the client

    3. round on the client as often as possible since there are no alternatives

    4. utilize a call light adapter that will allow the client to call for help by turning his head to activate a special button

81. A nurse is educating a group of student nurses about proper body mechanics to prevent injury to the nurse. Which of the following would the nurse include in her teaching?

    1. bend over from the waist to pick up objects

    2. hold weight as close to the body as possible when carrying something heavy

    3. when pulling a client up in bed, position the bed as low as possible to the floor

    4. try to lift clients with only one nurse to assist to avoid taking too many nurses off the floor

82. A nurse is preparing to start an IV on a client. Which action by the nurse increases the risk of infection in this client?

    1. The nurse washes his hands and applies gloves before starting the IV.

    2. After placing the IV, the nurse removes his gloves and washes his hands.

    3. The nurse prepares strips of tape to secure the IV and sticks them to the tray table.

    4. The nurse cleans the area with alcohol or another approved skin cleanser and allows it to dry.

83. The nurse is teaching a group of parents with infants and toddlers about poisoning. Which information would the nurse include in her teaching? **Select all that apply.**

    1. place all chemicals on a high shelf out of reach

    2. do not induce vomiting if the child is unconscious

    3. call the Poison Control Center before inducing vomiting

    4. keep the number of the Poison Control Center near the phone

    5. if the child ingests household cleaners or grease, induce vomiting

84. A home health nurse is visiting a client who is due for a dressing change for a diabetic foot ulcer. While at the client's home, the nurse notes open cleaning products sitting on the counter next to a plate of chicken. Which is the best response by the nurse?

    1. notify the health care provider about the hazardous conditions found in the client's home

    2. explain to the client that this situation is unsafe, then offer to check her home for other hazards she may not be aware of

    3. perform the dressing change without commenting on the chemicals, then notify social services to intervene

    4. do not say anything; the nurse is there to address the client's dressing change and not criticize the client's housekeeping

85. The nurse is teaching a family about safety from poisons. The nurse would include which statements in her teaching? **Select all that apply.**

    1. "If someone accidentally ingests poison, try to induce vomiting unless the person is unconscious."

    2. "If the person vomits, save the vomitus in case it is requested by the Poison Control Center or emergency department."

    3. "Post the phone number of the Poison Control Center near the phone if you have small children."

    4. "If the Poison Control Center recommends going to the hospital, drive as fast as you can safely do so."

    5. "Older adults are at risk of accidentally overdosing on prescription medications due to poor eyesight or memory loss."

86. A nurse in the emergency department is notified that several critically injured clients will be coming in following the collapse of a high-rise apartment building. Which action by the nurse is the **priority**?

    1. notify the charge nurse to call in extra staff

    2. activate the facility's emergency response plan

    3. check the crash cart supplies and restock extra items

    4. determine which current clients can be sent back to the waiting area

87. The nurse is preparing to review transmission-based precautions with other nurses on the unit. Which statement regarding transmission-based precautions would the nurse include in her teaching?

    1. "Measles and adenovirus require airborne precautions."

    2. "Barrier protection requires a private room for the client."

    3. "Droplet precautions are used for clients with meningitis."

    4. "Contact precautions are used for clients with disseminated varicella zoster."

88. A group of nurses are reviewing surgical asepsis. Which statement by one of the nurses requires further teaching on the topic?

   1. "Full-strength chlorhexidine will sterilize the skin."

   2. "The edges of a sterile field are considered unsterile."

   3. "If a sterile object touches an unsterile object, the sterile object is considered contaminated."

   4. "Sterile objects that are out of view or below waist level are considered unsterile."

   5. "Airborne microorganisms can contaminate sterile objects and make them unsterile."

89. The nurse is instructing a student nurse about proper donning and doffing of personal protective equipment (PPE). Which statement by the student nurse indicates an understanding of the order in which to apply PPE?

   1. "When removing PPE, gloves are removed last."

   2. "When removing PPE, the mask is removed before the gown."

   3. "The PPE should be applied just inside the door of the client's room."

   4. "The gown is put on first, then the gloves, then eye protection, and the mask last."

90. The nurse is caring for an elderly client with a history of Alzheimer's and falls. The nurse understands which to be the **priority** nursing diagnosis for this client?

   1. risk for injury

   2. impaired skin integrity

   3. altered body image due to confusion

   4. impaired physical mobility due to dementia with Lewy bodies

91. The nurse is preparing to administer an antihypertensive and an anticoagulant to a client. Which should the nurse do **first** before administering the medication?

   1. verify the client's allergies

   2. verify the client's name and room number

   3. ask the client to state her name and date of birth

   4. scan the client's wristband and medication barcode

   5. verify the client's name, date of birth, and medical record number with the medication order

92. The nurse is performing discharge teaching to a client who gave birth to her first child. Which statement by the client indicates a need for further teaching?

   1. "I will put my baby to sleep on her tummy."

   2. "My baby's first visit to the doctor should be 3 to 5 days after birth."

   3. "I should keep my baby in an approved car seat while riding in the car."

   4. "I will keep the numbers of my pediatrician and the poison control center handy."

93. Mix and Match: Match the transmission-based precaution used with a disease.

Disease	Precaution
1. measles	contact
2. shingles	droplet
3. tuberculosis	droplet
4. mumps	contact
5. diphtheria	airborne
6. influenza	contact
7. herpes simplex	airborne
8. C. diff	droplet
9. MRSA	airborne

HEALTH PROMOTION AND MAINTENANCE

94. The nurse is teaching the client about smoking cessation. Which client statement indicates a need for further teaching by the nurse?

  1. "Social smoking can still be detrimental to my health."

  2. "E-cigarettes can help me wean off nicotine so I can quit."

  3. "Pack years are calculated by my packs per day multiplied by the number of years I've smoked."

  4. "Nicotine replacement therapy along with a smoking cessation program is the most successful treatment."

95. The nurse educator is teaching a group of newly hired nurses about hospice and palliative care. Which statement by the group requires further clarification?

  1. "Palliative care is not limited by specific time periods."

  2. "Hospice clients have a prognosis of 6 months or less to live."

  3. "Palliative care begins when curative treatments have been stopped."

  4. "Hospice care is provided in 60- and 90-day periods and may continue if the client is eligible."

96. The nurse is teaching a client about dietary modifications to control hypertension. Which statement by the client indicates a need for further teaching?

  1. "I can have a cup of fresh fruit as a snack."

  2. "Baked ham is a good dinner choice for me."

  3. "I need to check the label for sodium in ketchup."

  4. "I need to cut out frozen pizza as a fast meal option."

97. The nurse is caring for a pregnant client at 24 weeks. The client voids before the nurse measures the fundal height. Which finding by the nurse would be expected in assessment of this client?

  1. a fundal height of 22 to 26 cm

  2. a fundal height of 27 to 30 cm

  3. a fundal height of 29 to 33 cm

  4. a fundal height of 31 to 34 cm

98. A mother brings her 6-month-old baby to the nurse practitioner for a routine well-baby check. Which behavior reported by the mother is concerning to the nurse?

  1. looks at self in a mirror

  2. brings things to mouth

  3. does not laugh or make squealing sounds

  4. begins to sit without support

99. The nurse is teaching an HIV-positive client who just delivered an HIV-positive full-term infant. Which statement by the client indicates a need for further teaching?

   1. "The antiviral medicines will cure my baby in about six months."
   2. "There is a low risk of my baby transmitting the virus to household members."
   3. "I should completely avoid breastfeeding my baby and purchase formula instead."
   4. "Pneumonia and herpes simplex are common secondary infections my baby may develop."

100. The nurse is caring for a client with morning sickness who is 8 weeks pregnant with her first child. What should the nurse advise the client to do to manage nausea?

   1. eat an omelet for breakfast to ensure adequate protein intake
   2. eat foods served warm with moderate amounts of spices
   3. consume most of the daily fluid intake early in the day
   4. brush the teeth immediately after eating; this helps get the food taste out that may trigger nausea

101. Using Naegele's Rule, calculate the estimated date of birth for a client who reports the first day of the last menstrual period was August 7.

   1. May 7
   2. May 14
   3. October 31
   4. November 14

102. The nurse is caring for a client diagnosed with syphilis. The client presents with a widespread, symmetric maculopapular rash on the palms and soles. The nurse understands that the client is in which stage of the infection?

   1. primary syphilis
   2. secondary syphilis
   3. early latent syphilis
   4. latent phase syphilis

103. The labor and delivery nurse expects which clients to be at high risk for amniotic fluid embolus (AFE)? **Select all that apply.**

   1. a 27-year-old client with preeclampsia
   2. a healthy 23-year-old anticipating a vaginal delivery
   3. a 42-year-old expecting her second child via cesarean section
   4. a 32-year-old client with diabetes anticipating induced labor

104. A nurse is preparing staff education on the developmental stages and milestones in a normally developing fetus. Which information should be included?

   1. The testes at the inguinal ring descend to scrotum at 12 weeks.

   2. The bladder and urethra separate from the rectum at 12 weeks.

   3. The kidneys are in position at 16 weeks with typical shape and plan.

   4. The nostrils reopen and primitive respiratory-like movement begins at 24 weeks.

105. The nurse is monitoring fetal heart rate (FHR) on a laboring client. Which finding should be reported to the health care provider?

   1. FHR of 154 bpm with moderate variability

   2. FHR of 114 bpm with moderate variability

   3. FHR of 170 bpm lasting more than 10 minutes

   4. FHR of 156 bpm with minimal variability in a premature infant

106. The nurse is teaching a new mother about postpartum fatigue (PPF). Which information would the nurse include?

   1. PPF is more common in women with cesarean births.

   2. Fatigue usually improves over the first 6 weeks after birth.

   3. Fatigue can help reduce the incidence of postpartum depression.

   4. Nursing mothers can minimize fatigue by breastfeeding in the side-lying position.

107. The nurse is caring for a client with myasthenia gravis (MG) who is 14 weeks pregnant. Which of the following does the nurse understand about MG in the pregnant client?

   1. Most women with MG tolerate labor poorly unless they are in excellent physical health.

   2. Approximately 25% to 30% of neonates born to women with MG develop neonatal myasthenia.

   3. MG usually goes into remission with younger clients and causes exacerbation in older clients.

   4. Narcotics must be used with caution due to the risk of respiratory depression in clients who are already at risk for respiratory muscle weakness.

108. The nurse is preparing to assess cranial nerve VIII on a client. Which tests will the nurse perform? **Select all that apply.**

   1. Allen's test

   2. Phalen's test

   3. the Rinne test

   4. the Weber test

109. Which client does the nurse recognize as having the highest increased risk of developing breast cancer?

    1. a 68-year-old client with dense breasts

    2. a 34-year-old client pregnant with her first child

    3. an obese client with a body mass index of 30

    4. a client with two first-degree relatives with breast cancer

110. A nurse on the oncology unit is preparing to care for a client newly diagnosed with small cell lung cancer. Which statements would the nurse include in client teaching? **Select all that apply.**

    1. "Avoid aspirin-based products to reduce the risk of bleeding."

    2. "Avoid crowds and report low-grade fever, sore throat, or chills."

    3. "Keep vaccinations current, including live vaccines, to promote wellness."

    4. "Use a soft toothbrush and electric razor to minimize the risk of bleeding."

    5. "Inspect the mouth regularly for sores and ulcers and rinse the mouth after meals."

111. The nurse is teaching a client the proper technique for using a cane. Which statements should the nurse include in the teaching? **Select all that apply.**

    1. "Hold the cane on the affected side."

    2. "Hold the cane on the unaffected side."

    3. "Move the cane at the same time as the affected leg."

    4. "Move the cane at the same time as the unaffected leg."

    5. "Hold the cane 8 to 10 inches from the side of the foot."

112. A nurse is caring for a client with dumping syndrome. Which statement by the client indicates a need for further teaching?

    1. "I should lie down after I eat my meals."

    2. "I may experience weakness and dizziness."

    3. "I should eat a low-fat, high-protein, low-carbohydrate diet."

    4. "I should eat small meals and avoid drinking fluids with my meals."

113. The nurse is precepting a student nurse on the medical-surgical unit who is caring for a client with a T-tube. Which statement by the student nurse regarding the care of the tube indicates a need for further teaching?

    1. "I should report a sudden increase in bile output."

    2. "The client should be in a semi-Fowler's position to promote drainage."

    3. "The drainage system should be kept below the level of the gallbladder."

    4. "I will clamp the tube if the client becomes nauseated or begins to vomit."

114. The nurse is caring for a client with a non-rebreather mask. Which is the **priority** nursing action when caring for this client?

   1. maintain the mask snugly on the face
   2. adjust flow rate to keep the reservoir bag inflated
   3. ensure that the reservoir bag is not kinked or twisted
   4. ensure that valves open during expiration and close on inhalation

115. The nurse is talking to a 67-year-old client who has just retired from the job he's had since age 17—the only job he's ever had. The nurse understands that the client is in which of Erikson's stages?

   1. intimacy versus isolation
   2. ego integrity versus despair
   3. identity versus role confusion
   4. generativity versus stagnation

116. A community health nurse is lecturing students at a nearby community college about high-risk behavior. Which of the following should the nurse include in the lecture?

   1. Suicide is the most common cause of death in this age group.
   2. Cancer is the third most common cause of death in this age group.
   3. Homicide is the second most common cause of death in this age group.
   4. College-age students are more likely to die from unintentional injuries.

117. A client's wife tells the nurse, "I can't believe my husband has high blood pressure. He feels fine. What caused this?" The nurse's response should include which of the following? **Select all that apply.**

   1. "One-third of people with high blood pressure are not aware of it."
   2. "Clients over 50 years of age are at the highest risk of hypertension."
   3. "Hypertension is more common in Hispanics and Native Americans."
   4. "Hypertension is more prevalent in the southeastern United States."
   5. "Your husband works at a desk job all day, so he does not get as much physical activity as he should."

118. A mother brings her 6-month-old child to the clinic for a wellness checkup. The nurse anticipates that the health care provider will order which vaccinations for this client?

   1. DTaP and MMR
   2. Hib and varicella
   3. hepatitis B and DTaP
   4. hepatitis A and MMR

119. The nurse is working with a client who has just been diagnosed with pancreatic cancer. The client says, "I have so much left to do. I'm too young to die like this." Which of the following stages of Kübler-Ross's five stages of grieving does the nurse recognize in this client?

    1. anger

    2. denial

    3. bargaining

    4. acceptance

    5. depression

120. The clinic nurse is talking to a client who has just been prescribed hormone replacement therapy (HRT). Which statement about HRT by the nurse is correct?

    1. "HRT decreases the risk of stroke."

    2. "HRT increases the risk of osteoporosis."

    3. "HRT decreases the risk of deep vein thrombosis."

    4. "HRT increases the risk of coronary artery disease."

121. The nurse is educating a client who is 10 weeks pregnant about prenatal nutrition. The client is of normal weight. Which statement by the client indicates an understanding of weight gain during pregnancy?

    1. "I should gain 15 to 20 pounds."

    2. "I should gain 25 to 35 pounds."

    3. "I should gain 35 to 40 pounds."

    4. "I should gain 40 to 45 pounds."

122. The labor and delivery nurse notes that the health care provider has rated a newborn's Apgar score as 9. The nurse understands which to be true regarding Apgar scores?

    1. The optimum score is 10.

    2. A baby with poor activity would rate a 1 in that area.

    3. The highest score that each factor may receive is 3.

    4. Scores are obtained 5 minutes after birth and repeated 5 minutes later.

123. The nurse is discussing developmental stages with the mother of a six-month-old infant. Which statement indicates an unexpected deviation from normal development?

    1. The infant is walking alone by 15 months.

    2. The infant waves good-bye by 7 months.

    3. The infant rolls from the tummy to the side at 12 months.

    4. The infant transfers a toy from one hand to the other at age 9 months.

124. The nurse is teaching a 28-year-old male client about testicular cancer. Which statement by the client indicates understanding of the nurse's teaching?

   1. "Testicular cancer is one of the hardest cancers to treat and cure."

   2. "Testicular cancer is the most common cancer in men ages 25 – 35."

   3. "A lump larger than a quarter should be reported to my health care provider."

   4. "The best time to perform testicular self-examination is just after bathing because the scrotum is more relaxed."

125. The nurse is performing an admission assessment on a client. The client states that she has been smoking two packs of cigarettes a day for 20 years. The nurse would chart how many pack years for this client?

   1. 10 pack years

   2. 20 pack years

   3. 30 pack years

   4. 40 pack years

126. The nurse is providing teaching to a client newly diagnosed with hypertension. The nurse knows that the client understands the teaching when the client selects which menu option?

   1. frozen pizza and a spinach salad

   2. baked chicken with fresh green beans

   3. a ham sandwich with peas and carrots

   4. a can of chicken soup and a grilled cheese sandwich

127. The nurse is participating in a free community health screening with a group of student nurses. Which statement by a student nurse requires further teaching by the licensed nurse?

   1. "Colorectal cancer screening should begin at age 50."

   2. "Men should have a prostate-specific antigen test starting at age 55."

   3. "High-density lipoprotein should be greater than 50 mg/dL for women."

   4. "Risk factors for hypertension include being over age 60 and leading a sedentary lifestyle."

128. The nurse is teaching a newly diagnosed client about Crohn's disease. The nurse understands which barriers may prevent effective client learning? **Select all that apply.**

   1. language barriers

   2. motivation to learn

   3. lack of a support system

   4. adequate financial resources

   5. cognitive dysfunction, such as schizophrenia

129. The nurse is conducting a health fair at a local high school on reducing high-risk behaviors. Which teaching should the nurse include in the presentation? **Select all that apply.**

   1. Always buckle up, even for a short trip.
   2. Use approved bike helmets for bike riding.
   3. Do not drive for one hour after drinking alcohol.
   4. Condoms offer full protection against sexually transmitted infections.
   5. Dive into untested waters with the hands fully extended over the head.

130. A first-time parent is discussing developmental milestones with a nurse. The nurse tells the client she can reasonably expect her child to achieve which of the following by the time the child is 2 years old?

   1. is left-hand dominant
   2. clings to caregivers in new situations
   3. walks with assistance of another
   4. says several single words

131. The nurse is teaching a group of student nurses about principles of teaching. Which statement by a student nurse requires further instruction from the licensed nurse?

   1. "A client's living situation can affect his readiness and ability to learn."
   2. "The client's age and developmental stage must be considered when teaching clients."
   3. "Tactile or kinesthetic learners prefer to learn by watching a video or reading a handout."
   4. "I should allow clients to demonstrate their understanding of what they have learned and practice skills."
   5. "Some barriers to learning include financial resources, lack of support systems, and a low level of literacy."

132. The nurse is reviewing the medication history for a 24-year-old client in the fertility clinic. Which medication does the nurse understand to be a Category X medication in pregnancy?

   1. metformin
   2. amoxicillin
   3. gabapentin
   4. simvastatin

133. A community health nurse is preparing a lecture on lifestyle and risk factors for a college-age audience. The nurse understands that which causes of death are the most common among this age group?

   1. HIV, suicide, unintentional injuries
   2. suicide, cancer, unintentional injuries
   3. suicide, unintentional injuries, homicide
   4. homicide, unintentional injuries, heart disease

134. The nurse is caring for a client who is 38 weeks pregnant and plans to breastfeed. This is the client's first child, and she expresses concern about lactation. The nurse tells the client that which measures stimulate lactation? **Select all that apply.**

   1. breast massage
   2. frequent breastfeeding
   3. pumping breasts between feedings
   4. vigorous exercise one week after birth
   5. applying cold compresses to the breasts

135. A nurse is preparing to talk about hormone replacement therapy (HRT) to a group of women at a women's fair at the local hospital. Which statements regarding HRT are correct? **Select all that apply.**

   1. HRT decreases the risk of breast cancer.
   2. HRT decreases the risk of stroke in postmenopausal women.
   3. HRT lowers the risk of bone fractures caused by osteoporosis.
   4. HRT increases the risk of bone fractures caused by osteoporosis.
   5. HRT decreases the risk of coronary artery disease (CAD) in women who do not smoke.

136. A pediatric nurse in an ambulatory care clinic is admitting a neonate for the 2-week office visit. Which comment by the mother should alert the nurse to suspect colic?

   1. "My baby looks yellow."
   2. "After feedings, my baby pulls his legs up and cries."
   3. "My baby is quiet and doesn't cry much."
   4. "My baby is alert for brief periods of 10 – 20 minutes at a time."

137. A normal, healthy 35-year-old male client visits the doctor's office for a routine annual physical. When auscultating between the first and second interspaces on the anterior chest, the nurse anticipates which type of breath sound?

   1. bronchovesicular
   2. vesicular
   3. bronchial
   4. tracheal

138. A mother infected with hepatitis B asks the nurse about the possibility of breastfeeding her neonate. Which response by the nurse would be **most** appropriate?

   1. "Yes, breastfeeding is an acceptable option."
   2. "No, you should not breastfeed your baby."
   3. "Yes, breastfeeding is an acceptable option once your baby is immunized with the hepatitis B vaccine."
   4. "Bottled formula is just as nutritious for your baby."

PSYCHOSOCIAL INTEGRITY

139. A client is discussing her problematic marital relationship with the nurse. Which statement by the nurse is an example of the nontherapeutic communication technique of giving reassurance?

    1. "I think you should try marital counseling. I've had to do that myself once and it helped."

    2. "Why don't you see a conflict resolution specialist? I can give you that information."

    3. "I agree with you. He should not argue with you when he has problems at work that are not your fault."

    4. "Everything will be okay if you talk to him about how it makes you feel."

140. The nurse is caring for a client with a history of schizophrenia. The nurse asks the client if he is ready to eat his lunch. The client responds, "Rain, train, down the drain, Jane's brain." The nurse recognizes this type of speech pattern as which type?

    1. echolalia

    2. word salad

    3. neologisms

    4. clang association

141. The nurse is talking to a group of student nurses about content of thought in clients with schizophrenia. The nurse gives an example of a client stating that her new tooth filling allows her to communicate with the Secret Service and follow their directives. Which response correctly identifies this content of thought?

    1. somatic delusion

    2. delusion of grandeur

    3. delusion of persecution

    4. delusion of control or influence

142. A 79-year-old client with moderate dementia and limited mobility is being cared for at home by her son who lives with her. She has been receiving home health for care of a nonhealing diabetic foot ulcer. The home health nurse encourages the son to bring his mother to the ED for more aggressive treatment in an in-patient setting. The son responds that he cannot afford to pay for the medical bills and prefers to care for her at home. The nurse then notices a stage 2 decubitus ulcer on the client's sacrum. The son claims to have his sister come every day and assist with bathing and turning in the bed. Which type of violence is the son guilty of?

    1. physical neglect

    2. physical violence

    3. emotional violence

    4. economic exploitation

143. The nurse is caring for a client scheduled to receive electroconvulsive therapy (ECT). Which is the **priority** nursing action while caring for this client during the treatment?

   1. monitor the airway and be prepared to provide suction if needed

   2. continuously observe vital signs and cardiac function on the monitor

   3. provide support and safe positioning to the client's arms and legs during the seizure

   4. record the type, frequency, duration, and amount of movement induced by the seizure

144. The nurse is caring for a client for whom English is a second or other language and who is very reluctant to disclose personal information. Which statement reflects an understanding of culturally or socially competent care for this specific client?

   1. Making direct eye contact with the client may be viewed as disrespectful.

   2. Care and activities should be scheduled around designated prayer times whenever possible.

   3. The patient may be undocumented, fearful of disclosing his or her status, and therefore cautious in institutional settings.

   4. The patient may not be well educated.

145. The nurse is caring for a client diagnosed with bipolar disorder. During the morning assessment, the client tells the nurse that she hears people in the room behind her bed talking about her. Which response by the nurse **best** reflects therapeutic communication?

   1. "What do you hear them saying?"

   2. "I will see if we can move you to another room."

   3. "I will notify your doctor in case he wants to change your medications."

   4. "I understand that the voices seem real to you, but I don't see or hear anyone else in here."

146. A nurse on the mental health unit is preparing a presentation on suicide for a group of student nurses. Which information would be included in this presentation? **Select all that apply.**

   1. Chronic pain or serious, disabling illness has little to no effect on suicide risk.

   2. Hispanic Americans attempt suicide at a greater rate than whites or African Americans.

   3. Suicide risk declines sharply once antidepressant medication has been taken for a few weeks.

   4. White males over the age of 80 are at the greatest risk among all age, race, and gender groups.

   5. Threatened suicide and/or gestures should be taken seriously and handled by trained professionals.

147. The nurse is caring for a client who is taking tricyclic antidepressants. Which statement by the client indicates that the medication is working properly?

  1. "I haven't felt like going to work this week."
  2. "I've joined a bridge club in my neighborhood."
  3. "I sleep 12 hours a night and take a nap during the day."
  4. "I have felt my heart racing since I started the medicine."

148. The ED nurse is caring for a female client who was just brought in following a sexual assault. Which interventions by the nurse are appropriate for this client? **Select all that apply.**

  1. help the client bathe and change into fresh clothing before the examination begins
  2. preserve any evidence, including clothing, and take photographs of injuries as appropriate
  3. assure the client that surviving the assault is most important, and she did what was needed to stay alive
  4. take the client to a quiet, private room for assessment to assess stress levels before beginning examination or treatments
  5. tell the client that she should avoid wearing skimpy clothing in questionable areas of the city to avoid another incident

149. A nurse has admitted a client to the mental health unit following an attempted suicide. The client also attempted suicide four months earlier. Which is the **best** way to ensure client safety?

  1. give the client a task to do, such as folding towels, to distract him
  2. assign a staff member to remain with the client one-on-one at all times
  3. obtain an order for chemical and physical restraints to be used as needed
  4. keep the client in the day room around other clients who can help watch the client
  5. place the client in isolation after removing potentially unsafe articles, such as shoelaces and belts

150. The nurse is caring for a client who is a victim of domestic violence. Which of the following would the nurse expect to find in the client's social history? **Select all that apply.**

  1. The client is under 30 years old.
  2. The client is active in a local charity.
  3. The client has a history of child abuse.
  4. The client has been in past abusive relationships.
  5. The client is employed as a college professor.

151. The nurse is caring for a client who presented to the ED with a blood alcohol level of 208 mg/dL. The client states that his last drink was about 8 hours ago. He exhibits coarse tremors of the hands, anxiety, and elevated blood pressure. Which of the following would the nurse expect if his condition progresses to withdrawal delirium? **Select all that apply.**

1. fever of 100°F to 103°F

2. increased appetite, especially for sweets

3. excessive sleeping of 14 hours or more daily

4. onset of delirium 12 to 24 hours after the last drink

5. onset of delirium 48 to 72 hours after the last drink

6. disorientation and fluctuating levels of consciousness

152. The nurse in a mental health facility is teaching a group of student nurses about schizophrenia. Which is true regarding the phases of schizophrenia? **Select all that apply.**

1. The average length of the prodromal phase in most clients is from 2 to 5 years.

2. Clients in the premorbid phase tend to do well in school and have more outgoing personalities early in the disorder.

3. In the active phase of schizophrenia, physiological causes such as drug abuse or a medical condition must be considered as a cause.

4. During the residual phase, negative symptoms can remain and the client commonly has a flat affect and impaired role functioning.

5. During the prodromal phase, treatment includes family interventions to improve coping, cognitive therapy, and therapeutic support for identified problems.

153. The nurse is caring for an elderly female client who presents as being alert and oriented. In the late afternoon, the client becomes extremely agitated and confused. Which of the following responses by the nurse is **most** appropriate?

1. call a family member to come and stay with the client

2. call the health care provider and ask for an order for Xanax

3. reorient the client and offer distraction and reassurance in a soft voice

4. tell the client that if she does not cooperate, she will be placed in restraints

154. The nurse is caring for a teenage client diagnosed with anorexia nervosa. The client's mother asks the nurse about eating disorders in general. Which information would the nurse provide? **Select all that apply.**

1. Anorexia nervosa is more common than bulimia.

2. Clients with bulimia may have erosion of the tooth enamel.

3. Binging and purging can occur in both anorexia nervosa and bulimia.

4. Extreme exercising and calorie restriction is common with anorexia nervosa.

5. Clients with eating disorders may develop the disorders because of issues of power and control.

6. Clients with anorexia have a distorted body image and think that they are fat even if they are very thin.

155. The nurse is seeing a client in the clinic with her 18-month-old daughter. The client asks the nurse when her child should start going to the dentist. Which response by the nurse is correct?

    1. "She should go by her first birthday."
    2. "She should start receiving oral exams at 2 years of age."
    3. "She should go to a dentist once a year beginning at age 3."
    4. "You don't need to worry about it until she starts kindergarten."

156. The nurse is caring for a client in the psychiatric unit who has issues with coping and defense mechanisms. The nurse understands that which is true regarding coping and defense mechanisms? **Select all that apply.**

    1. Coping mechanisms are destructive ways to avoid dealing with reality.
    2. Physical symptoms, general irritability, and self-destructive behaviors are some of the signs of inadequate coping.
    3. Criticizing ineffective defense mechanisms will guide the client toward better coping techniques.
    4. Ineffective coping mechanisms allow anxiety to increase, triggering the client to utilize defense mechanisms in order to protect himself from the anxiety.
    5. The inability to cope can be caused by a lack of an adequate support system, a serious medical diagnosis, situational crises, or a lack of psychological resources.

157. The nurse is caring for a client whose family brought him to the hospital because they were worried about his personal safety. Which of the following statements by the client during the admission assessment indicates the need for immediate intervention by the nurse?

    1. "Things are so bad that sometimes I don't know what to do make them better."
    2. "My family normally supports my goals and helps me when I have a difficult time."
    3. "I wish that everyone would leave me alone and quit trying to give me advice all the time."
    4. "I keep a gun in my nightstand and sometimes I fall asleep holding it, trying to decide if I should pull the trigger or not."

158. The nurse is caring for a client with schizophrenia who is having active hallucinations. The nurse implements which actions to manage the client during the episode? **Select all that apply.**

    1. administers medications as ordered
    2. uses gentle touch to reassure the client
    3. tells the client that others see or hear what he does
    4. distracts the client by placing him in the dayroom with others
    5. asks the client if he hears voices telling him to harm himself or others
    6. goes along with what the client says to decrease the risk of increasing the client's anxiety

159. A client suffering from visual hallucinations calls the nurse to her room and says, "You need to hurry up and kill all these bugs on the wall before they get on me." Which response by the nurse is **most** appropriate?

1. "Why don't you lay down and take a nap?"

2. "I don't see them. Can you show me where they are?"

3. "I will call maintenance and have them come take care of this right away."

4. "I know the bugs seem real to you, but I don't see anything on the walls."

160. The nurse is in the dayroom of the psychiatric unit observing the clients. Which client behavior would the nurse interpret as exhibiting inadequate coping?

1. A client is sitting in a chair coloring in a coloring book.

2. A client is arguing about a TV program with another client.

3. A client is playing a new card game with a group for the first time.

4. A client is in the corner alone, rocking and pulling out her eyelashes.

161. The nurse is working in a mental health facility that uses group therapy with the clients. The nurse understands which to be correct regarding group therapy?

1. The termination stage begins with the initial group meeting.

2. Members' feelings about their accomplishments are explored in the working stage.

3. During the working stage, members may be unclear about the purpose of the group.

4. Group roles and responsibilities are established in the working stage of group therapy.

162. The nurse is admitting a client with schizophrenia. The client is extremely socially withdrawn, is unable to perform activities of daily living, has an inappropriate affect, and has grimacing mannerisms. The nurse understands that this client is experiencing which type of schizophrenia?

1. residual schizophrenia

2. paranoid schizophrenia

3. catatonic schizophrenia

4. disorganized schizophrenia

5. undifferentiated schizophrenia

163. A client is having a panic attack. Which nursing intervention has priority for this client?

1. have the client recount a positive childhood memory

2. provide the client with a glass of water

3. tell the client to take deep breaths

4. ask the client to identify the source of his anxiety

164. The nurse is precepting a new nurse in the psychiatric unit. The nurse is discussing interventions for schizophrenia. Which statement by the student nurse indicates an understanding of management of schizophrenia? **Select all that apply.**

    1.   "I should be warm and friendly to put the client at ease."

    2.   "I can reassure the client that he is in a safe environment."

    3.   "Puzzles or word games are good activities to engage in."

    4.   "I can help the client use art or writing to express his feelings."

    5.   "I won't tell the client when I'm leaving him so he won't get upset."

165. The mental health nurse is caring for a client with Cluster B personality disorder. The nurse would expect the client to exhibit which behaviors? **Select all that apply.**

    1.   suspicious of others, magical thinking, eccentric behavior, paranoia, relationship deficits

    2.   preoccupation with rules and details, hoarding, ritualistic behavior, extremely devoted to work

    3.   easily bored, poor and shallow interpersonal relationships, enjoys being the center of attention

    4.   impulsivity, unpredictable behavior, extreme mood shifts, easily angered, playing people against each other

    5.   suspicious and untrusting of others, argumentative, controlling of others, thoughts of grandiosity

166. The nurse suspects a client is experiencing alcohol withdrawal syndrome. Which action is **most** appropriate?

    1.   record suspicions in the medical record

    2.   question the family about his drinking

    3.   notify the physician

    4.   ask the client about his drinking

167. A client is suspected of having posttraumatic stress disorder. Which problem is the **most** important for the nurse to assess?

    1.   panic attacks

    2.   anorexia

    3.   suicide

    4.   short-term memory loss

168. The nurse is caring for a client whose cultural background is different from her own. Which nursing action is appropriate?

    1.   understand that fear of death is universal

    2.   know that dietary habits are equally important to all cultures

    3.   respect the client's cultural beliefs

    4.   explain the nurse's cultural beliefs to the client

169. The nurse discovers a hospice client has expired. The family members are assembled in the facility's waiting room. Which of the following statements by the nurse would be the **most** appropriate?

    1. "My condolences on the passing of your family member. You may visit him if you wish."

    2. "I will give you some time to spend with your loved one. Let me know if you need anything."

    3. "You should view your loved one as a way of saying farewell."

    4. "It would be best if you not view your loved one just yet."

170. A 17-year-old female with a self-admitted opioid addiction is seen by the nurse in a mental health clinic. Which intervention would the nurse **not** consider in establishing a therapeutic relationship?

    1. discuss the impact of substance use

    2. require the client to attend all therapy sessions

    3. explore alternative approaches to managing stress

    4. assess the presence of other psychiatric disorders

171. A nurse is caring for a client with agoraphobia. Which signs and symptoms would the nurse anticipate? **Select all that apply.**

    1. panic attacks

    2. impaired short-term memory

    3. auditory hallucinations

    4. inability to leave home

172. The nurse is caring for a client who has been diagnosed with terminal pancreatic cancer. The family is asking what to expect when the end draws near. Which response by the nurse is **most** appropriate?

    1. "I will have the doctor talk to you about that."

    2. "The hospice nurse is the best person to answer your questions. I can put in a consult for you."

    3. "Don't worry about that right now. You don't know if there is another treatment option that will work."

    4. "I can tell you what to look for when the time comes. In the meantime, what are your wishes and goals for care?"

173. The nurse is educating a group of student nurses about perceived loss. The nurse knows that the students understand when one of them verbalizes which example?

    1. a single mother loses her job

    2. a student fails his college chemistry class

    3. a husband is grieving the loss of his wife of 40 years

    4. a first-time mother is disappointed that she had a boy instead of a girl

174. The nurse is teaching a group of women at a community center about risk factors for spousal abuse. Which would the nurse identify as risk factors? **Select all that apply.**

   1. alcohol or drug use
   2. low income or poverty
   3. being over the age of 40
   4. a higher level of education
   5. having a large circle of friends
   6. pregnancy, especially if it is unplanned

175. During the nurse's shift in the emergency department, a nurse assesses a client who is suspected of being under the influence of opioids. Which symptom is indicative of opioid use?

   1. hypotension
   2. diaphoresis
   3. shallow respirations
   4. outbursts of anger

176. A client is prescribed diazepam (Valium) as needed to control the symptom of alcohol withdrawal. Which symptom may indicate the need for the nurse to administer phenytoin (Dilantin) to supplement the effect of Valium?

   1. disturbed heart rate
   2. hallucinations
   3. drowsiness
   4. seizures

177. The nurse is assessing a client who is a polysubstance abuser, with fentanyl being one of the drugs most frequently used. Which physiological symptoms are suggestive of fentanyl intoxication? **Select all that apply.**

   1. diarrhea
   2. nausea
   3. urge to urinate
   4. anxiety

178. A client is telling the nurse about his perception of his thought patterns. Which of the following statements by the client would validate the diagnosis of bipolar disorder?

   1. "Sometimes I'm ready to take on the world, but other times I'm too tired to get out of bed."
   2. "I need to check and then recheck all the kitchen appliances several times to make sure they are off before I feel comfortable leaving my home."
   3. "My neighbors hold sacrificial rites in their backyard."
   4. "I keep on patrol all night so the enemy won't invade my home and hurt me or my family."

PHYSIOLOGICAL INTEGRITY—BASIC CARE AND COMFORT

179. The nurse is providing dietary instruction to a client with diabetes who has normal kidney function. Which statement by the client requires intervention by the nurse?

    1. "I should limit cholesterol intake to 200 mg/day."

    2. "I should eat very low or no carbohydrates when possible."

    3. "My protein intake should be 15% to 20% of my daily calories."

    4. "Fiber will improve my carbohydrate metabolism and lower cholesterol."

180. A client with gastroesophageal reflux disease (GERD) is talking to the nurse about ways to manage her condition. Which statement reflects an understanding of management of GERD?

    1. "I can elevate the head of my bed 6 to 12 inches to help prevent nighttime reflux."

    2. "I can eat a large breakfast and smaller meals for lunch and dinner to help me feel better."

    3. "Lying on my left side will promote oxygenation and frequent swallowing to help clear my esophagus."

    4. "I should take liquid antacids to coat my esophagus and buffer acid 2 hours before I eat and 1 hour after meals."

181. The nurse is caring for a client who adheres to a lacto-vegetarian diet. Which meal tray would the nurse deliver to the client?

    1. chicken sandwich, brown rice, yogurt, and milk

    2. steamed vegetables with rice and apple slices

    3. scrambled eggs, cottage cheese, dry toast, and milk

    4. baked zucchini, spinach salad with cheese, and yogurt

182. The nurse is caring for a client who just returned from an above-the-knee amputation of the left leg. Which position should the nurse place the client in?

    1. supine, with the affected limb flat on the bed

    2. supine, with a wedge pillow between the thighs

    3. supine, with the affected limb elevated on a pillow

    4. on the left side with the head of the bed at 30 degrees

183. A client has orders for placing a nasogastric tube. In which position should the nurse place the client for insertion?

    1. low Fowler's

    2. high Fowler's

    3. reverse Trendelenburg's

    4. on the side opposite of the nare used for insertion

184. The nurse is assisting the health care provider performing a liver biopsy on a client. How should the nurse position this client? **Select all that apply.**

1. position the client supine with the left upper abdomen exposed
2. position the client supine with the right upper abdomen exposed
3. position the client in a low Fowler's with the right upper abdomen exposed
4. raise the client's right arm and extend it behind the head, over the left shoulder
5. raise the client's right arm and extend it across the front of the chest touching the left shoulder

185. The unit nurse is precepting a nursing student who is assisting a client with a femur fracture onto a fracture bedpan. Which action by the student nurse requires intervention by the unit nurse? **Select all that apply.**

1. The student nurse tries to lift the client onto the bedpan.
2. The student nurse positions the head of the bed between 30 and 45 degrees.
3. The student nurse places the call light within reach and tells the client she will return shortly.
4. The student nurse places the bedpan with the shallow end under the buttocks toward the sacrum.
5. The student nurse places the bedpan with the deeper end under the buttocks toward the sacrum.

186. The nurse is caring for a client who just had a laparoscopic appendectomy. The client tells the nurse that she does not want "drugs" for pain management, but prefers alternative therapy and/or complementary therapy. Which is the **best** response by the nurse?

1. "I know of some herbs and supplements that you can take to manage the pain."
2. "Tell me what works for you, and I will see what we can provide for your comfort."
3. "We use real medicine here in the hospital, so I will bring you hydrocodone for pain when you need it."
4. "Yoga always relaxes me. I will get you a foam mat from physical therapy so you can practice when you want."

187. The nurse is caring for a client with fluid overload who is on strict I's and O's. The nurse understands that which is the **best** way to ensure accurate I's and O's?

1. clear any IV pumps and reset to zero for accurate IV fluid intake
2. ask the client to keep up with how many cups of fluid he drinks at meals
3. ask the client to report how much urine is in the urinal each time he uses it
4. tell the client not to ask for any extra water or drinks that are not on the meal tray

188. A client has just returned from a cardiac catheterization with access via the femoral artery. Which position or activity should the nurse anticipate the health care provider will order for this client?

    1. bed rest with bathroom privileges

    2. bed rest with head of bed at 45 degrees

    3. ambulation to prevent blood clot formation

    4. bed rest with head of bed at 30 degrees or less

    5. up to chair with assistance if the client is steady on his feet

189. Mix and Match: Match the nursing intervention to the pulmonary disorder.

Pulmonary Disorder	Nursing Intervention
1. emphysema	hydration of at least 2L/day to thin and loosen pulmonary secretions
2. asthma	teach controlled coughing
3. cystic fibrosis	prevent spread of infection to others
4. chronic bronchitis	identify and minimize pulmonary irritants
5. pneumonia	teach diaphragmatic, pursed-lip breathing
6. influenza	provide frequent mouth care to reduce chances of infection from mucus being present
7. pulmonary embolus	monitor drainage from chest tube system
8. pneumothorax	monitor for right-sided heart failure

190. Mix and Match: Match the nursing intervention to the endocrine disorder.

Endocrine Disorder	Nursing Intervention
1. tumor posterior pituitary gland	measure urine specific gravity
2. hypoparathyroidism	monitor airway
3. Addison's disease	instruct on high-sodium, low-potassium diet
4. Cushing's disease	instruct on low-sodium, high-potassium diet

191. Mix and Match: Match the nursing intervention to the location of injury to the portion of the client's brain.

Injured Brain Area	Nursing Intervention
1. frontal lobe	assist with ADL due to visual disturbances
2. temporal lobe	assist with walking
3. occipital lobe	monitor vital signs
4. brain stem	give simple instructions; reorient as needed
5. parietal lobe	provide simple, one-step instructions
6. cerebellum	speak clearly due to impaired hearing

PHYSIOLOGICAL INTEGRITY— PHARMACOLOGICAL AND PARENTERAL THERAPIES

192. The nurse is caring for an elderly client who has been taking cimetidine (Tagamet) for a year. The nurse should monitor for which central nervous system side effects? **Select all that apply.**

1. tetany
2. agitation
3. confusion
4. constipation
5. disorientation

193. The nurse is caring for a client scheduled to receive cyclopentolate HCl preoperatively. Which finding in the client's history would prompt the nurse to notify the health care provider?

1. osteoporosis
2. hypothyroidism
3. renal insufficiency
4. cardiac dysrhythmias

194. The nurse is providing discharge teaching to a client who has been prescribed prednisone. The nurse instructs the client to report which symptom to the health care provider?

1. increased appetite
2. anxiety or confusion
3. strong, bounding pulses
4. weight gain of 3 pounds

195. A client with asthma has orders for terbutaline. Which finding in the medical history would the nurse be **most** concerned about?

1. diabetes
2. migraines
3. osteoarthritis
4. coronary artery disease

196. The nurse is caring for a client with multiple IV medications. Which of the following drugs are compatible?

1. vancomycin and heparin
2. nitroglycerin and dopamine
3. sodium bicarbonate and dobutamine
4. furosemide (Lasix) and ondansetron (Zofran)

197. The nurse is preparing to administer pilocarpine hydrochloride eye drops to a client with glaucoma. Which is the correct technique to administer eye drops? **Select all that apply.**

   1. instruct the client to tilt the head back and look up
   2. pull the upper lid up and place the drops just above the pupil
   3. pull the lower lid down and place the drop into the conjunctival sac
   4. to instill multiple drops, wait 3 to 5 minutes between drops to allow maximum absorption
   5. instruct the client to close the eyes and gently rub the eyelids to ensure maximum absorption

198. The nurse is teaching a client about alendronate sodium (Fosamax). Which statement by the client indicates a need for further teaching?

   1. "I should take this with a meal."
   2. "I will call my doctor if I develop a fever."
   3. "I should not lie down for at least 30 minutes."
   4. "Dairy products reduce the absorption of this medicine."

199. The ED nurse admits a client with second-degree burns to the arms and third-degree burns to the legs. Based on the Parkland formula, which IV fluid would the nurse anticipate for this client during the first 24 hours?

   1. D5W
   2. colloid solutions
   3. crystalloid solutions
   4. 5% albumin in isotonic saline

200. A 12-year-old client has new orders for amphetamine and dextroamphetamine (Adderall) for attention-deficit/hyperactivity disorder. The nurse should alert the client's caregivers about which adverse effect?

   1. nausea
   2. seizures
   3. weight gain
   4. constipation

201. A client with suspected vitamin C toxicity presents to the ED. Which manifestations of toxicity would the nurse expect in this client? **Select all that apply.**

   1. muscle weakness
   2. halos around objects
   3. occult rectal bleeding
   4. dry mucous membranes
   5. increased estrogen levels

202. The nurse is working in the mental health unit and is educating a group of student nurses about atypical antipsychotics. Which statement by one of the student nurses requires further teaching about this class of drugs?

1. "These drugs can cause bradycardia."

2. "This class of drugs can cause diabetes."

3. "Weight gain and obesity are side effects of these drugs."

4. "Rarely, neuroleptic malignant syndrome can occur and may be fatal."

203. The nurse is preparing to administer a calcium channel blocker to a client with hypertension. The nurse understands that the mechanism of action of these drugs is to

1. cause vasodilation and increase total peripheral resistance.

2. cause vasodilation and decrease total peripheral resistance.

3. cause vasoconstriction and decrease total peripheral resistance.

4. cause vasoconstriction and increase total peripheral resistance.

204. The charge nurse is working with a student nurse who reports that her assigned client has severe flushing of the upper body following an IV antibiotic infusion. The charge nurse understands that the antibiotic likely responsible for this "red man syndrome" is which medication?

1. cephalexin

2. amoxicillin

3. gentamicin

4. vancomycin

205. The nurse is educating a client who is newly diagnosed with angina about his newly prescribed nitroglycerin. The nurse understands that teaching is effective when the client makes which statement?

1. "It is safe to take one dose of nitroglycerin if I am taking sildenafil."

2. "I should chew up three tablets at once, and then call 9-1-1 if I still have chest pain in 15 minutes."

3. "I can take up to three tablets, 5 minutes apart, under my tongue as needed for chest pain."

4. "I can keep the pills in a glass cup on my nightstand so I can reach them easily in an emergency."

206. A client is ordered to receive 1,000 ml of D5W over 6 hours. The infusion set administers 10 gtt/mL. At what rate (gtt/min) should the nurse set the flow?

1. 24 gtt/min

2. 26 gtt/min

3. 28 gtt/min

4. 30 gtt/min

207. The nurse is caring for a client who presents with increased ammonia levels, elevated BUN, and altered mental status. Which medication would the nurse anticipate the health care provider ordering for this client?

   1. lactulose
   2. sucralfate
   3. lamotrigine
   4. gabapentin

208. The nurse is caring for a client with AIDS who is diagnosed with thrush. Which instruction should the nurse give to the client's caretaker, who will be administering nystatin (Mycostatin) oral solution?

   1. take the medication before meals
   2. take the medication after meals
   3. mix the medication with orange juice
   4. take the medication at bedtime

209. An adolescent client ingests a large number of acetaminophen tablets in an attempt to commit suicide. Which laboratory result is associated with acetaminophen overdose?

   1. metabolic alkalosis
   2. increased blood urea nitrogen level
   3. decreased hemoglobin and hematocrit
   4. elevated liver enzyme levels

210. A client diagnosed with bipolar disease is receiving a maintenance dosage of lithium carbonate. His wife calls the community mental health nurse to report that her husband is displaying mild aggression and poor judgment. Which intervention is appropriate?

   1. administer an extra dose of lithium carbonate
   2. take client to the closest emergency department
   3. measure lithium blood level
   4. arrange for hemodialysis

211. Which instruction is correct for a client receiving lithium carbonate for bipolar disorder?

   1. breastfeeding may be done
   2. driving or using machinery is acceptable
   3. drugs containing ibuprofen should be avoided
   4. fluid intake should be limited to eight 8-oz glasses per day

212. The mental health unit nurse is precepting a student nurse. Together they are caring for a client with schizophrenia. The nurse asks the student nurse to select the atypical antipsychotic from the client's medication list. The nurse anticipates the student nurse to select which medication?

    1. loxapine
    2. thioridazine
    3. risperidone
    4. haloperidol

213. The nurse is educating a client about MAOI and diet. Which dietary selection by the client indicates that the nurse's teaching was effective?

    1. egg-white omelet with a cup of yogurt
    2. baked chicken breast with green beans
    3. scrambled eggs with sausage and toast
    4. hot dog with sauerkraut, beans, and a fruit cup

214. The clinic nurse is seeing a client who is taking duloxetine hydrochloride. When updating the client's medical history, for which condition mentioned by the client would the nurse notify the health care provider?

    1. recent worsening of insomnia
    2. unplanned weight loss of 6 pounds
    3. uncontrolled narrow-angle glaucoma
    4. removal of a benign skin cancer on the leg

215. The ED nurse has admitted a client with suspected overdose of tricyclic antidepressants. Which signs and symptoms does the nurse expect to find in this client? **Select all that apply.**

    1. confusion
    2. dry mouth
    3. bradycardia
    4. dysrhythmias
    5. constricted pupils
    6. flushing of the skin

216. The nurse is training persons enrolled at a community center information session on administering naloxone (Narcan) to opioid overdose victims. Which information should the nurse include when teaching this group? **Select all that apply.**

    1. is administered by subcutaneous injection in the abdomen, thigh, or arm
    2. works instantly
    3. lasts 30 minutes
    4. can be administered by lay persons, provided they have had training

PHYSIOLOGICAL INTEGRITY— REDUCTION OF RISK POTENTIAL

217. The nurse is caring for a client with seizure disorder. Which statement regarding seizure precautions is correct?

    1. Padded tongue blades should be at the bedside.

    2. Oxygen and suctioning should be at the bedside.

    3. Padding bed rails with blankets can help prevent injury.

    4. Restraint mitts will help keep the client from removing tubes or IVs.

218. The nurse is assessing a client with a diagnosis of chronic obstructive pulmonary disease (COPD) exacerbation. Which finding would be expected for this client?

    1. hypoxemia and hypocarbia

    2. hyperoxemia and hypocarbia

    3. hypoxemia and hypercarbia

    4. hyperoxemia and hypercarbia

219. The nurse is assessing a client with a stage 3 pressure ulcer. Which finding is consistent with this type of pressure ulcer?

    1. Eschar is present on at least part of the wound.

    2. Full-thickness skin loss is present with undermining.

    3. Partial-thickness skin loss of the epidermis is present.

    4. The area is red and does not blanch with external pressure.

220. The nurse is caring for a client who just returned from a total hip arthroplasty. A student nurse is helping provide care for this client. Which action by the student nurse requires intervention by the nurse?

    1. The student nurse floats the client's heels with a pillow.

    2. The student nurse positions the client with the legs adducted.

    3. The student nurse applies the sequential compression device (SCD) per orders.

    4. The student nurse encourages deep breathing and incentive spirometer use every 2 hours.

221. The nurse is caring for a homeless client brought to the emergency department with a diagnosis of heat stroke. Which key features of heat stroke would the nurse expect to note upon assessment? **Select all that apply.**

    1. a body temperature of 104.2°F

    2. heart rate of 116 and blood pressure of 78/52

    3. heart rate of 49 and blood pressure of 152/90

    4. heart rate of 120 and respiratory rate of 9 breaths per minute

    5. blood pressure of 82/48 and respiratory rate of 26 breaths per minute

222. A college student presents at the emergency department after being thrown off a horse. Head injury with increased intracranial pressure (ICP) is suspected. The nurse understands that *late* signs of increased ICP include which manifestations? **Select all that apply.**

1. seizures
2. irritability
3. restlessness
4. disorientation
5. severe headache
6. nausea and vomiting

223. The nurse is performing discharging instruction for a female client with cystitis. Which statement by the client indicates a need for further teaching?

1. "I should void before and after intercourse."
2. "I should wear loose-fitting cotton underwear."
3. "I can continue using spermicide for birth control."
4. "If I have burning when I urinate, I will contact my physician."

224. A client in the emergency department is complaining of abdominal pain after an episode of nausea and vomiting. Which statement by the client to the nurse necessitates prompt notification of the health care provider?

1. "I started hurting when I got up this morning to go to work."
2. "My grandmother had to have her appendix out many years ago."
3. "I haven't eaten anything because I've been so nauseated and throwing up."
4. "The pain is worse when I cough or move but feels better when I bend my right hip."

225. The nurse is preparing to perform a focused abdominal assessment on a client. Which is the correct order of this assessment?

1. inspection, auscultation, palpation, percussion
2. inspection, palpation, percussion, auscultation
3. inspection, percussion, auscultation, palpation
4. inspection, percussion, palpation, auscultation

226. The nurse is caring for a client who has just returned from the cardiac catheterization lab. Which complications of cardiac catheterization require immediate intervention by the nurse? **Select all that apply.**

1. chest pain
2. decreased appetite
3. difficulty swallowing
4. hematoma formation
5. decreased pulses in the affected extremity

227. The nurse is preparing to remove a peripheral IV from a client. Which nursing action is the **priority** with this procedure?

    1.   checking for an intact catheter tip

    2.   washing the hands and donning gloves

    3.   charting the client's tolerance to the procedure

    4.   removing catheter slowly using the dominant hand

    5.   holding pressure on the site until hemostasis is achieved

228. The nurse has received shift report on the assigned client. Which client would the nurse anticipate to be at **highest** risk for skin breakdown?

    1.   an elderly client who is up to the chair for meals with assistance

    2.   a 24-year-old client with diabetes whose hemoglobin A1C is 6.4%

    3.   a client who is legally blind and lives independently, except for driving

    4.   a client with severe right-sided weakness from a stroke and residual peripheral neuropathy

    5.   a client who had a right pneumothorax and has a chest tube and can reposition independently

229. The nurse is teaching a client and her family about home care following a laryngectomy. Which statement by the client indicates a need for further teaching from the nurse?

    1.   "I will purchase a Medic-Alert bracelet."

    2.   "I can wear loose-fitting turtlenecks to cover the stoma."

    3.   "I can resume water aerobics once my doctor says it is okay."

    4.   "I have a lot of green houseplants year-round throughout my home."

230. A student nurse is discussing fluid overload with the staff nurse. Which statement by the student nurse indicates a need for further explanation by the staff nurse?

    1.   "Pitting edema is the best indicator of fluid overload."

    2.   "The client may have distended veins in the hands and neck."

    3.   "I may hear moist crackles in the lungs during my respiratory assessment."

    4.   "The client may need drug therapy and sodium restriction to treat the overload."

231. The nurse is teaching a newly admitted client about fall prevention. The nurse understands that which of the following interventions can help prevent client falls? **Select all that apply.**

    1.   keep personal articles within reach

    2.   explain the use of the call light system

    3.   keep the bed in the lowest position with all side rails up

    4.   dim the room lights so that the client can get adequate rest

    5.   remind the client to call for assistance when getting out of bed

232. The nurse is caring for a client in the cardiac unit and notices the client's rhythm changes from normal sinus rhythm to coarse ventricular fibrillation. Which is the **priority** nursing action?

   1. call a code blue

   2. check the client and check the leads

   3. initiate CPR while waiting on help to arrive

   4. prepare to start the client on a diltiazem (Cardizem) drip

   5. clear the room of unnecessary items to allow room for the crash cart and team

233. The nurse is teaching a group of student nurses about radiation therapy. Which would the nurse include in the teaching? **Select all that apply.**

   1. The dose is always more than the exposure.

   2. Clients receiving brachytherapy are radioactive.

   3. Clients receiving teletherapy are not radioactive.

   4. Beta particles are the most common type of radiation therapy.

   5. Bodily waste from a client receiving brachytherapy does not require special handling.

234. A 2-month-old infant has been brought to the ED. Which finding by the nurse would raise suspicion for shaken baby syndrome?

   1. failure to track with the eyes

   2. crying without tear production

   3. bruising to the arms and shoulders

   4. greater-than-expected head circumference and bulging fontanels

235. The nurse is evaluating clients for risk of heparin-induced thrombocytopenia (HIT). Which client is at **greatest** risk for HIT, based on the nurse's assessment?

   1. a male client who just completed a 1-week course of heparin

   2. a male client taking enoxaparin for management of unstable angina

   3. a female client receiving heparin for postsurgical thromboprophylaxis

   4. a female client taking enoxaparin to prevent clots following a mild myocardial infarction

236. The nurse is caring for a client who just arrived in the PACU following a colonoscopy with polyp removal. The client's level of sedation is assessed using the Ramsay Sedation Scale (RSS). The client responds quickly, but only to commands. What Ramsay score would the nurse chart for this client?

   1. RSS 1

   2. RSS 2

   3. RSS 3

   4. RSS 4

   5. RSS 5

   6. RSS 6

237. The nurse is caring for a client who has a lithium level of 2.2 mEq/L. Based on this lab value, what would the nurse anticipate to do in order to care for this client? **Select all that apply.**

    1. prepare to administer IV fluids

    2. notify the health care provider

    3. order a mechanical soft diet for the client

    4. administer the next dose of lithium when it is due

    5. observe the client for confusion and slurred speech

238. The nurse is caring for a client receiving hemodialysis. During hemodialysis, the client becomes anxious, experiencing tachypnea and hypotension. The nurse suspects which complication of hemodialysis?

    1. air embolism

    2. clotting of the graft site

    3. dialysis encephalopathy

    4. disequilibrium syndrome

239. The nurse is assisting the health care provider to perform a renal biopsy. Which position should the nurse place the client in?

    1. in the semi-Fowler's position

    2. on the same side of the kidney to be biopsied

    3. on the side opposite of the kidney to be biopsied

    4. prone with a pillow under the shoulders and abdomen

240. The nurse is reviewing labs of a newly admitted client. Which lab result would prompt the nurse to contact the health care provider?

    1. ALT 33 units/L

    2. BNP 760 pg/mL

    3. WBC 10,450 mcL

    4. direct bilirubin 0.2 mg/dL

241. The nurse is caring for an adult client with a total bilirubin of 2.1 mg/dL. Which signs and symptoms would the nurse expect to find? **Select all that apply.**

    1. itchy skin

    2. nausea

    3. pale stools

    4. colorless urine

    5. none; this is a normal lab value

242. The nurse is caring for a client with hypoparathyroidism. The nurse understands that this client is at risk for which problem?

1. hypercalcemia
2. hypermagnesemia
3. decreased phosphorus levels
4. low parathyroid hormone levels

243. The nurse is performing an admission assessment on a client with thrombocytopenia. Which signs and symptoms and lab findings would the nurse expect to see in this client? **Select all that apply.**

1. epistaxis
2. petechiae
3. vomiting blood
4. elevated hematocrit
5. increased platelet count

244. The nurse is educating a client newly diagnosed with gout regarding dietary choices. The nurse understands that further teaching is needed if the client orders which foods for lunch?

1. fruit cup with corn bread and tea
2. tuna fish sandwich with green peas
3. a peanut butter sandwich with 1 percent milk
4. low-fat cheese and crackers with blueberries

245. A client is scheduled for a CT of the brain with and without IV contrast dye to evaluate a possible hemorrhage. Which finding in the client's history should the nurse report immediately to the health care provider?

1. allergy to shellfish
2. history of schizophrenia
3. allergy to cephalosporins
4. presence of a pacemaker

246. The nurse is caring for a client scheduled to receive electroconvulsive therapy (ECT). Following the procedure, the nurse should be watching for which serious complications? **Select all that apply.**

1. skin burns
2. airway compromise
3. cardiac dysrhythmias
4. loss of bladder control
5. neurological complications

247. The nurse is reviewing arterial blood gases (ABGs) on a client. Which finding would prompt the nurse to notify the health care provider?

    1. pH 7.42

    2. pH 7.67

    3. hCO3 24 mEq/L

    4. paCO2 41 mmHg

    5. paCO2 44 mmHg

248. The nurse is preparing the client for a liver biopsy. Which statement by the client indicates a need for further instruction regarding the procedure?

    1. "I can resume strenuous activity in 2 to 3 days."

    2. "I will have to lay on my right side after the procedure."

    3. "I will have a small bandage instead of stitches afterward."

    4. "My right shoulder may begin to hurt as the anesthesia wears off."

    5. "I may have a small amount of pain or discomfort during the procedure."

249. The nurse is caring for a client receiving warfarin therapy for atrial fibrillation. Laboratory results show an INR of 3.9. The nurse would expect which order from the health care provider?

    1. an order to increase the warfarin dose

    2. an order to decrease the warfarin dose

    3. an order for protamine sulfate

    4. no new order; the INR is therapeutic

250. The nurse is educating a client who has been ordered to wear a Holter monitor. Which statement by the client indicates a need for further education by the nurse?

    1. "I can wear the monitor while I shower."

    2. "I should keep the monitor on when I sleep."

    3. "I should avoid metal detectors and electric razors while wearing the monitor."

    4. "I should keep a log of any chest pain, shortness of breath, or skipped beats while wearing the monitor."

251. The nurse is caring for a client with diabetes whose HgbA1C level is 6.9. The client asks the nurse what this means. Which response by the nurse is appropriate?

    1. "Your level is within target range and indicates good glycemic control."

    2. "Your level is too high, and you will need to increase your medications."

    3. "Your level is too low, and you will need to decrease your medications."

    4. "Your health care provider may want to place you on an insulin pump."

252. The nurse is caring for a client who just had an arteriovenous (AV) fistula placed for dialysis. The nurse is providing home care instructions to the client. Which statement by the client indicates a need for further teaching by the nurse?

   1.   "I should avoid wearing a watch on my arm with the fistula."

   2.   "It may take several weeks before the fistula is ready to use."

   3.   "I should not have my blood pressure taken in my access arm."

   4.   "I should wear tight sleeves to protect and support the fistula so I don't bend it."

253. The nurse is caring for a client who is undergoing a pharmacological stress test because she cannot use the treadmill. The nurse administers the prescribed dose of adenosine. Which physiological response indicates an adverse effect of the adenosine requiring intervention by the nurse? **Select all that apply.**

   1.   nausea

   2.   RR of 18

   3.   HR of 97

   4.   chest pain

   5.   facial flushing

254. The nurse is caring for a client who was admitted with an upper respiratory infection. The client's temperature is 102.4°F, and he is confused. In the last 2 hours, systolic blood pressure has dropped from 138 to 90. The nurse should perform which intervention? **Select all that apply.**

   1.   obtain blood cultures

   2.   place the client on NPO status

   3.   administer supplemental oxygen

   4.   administer antipyretics as ordered

   5.   encourage rest and limit physical activity

   6.   provide a warming blanket to alleviate chills

255. Mix and Match: Match the laboratory test to the abnormal value.

Laboratory Test	Abnormal Value
calcium	8.1 mg/L
pH	7.56
specific gravity	1.000
potassium	5.8
LDL	160 mg/dL
HDL	34 mg/dL

256. The nurse is caring for a client with dementia who has pulled out three peripheral IVs. Which intervention by the nurse is the **best** way to manage this client?

   1. place the client in restraints or mitts

   2. tell the family that they need to stay with the client

   3. replace the IV and wrap it in gauze to hide it from view

   4. tell the client that if she pulls another IV out, she will have to have a PICC line placed

PHYSIOLOGICAL INTEGRITY— PHYSIOLOGICAL ADAPTATION

257. The nurse is preparing to extubate a client. Arrange in order of priority the actions that the nurse should take to perform this procedure.

1. hyperoxygenate the client
2. explain the procedure to the client
3. immediately instruct the client to cough
4. apply oxygen by nasal cannula or face mask
5. thoroughly suction the ET tube and the oral cavity
6. teach the client how to use an incentive spirometer every 2 hours
7. rapidly deflate the ET tube cuff and remove tube at peak inspiration
8. set up the prescribed oxygen delivery system and bring in equipment for emergency reintubation

258. The nurse is reviewing labs on a client with second- and third-degree burns from a house fire. Which abnormal lab value would the nurse expect to find with this client?

1. pH of 7.41
2. albumin of 3.9 g/dL
3. hemoglobin of 15 g/dL
4. potassium of 5.9 mEq/L

259. The nurse is teaching a newly diagnosed client about Guillain-Barre syndrome (GBS). What information would the nurse provide in her teaching? **Select all that apply.**

1. GBS affects females more often than males.
2. The acute period lasts several days to 2 weeks.
3. GBS tends to be self-limiting with temporary paralysis.
4. Common symptoms include muscle weakness and paralysis.
5. Infections such as Epstein-Barr virus have been associated with GBS.

260. The nurse is caring for a client who just had a bone marrow biopsy. The nurse understands that which statement is the nursing **priority** for this client?

1. keeping the client NPO for 2 hours
2. avoiding contact sports for 24 hours
3. monitoring the client for excessive bleeding
4. applying alcohol to the site every 4 hours to prevent infection

261. A client newly diagnosed with gout asks the nurse about the condition. Which statement should the nurse include in teaching for this client?

   1. "Aspirin can be used for mild pain when you have a flare-up."
   2. "Avoid foods high in purines such as organ meats and shellfish."
   3. "Lasix can help keep your urine flushed out to lessen the chance of an attack."
   4. "A few glasses of wine every week will help you reduce stress, which can trigger an attack."

262. The nurse is caring for a client with a diagnosis of upper GI bleeding. Which findings on physical assessment are consistent with this diagnosis?

   1. increased heart rate
   2. decreased heart rate
   3. increased hemoglobin
   4. bounding peripheral pulses

263. The nurse notes irritability, microcephaly, and short palpebral fissures in a newborn in the nursery. The nurse suspects which diagnosis for this infant?

   1. syphilis
   2. TORCH syndrome
   3. brachial plexus injury
   4. fetal alcohol syndrome (FAS)

264. The nurse is providing dietary teaching to the parents of a 7-year-old child with celiac disease. Which statement by the parents indicate that dietary teaching was successful?

   1. "We will serve rice more often."
   2. "We will serve pretzels as a snack."
   3. "I will use rye bread for sandwiches."
   4. "We will start having steel-cut oatmeal for breakfast."

265. The nurse is caring for a client with a T-tube following a cholecystectomy. Which statement is correct regarding management of these tubes? **Select all that apply.**

   1. keep the drainage system at the level of the heart
   2. report foul order and purulent drainage to the health care provider
   3. remove the tube when drainage slows to less than 50 mL every 8 hours
   4. do not clamp or irrigate the T-tube without orders from the health care provider
   5. clamp the tube before meals and observe the client for abdominal distention or discomfort

266. The nurse is precepting a student nurse on leukemia classifications. Which statement by the student nurse reflects an understanding of classifications of leukemia?

    1.   "Acute lymphocytic leukemia has an average age of onset of 15 to 39 years."

    2.   "Chronic myelogenous leukemia contains mostly granulocytes in the bone marrow."

    3.   "Chronic myelogenous leukemia has mostly lymphocytes found in the bone marrow."

    4.   "Acute myelogenous leukemia has primarily granulocytes present in the bone marrow."

267. The nurse is caring for a client who is HIV positive and gave birth to a full-term infant. The nurse is teaching the client about infections in HIV-positive infants. Which infection does the nurse understand is the **most** common opportunistic infection in children and infants with HIV?

    1.   hepatitis C

    2.   strep throat

    3.   cytomegalovirus infection

    4.   *Pneumocystis jiroveci* pneumonia

268. The nurse is caring for a client who just returned from a right mastectomy. Which position does the nurse anticipate for the client?

    1.   high Fowler's with the unaffected arm elevated on a pillow

    2.   flat with the client positioned on the affected side or back

    3.   semi-Fowler's with the affected arm supported on a pillow

    4.   reverse Trendelenburg's with the arm on the affected side supported on a pillow

269. The nurse is caring for a client in the ICU who has an arterial line for hemodynamic monitoring. Which action will the nurse take in caring for this client?

    1.   position the client with the transducer at the level of the right atrium

    2.   position the client with the transducer at the level of the left ventricle

    3.   position the client with the transducer at the level of the right clavicle

    4.   position the client with the transducer at the level of the right ventricle

270. A 47-year-old client presents to the emergency department with severe hypotension, muscle weakness, fatigue, and vomiting. Labs reveal a potassium level of 6.1 mEq/L and a sodium level of 128 mEq/l. Which of the following should the nurse anticipate for this client?

    1.   administration of IV spironolactone

    2.   boluses of Lactated Ringer's to increase blood pressure

    3.   administration of IV saline, dextrose, or hydrocortisone

    4.   boluses of 0.45% normal saline with 40 mEq/L of potassium

271. The nurse is precepting a student nurse. The primary nurse asks the student nurse to figure the client's intake and output for the shift. Which statement by the student nurse indicates an understanding of this procedure?

　　1.　"Wound drainage is not included in output measurement."

　　2.　"I only need to count urinary output for my output total."

　　3.　"I don't need to count the client's emesis since it was a small amount."

　　4.　"I will include all IV fluids, liquids the client drank, IV flushes, and IV antibiotics in my intake total."

272. The nurse is caring for a client who is on 2 L/minute of oxygen via nasal cannula. The nurse understands that this flow rate corresponds to which FiO2?

　　1.　24% FiO2

　　2.　28% FiO2

　　3.　32% FiO2

　　4.　36% FiO2

273. The nurse is discussing various oxygen delivery systems with a newly graduated nurse who has just begun working on the medical floor. Which statement by the student nurse indicates an understanding of the different oxygen delivery systems?

　　1.　"A tracheostomy collar requires a flow rate of at least 6 L/minute to be effective."

　　2.　"High-flow oxygen delivery systems include the venturi mask, face tent, and non-rebreather masks."

　　3.　"The non-rebreather mask should receive a high enough flow rate to keep the reservoir bag completely full."

　　4.　"Nasal cannulas, non-rebreather masks, simple face masks, and partial rebreather masks are examples of low-flow oxygen delivery systems."

274. A nurse is providing pre-op teaching to a client who will be undergoing a coronary artery bypass graft. Which of the following should the nurse include in the teaching? **Select all that apply.**

　　1.　"Your medications will be changed after surgery."

　　2.　"You will be on strict bed rest for the first 48 hours."

　　3.　"You will be using a bedpan after surgery to urinate."

　　4.　"You will need to splint the chest incision when you cough or breathe deeply."

　　5.　"You will be on the ventilator after surgery and have one or more chest tubes."

275. The nurse is caring for a client with vitamin B12 deficiency anemia. Which physical assessment finding would the nurse expect to note in this client?

1. glossitis
2. paresthesias
3. weakness and pallor
4. dark purple or cyanotic skin on the face and mucous membranes

276. The nurse is caring for a client in the cardiac unit who has a systolic murmur. Which assessment finding would the nurse expect when auscultating this client's heart sounds?

1. The murmur can be heard between S3 and S4.
2. The murmur can be heard between S4 and S1.
3. The murmur can be heard between S2 and S1.
4. The murmur can be heard between S1 and S2.

277. A student nurse is precepting on the cardiac unit with the charge nurse. The charge nurse is educating the student about heart sounds and asks the student nurse to describe what causes the S1 sound. Which response by the student nurse reflects an understanding of cardiac sounds?

1. "It is caused by the mitral and tricuspid valves closing."
2. "It is caused by the mitral and pulmonic valves closing."
3. "It is caused by the pulmonic and aortic valves closing."
4. "It is caused by the aortic and tricuspid valves closing."

278. The nurse is seeing a client in the clinic who complains of a sore throat. The client asks for an antibiotic. How should the nurse respond? **Select all that apply.**

1. "You can try gargling with warm saline to relieve the discomfort."
2. "You should use a dehumidifier to dry out the air, which will soothe the throat."
3. "Most sore throats are caused by viruses, which cannot be treated with antibiotics."
4. "There are three or four antibiotics that we prescribe for a sore throat, so the doctor will decide which one you need."
5. "You should increase your fluid intake. Drink lots of water and try warm soup to help with the discomfort."

279. A client with third- and fourth-degree burns is in the burn unit. The nurse understands that which of the following is true regarding fluid shift in burn clients?

1. The fluid shift can cause hypokalemia and hypovolemia.
2. Hemoconcentration increases blood flow and reduces blood viscosity.
3. Excessive weight loss can occur during the first 12 hours post burn due to the fluid shift.
4. Severe edema can occur in areas that were not burned, due to the leakage of electrolytes and fluids from the vascular space.

280. A client is 2 hours post-op for a right total knee replacement. Upon assessment by the nurse, which information requires notification of the doctor?

1. hemoglobin is 10.2 grams per liter

2. bleeding on the dressing of 2 cm

3. oral temperature of 100.4°F

4. complaint of pain at incision site

281. A client is brought to the ED following a drowning event. The nurse assigned to the client understands that which is true regarding drowning?

1. Drowning in very cold water causes a worse outcome for the client than drowning in warmer water.

2. Aspiration of both salt and fresh water increases surfactant in the lungs and leads to increased lung compliance.

3. If possible, the cause of drowning should be determined in order to know if the client suffered a medical condition such as a seizure that requires follow-up treatment.

4. Contaminants in the water such as microbes, mud, chemicals, and algae do not affect the degree of injury to the lungs.

282. The nurse is caring for a client in ICU diagnosed with rabies following a bite from an infected raccoon. The nurse understands which to be true regarding rabies? **Select all that apply.**

1. The client should not be bathed, and no running water should be present within hearing of the client.

2. Current treatment includes two doses of immunoglobulin and six doses of rabies vaccine over a period of 21 days.

3. Nuchal rigidity, convulsions, and tonic or clonic muscle contractions can occur during the neurological phase.

4. In the prodromal phase, the client can have irritability, extreme salivation, sore throat, fever, and hyperexcitability.

5. During the neurological phase, the client may have aches and pains in different parts of the body, along with sensitivity to light.

6. During the paralytic phase, the client becomes unconscious, has loss of bowel and urinary control, and has irregular or labored breathing.

283. The nurse is caring for a client who had a basilar artery stroke. The nurse would expect which signs and symptoms in this client?

1. memory problems, visual hallucinations, visual deficits, hemisensory disturbances

2. weakness in the foot and leg, sensory loss in the foot and leg, incontinence, ataxia, lack of spontaneity

3. impaired consciousness, visual loss, bilateral sensory and motor dysfunction, and pupil abnormalities

4. ataxia, contralateral facial weakness, contralateral hemiplegia, visual deficits, speech impairments, perceptual impairments

284. A client presents to the ED with complaints of sweating, heart palpitations, vertigo, and the urge to lay down shortly after eating. The nurse anticipates which diagnosis for this client?

1. appendicitis
2. cholecystitis
3. ulcerative colitis
4. dumping syndrome

285. The oncology nurse is assessing a client diagnosed with cancer of the tongue. Upon examination, which signs and symptoms would the nurse expect to find? **Select all that apply.**

1. weight gain
2. well-fitting dentures
3. a black, hairy tongue
4. difficulty swallowing
5. a sore that bleeds or does not heal
6. difficulty chewing or pain with chewing

286. The nurse is caring for a 52-year-old African American male newly diagnosed with hypertension. He has a history of chronic kidney disease and diabetes. The nurse would expect to see which medication order for this client?

1. enalapril 5 mg PO QD
2. enalapril 5 mg PO QD and amiloride 5 mg PO QD
3. enalapril 5 mg PO QD and atenolol 50 mg PO QD
4. enalapril 5 mg PO QD and amlodipine 2.5 mg PO QD

287. The nurse is performing discharge teaching to a client diagnosed with chronic pancreatitis. Which statement by the client indicates an understanding of home management of the condition? **Select all that apply.**

1. "I should avoid large, heavy meals."
2. "I can have an occasional glass of red wine."
3. "I can resume my daily jogging once I get home."
4. "I should avoid smoking and caffeinated beverages."
5. "I should add extra spices to my food to make it taste better."

288. The nurse is caring for a client with suspected connective tissue disease. Assessment findings include chronic back pain, weight loss, joint pain and itching, and visual disturbances. The nurse anticipates a diagnosis of which disorder for this client?

1. Reiter syndrome
2. Marfan syndrome
3. ankylosing spondylitis
4. systemic necrotizing vasculitis

289. Which assessment finding in a client with chronic kidney disease indicates late-stage symptoms?

   1. shortness of breath

   2. oliguria

   3. tea-colored urine

   4. edema in lower extremities

290. The ED nurse has admitted a client who is homeless and was found unresponsive in the street during below freezing temperatures. The client is diagnosed with severe hypothermia. The nurse should implement which measures for this client? **Select all that apply.**

   1. apply a heating blanket

   2. obtain an oral temperature

   3. assess level of consciousness

   4. position in the supine position

   5. massage the extremities vigorously

   6. prepare to administer CPR if indicated

291. Which of the following is **not** a recommended preparation for electroconvulsive therapy (ECT)?

   1. premedication with an anticholinergic agent

   2. morning bath, NPO after midnight

   3. informed consent in writing

   4. administration of an anticonvulsant 30 minutes before ECT

292. While in a restaurant the nurse notices a woman clutching her throat. The woman is unable to speak. The nurse asks the woman if she's choking, and she indicates yes. Which response by the nurse should be done **first**?

   1. establish an airway by tilting the chin back

   2. administer five quick chest compressions

   3. administer two rescue breaths

   4. perform the Heimlich maneuver

293. Which nursing action is **most** appropriate to initially relieve pain related to a recent soft tissue injury?

   1. administer an over-the-counter (OTC) medication for pain

   2. apply heat

   3. massage the area

   4. apply ice pack

294. What physical activity is recommended for a school-age child with asthma?

1. distance running
2. indoor swimming
3. soccer
4. basketball

295. A client has arterial blood gases drawn. The results are as follows: pH, 7.58; P_aCO2, 48 mm Hg; HCO3, 44 mEq/L, Base Excess, +13 mEq/L. Which condition is indicated?

1. respiratory alkalosis
2. respiratory acidosis
3. metabolic alkalosis
4. metabolic acidosis

296. The nurse is assessing a client with Parkinson's disease. Which sign of primary motor symptom involvement would the nurse expect to observe?

1. resting tremor
2. sleep disturbance
3. constipation
4. fatigue

297. A nurse is reviewing the laboratory reports prior to physician rounds. The serum calcium level of a client with hyperparathyroidism is 14.6 mg/dl. Which treatment should the nurse anticipate?

1. corticosteroids
2. renal dialysis
3. calcitonin
4. intravenous bisphosphonates

298. A nurse is employed on an oncology unit. A 62-year-old client is admitted for surgical treatment of a meningioma. The nurse would anticipate modifying the environment for which symptom?

1. difficulty swallowing
2. seizures
3. poor concentration
4. impaired mobility

299. A client presents to the emergency room with severe pain in the upper right abdomen. The client is nauseated and has a temperature of 102.2°F. Which nursing action would be a **priority** at this time?

1. relieve pain

2. obtain vital signs

3. administer IV fluids

4. prepare for surgery

300. The nurse is preparing to administer cefazolin to a client who is allergic to penicillin. The client states that penicillin causes him to itch and be slightly short of breath. Which response by the nurse is correct?

1. administer the cefazolin as ordered

2. call the pharmacy to substitute another medication

3. hold the medication and notify the health care provider

4. give the client diphenhydramine and then administer the cefazolin

301. The nurse is caring for a client who has shortness of breath, +2 pitting edema bilaterally of the lower extremities, crackles in the bases of the lungs, and a weight gain of 7 pounds in 1 week. The nurse administers furosemide 40 mg IV as ordered. Which would the nurse anticipate to indicate that the furosemide was effective? **Select all that apply.**

1. pitting edema of +3

2. pitting edema of +1

3. less shortness of breath

4. an increase in urine output of 250 mL/hr

5. a decrease or absence of crackles in the lungs

302. The nurse is caring for a client with left-sided heart failure. Which assessment findings does the nurse anticipate for this client? **Select all that apply.**

1. dyspnea

2. engorged spleen

3. dependent edema

4. jugular vein distention

5. weak peripheral pulses

6. crackles or wheezes in the lungs

303. The nurse is providing teaching to a client newly diagnosed with type 2 diabetes. Which should the nurse include in her teaching?

1. check the feet daily

2. have eye examinations every 2 years

3. use a heating pad to keep the feet warm

4. take extra insulin before consuming sweets

304. The nurse is caring for a client who had an inguinal hernia repair. Which interventions by the nurse are appropriate for this client? **Select all that apply.**

   1. encouraging fluid intake
   2. relieving urinary retention
   3. applying heat to the scrotum
   4. teaching turning, coughing, and deep breathing
   5. keeping the client on bed rest for the first 12 hours after surgery
   6. teaching the client to avoid lifting more than 20 pounds until approved by the health care provider

305. The nurse is caring for a client experiencing an acute flare-up of diverticular disease. Which interventions by the nurse are appropriate for this client? **Select all that apply.**

   1. encourage a diet high in fiber
   2. insert a nasogastric (NG) tube
   3. administer enemas as ordered
   4. administer IV fluids as ordered
   5. encourage coughing and deep breathing
   6. check stools for frank or occult bleeding

306. The nurse is caring for a two-year-old client who presented to the ER with vomiting, currant jelly-like stools, and abdominal pain that causes the child to draw the knees up to the abdomen in a fetal position. Which interventions does the nurse anticipate for this client?

   1. assessing for respiratory distress
   2. orders for a soft diet as tolerated
   3. monitoring for a normal, brown stool
   4. preparing the client for a barium enema
   5. placement of a nasogastric (NG) tube
   6. monitoring for fever and changes in blood pressure

307. The nurse comes upon a client in the clinic who appears to have experienced a sudden cardiac arrest. After retrieving the automated external defibrillator (AED), the nurse knows to use the equipment in the following manner, as per the American Red Cross. List the steps in order. Use all the steps.

   1. Make sure no one is touching the client. Tell everyone to "stand clear."
   2. Open the person's shirt and wipe the chest dry. Remove any visible patches.
   3. Attach the AED pads and plug in the connector.
   4. Push the "analyze" button to analyze the client's heart rhythm.
   5. Turn on AED. Follow visual and/or audio prompts.
   6. Begin CPR.
   7. As prompted, press the "shock" button after clearing the client.

308. The nurse is caring for a client with a gastric ulcer. Which menu choice by the client indicates an understanding of the nurse's dietary teaching?

   1. yogurt with fresh berries
   2. dry wheat toast with water
   3. coffee with cream and a bagel
   4. a grilled cheese sandwich with milk

309. The nurse is caring for a client with veno-occlusive disease. Which manifestations of this condition would the nurse expect to find? **Select all that apply.**

   1. jaundice
   2. weight loss
   3. weight gain
   4. right lower quadrant pain
   5. enlargement of the spleen
   6. right upper quadrant pain

310. The nurse is preparing to remove a client's abdominal stitches as ordered by the health care provider. Which is the correct action by the nurse?

   1. clean the stitches with soap and water before removing
   2. wash the hands and use gloves while removing the stitches
   3. wash the hands and use sterile technique when removing the stitches
   4. wear a gown, gloves, a mask, an eye shield, and shoe covers during the procedure

311. The ED nurse receives a client who is bleeding profusely from a gunshot wound. Which action by the nurse will **best** help this client avoid complications of extreme blood loss?

   1. draw a type and match
   2. administer type O blood
   3. administer type AB+ blood
   4. ask the family to donate blood

QUESTION BANK ANSWER KEY

1. Number 3 is correct.

Rationale: An uncomfortable feeling of pressure, squeezing, fullness, or pain in the center of the chest is the predominant symptom of an MI in women. Palpitations indicate an arrhythmia. Edema in the lower extremities is a later sign of cardiac failure. A feeling of nausea is less common when experiencing an MI.

2. Numbers 1 and 3 are correct.

Rationale: Anything below the level of the table surface is considered unsterile. After opening a bottle of sterile solution (betadine), the contents must be used or discarded but not returned to the sterile field. The edges and sides of the towel extending below the side of the table are routinely considered unsterile. Sterile packages are routinely opened with the first edge away while the last flap is pulled toward the person opening the package.

3. Correct response: Accountability

Rationale: Accountability is the ethical principle that states that the nurse is responsible for his own actions while providing client care.

4. Number 2 is correct.

Rationale: The ability to navigate a flight of stairs is a requirement for discharge after a total knee replacement. The client needs to be able to ambulate 75 feet. There is no set amount of flexion of the knee for discharge. Preparing a snack is not a standard requirement for discharge.

5. Numbers 1 and 2 are correct.

Rationale: After surgery, the client should avoid getting in a pool or tub as infection may occur. Long-term pain will be reduced, hopefully eliminated. Short-term pain will require pain medication to be administered as ordered. The client should be encouraged to take pain medication as frequently as needed. Physical therapy begins soon after surgery and may continue for several weeks, until full recovery occurs. Walking is considered a low-impact activity and would be encouraged after surgery.

6. Number 1 is correct.

Rationale: The ECG is most commonly used to initially determine the location of myocardial damage. An echocardiogram is used to view myocardial wall function after an MI has been diagnosed. Cardiac enzymes will aid in diagnosing an MI but not the location. While not performed initially, cardiac catheterization determines coronary artery disease and would suggest the location of myocardial damage.

7. Number 2 is correct.

Rationale: Pharyngeal diphtheria is a bacterial respiratory infection, not viral. Mumps is a viral infection that requires droplet precautions. Pertussis and mycoplasma pneumonia are both bacterial respiratory infections that require droplet precautions. Droplets usually travel no farther than 3 feet from the client. Standard precautions along with a surgical mask must be worn when working within 3 feet of a client who is on droplet precautions.

8. Number 4 is correct.

Rationale: The client who is post-op day 2 following a hernia repair and getting up to the chair is the most stable client for the UAP. Clients with internal radiation implants require special safety precautions, and all care personnel must be properly trained. Special handling procedures are required should the implant become dislodged and are beyond the scope of practice for a UAP. The client receiving blood for hypovolemic shock is potentially unstable and is at greater risk for an emergency than the more stable client who can get up to the chair. Wound dehiscence is a serious complication of abdominal surgery and requires special management, including dressing changes. The nurse may not delegate dressing changes to UAPs. The nurse is ultimately responsible for delegating tasks to the appropriate personnel and determining that the person is able to perform the task safely and correctly.

9.   Number 4 is correct.

Rationale: An interdisciplinary approach involves members from differing disciplines that are involved in attaining a common client outcome. Continuity of care, case management, and quality improvement are not related to the interdisciplinary approach.

10.   Number 2 is correct.

Rationale: Signing a consent form for a client with diminished capacity requires involvement of legal personnel with expertise on state regulations on these cases. The administrative personnel need to make a determination consistent with hospital policy. Allowing the client to sign the form violates the principles of informed consent. Involving the client's second cousin may be appropriate provided other more direct family members are unavailable. The physician is not able to sign for the client.

11.   Numbers 3 and 4 are correct.

Rationale: Inability of the myocardium to pump effectively will reduce the client's activity tolerance. Alternating activity with rest allows the client to function at her best. Assessment by the nurse is appropriate as pooling of fluid in the lower extremities results if the heart is unable to pump blood throughout the body. While clients with CHF need to be on strict intake and output, fluids do not necessarily need to be limited. Instead, the client's weight is a better assessment criteria of fluid overload. The client should be kept in a semi-Fowler's position.

12.   Number 2 is correct.

Rationale: Assessment of the insertion site for bleeding is a priority. Should bleeding occur, additional compression may be needed. Vital signs are monitored every 15 minutes for 2 hours after the procedure, every 30 minutes during the next 2 hours, and then every hour for 2 hours. The head of the bed may be elevated up to 30 degrees. Clients post-catheterization may eat and drink as tolerated.

13.   The correct order is 2, 3, 1, 4.

Rationale: A systematic approach to interpreting each strip is needed for consistency. Rate refers to frequency, determined by spaces between R and R. Rhythm is the interval of the pattern between R waves. The P wave is produced when the left and right atria depolarize. Regular intervals vary by less than 0.06 seconds. The P wave should occur regularly; be one for every QRS complex; be smooth, rounded, and upright in appearance; and look similar. The P-R interval measures the time from the onset of atrial contraction to onset of ventricular contraction. The normal interval is 0.12 – 0.20 seconds. The QRS complex presents depolarization (contraction) of the ventricles. The normal interval is 0.06 – 0.12 seconds.

14.   Numbers 3 and 4 are correct.

Rationale: Daily weight provides information about fluid balance and effectiveness of the therapy regime. Corticosteroids taken on a short-term basis are known to reduce the inflammation associated with Crohn's disease. A high-fat diet may exacerbate the diarrhea associated with Crohn's disease. Lactulose would promote peristalsis and would be contraindicated.

15.   Numbers 1, 2, and 3 are correct.

Rationale: Applying compression stockings will assist in preventing a deep vein thrombosis. Ambulation post-surgery with a walker is done to prevent complications of immobility. Coughing and deep breathing will facilitate oxygenation of the body after receiving anesthesia. Fluid intake need not be restricted post-op and may be encouraged depending on the client's medical history.

16. Number 4 is correct.

Rationale: Because of malabsorption, clients with cystic fibrosis (CF) need one and a half to two times as many calories as people without CF. Following a high-fat, high-calorie diet will help meet these clients' nutritional needs. Other options are not appropriate for clients with CF.

17. Number 2 is correct.

Rationale: As the client will require neurologic assessment, the RN should receive the client. The graduate nurse and certified nursing assistant both lack sufficient assessment skills. The charge nurse is needed to supervise the unit.

18. Number 3 is correct.

Rationale: An intervention by the mother is both distracting and comforting to the toddler. Painting a smiley face on the dressing covering the IV site may focus the child's attention further to the dressing. A puzzle is above the cognitive level of the toddler. Sedation may mask symptoms of distress.

19. Number 1 is correct.

Rationale: A student nurse would not be allowed to administer a blood transfusion without supervision. The remaining assignments are within the scope of practice of each health care practitioner.

20. Number 2 is correct.

Rationale: Continuity of care by the same nursing personnel helps build trust with the infant, an important developmental need at 4 months old. Playing music will influence the environment but is not the best choice for meeting the emotional needs of the infant. The gender of the nursing care provider is irrelevant. Placing the infant close to the nursing station will not address its emotional needs.

21. Numbers 1 and 3 are correct.

Rationale: Blood glucose levels should be closely monitored before exercise. If the level is below 70, the athlete should have a snack. If it is above 300, the athlete should inject insulin consistent with the personal plan and retest. The coach should know the athlete is a diabetic and what the signs/symptoms of hypoglycemia are so he can help if this occurs. Snacks high in carbohydrates should be carried in case of hypoglycemia. Insulin injections should be consistent with the athlete's schedule. Administering insulin prior to an athletic event will increase chances for hypoglycemia.

22. Number 3 is correct.

Rationale: Administering the IV antibiotic is the priority because it will treat the infection that is causing the fever. Giving an antipyretic should follow the IV antibiotic. Since the client has scheduled antibiotics, a wound culture is not necessary. The dressing change is important but should be performed after the antibiotic is administered.

23. Number 3 is correct.

Rationale: When performing a dressing change, the nurse first removes the old dressing while wearing clean gloves. The wound is assessed by noting drainage color, amount, and odor if any drainage is present. The color of the skin around the wound and in the wound bed is assessed, and the wound may be measured to ensure that the wound is healing as planned. Once the wound is thoroughly assessed, the gloves are discarded, hand hygiene is performed, and the sterile field is prepared for the dressing change. Charting the dressing change is the last step.

24. Number 3 is correct.

Rationale: The client with the negative heart catheterization is the most stable of this group of clients. The client will most likely be on telemetry, which allows early monitoring of any changes in heart rhythm before physical signs are present. A nonverbal client with seizures is more unstable and will have a more difficult time communicating needs to the nurse. Peritoneal dialysis is a more advanced skill and requires proper training and skill validation. An elderly client who just had a below-the-knee amputation is at greater risk of complications due to age, and is at higher risk of bleeding from the surgery.

25. Number 3 is correct.

    Rationale: The client with COPD exacerbation who can get up to the chair is the best choice for the UAP. Sitting upright in the bed or a chair allows for maximum ease of breathing and is the best position for coughing and clearing secretions. The nurse should perform oral care on clients with bleeding disorders due to the increased risk of bleeding. The client with a tibial fracture and external fixation must be positioned and turned in a specific manner so as to maintain fixation. Turning clients with special turning requirements should not be delegated to inexperienced personnel. The nurse must verify that the UAP is properly trained in turning these clients. Reinforcement of teaching is still considered teaching and may only be done by the licensed nurse. The nurse is responsible for all tasks that are delegated and must ensure that they are performed safely.

26. Number 3 is correct.

    Rationale: Administering enemas is within the scope of practice for LPNs. Administering blood and giving anything through any type of central line, including PICCs, is beyond the scope of practice for LPNs. Preoperative teaching must be done by the RN. The duties of an LPN may vary from state to state; it is the RN's responsibility to be familiar with the Nurse Practice Act of his state and to know the limitations of an LPN's duties.

27. Number 1 is correct.

    Rationale: In allowing the outside group to take a photo of the clients, the nurse committed a breach of confidentiality. Each client must give consent to be photographed and have the picture posted on social media. Failure to gain such consent is a serious violation. Had the nurse obtained administrative approval for the photograph, it would have been inadequate as only an individual may consent to have her image taken and shared with others. While the nurse failed to act in the best interest of the clients, the conduct is not necessarily unethical or unprofessional according to HIPAA.

28. Number 4 is correct.

    Rationale: Care coordination is limited in that the scope of work is based on a plan that is created with input from the client. The stakeholder in case management is an insurance company or a hospital. The main goal of care coordination is to promote a better quality of life for the client, while case management's goal also includes legal and financial issues that may involve stakeholders. Additionally, eliminating noncompliance and overutilization of resources is addressed. Care coordination is based on a holistic approach and an understanding of client-family dynamics, with less emphasis on issues that affect stakeholders. Advocating for client needs is emphasized over stakeholder interests.

29. Numbers 3, 4, and 5 are correct.

    Rationale: Responses 3, 4, and 5 are examples of how a nurse keeps the client's interest at the focus of care and maintains the role of client advocate. One of the duties is making sure that the client understands treatment options, including possible outcomes if the client refuses treatment. The nurse must also ensure that the client receives instruction in her native tongue if she does not speak English. This is especially important when obtaining consent for surgery and other invasive procedures. Copies of living wills, advance directives, and other legal health care documents should be placed in the client's chart if available. Only speaking to family members regarding the client's care is rude and does not show consideration for the client's wishes for her care. The nurse should not insist that any client become an organ donor. The nurse's opinion is secondary to the client's wishes. The nurse serves as a client advocate by following the client's wishes, not pushing what he thinks is best for the client.

30. Number 3 is correct.

Rationale: The Patient's Bill of Rights gives all clients the right to a quick and objective review of any claim that they levy against a health care facility, physician, or health care plan. Clients also have the right to view and receive copies of their medical records. Anyone presenting to an emergency department, whether insured or not, has the right to receive life-saving treatment and stabilization, or be transferred to another, more appropriate facility if required. It is against the law for an emergency department to refuse treatment to anyone, regardless of ability to pay. The client is responsible for providing correct information regarding past medical history, medications, and treatments. While the nurse is expected to make all reasonable efforts to corroborate client reports, the ultimate responsibility lies with the consumer of health care.

31. Numbers 1, 2, 4, and 5 are correct.

Rationale: Principles of triage include treating the least stable clients first. In this scenario, there are four clients requiring immediate attention. When a piece of equipment alarms, the first course of action is to check the client, and then troubleshoot the alarm. The nurse should never ignore any alarm for any reason. Clients who have just returned from surgery, especially an open surgical approach, are at risk for loss of airway due to anesthesia, bleeding from the site, and other potential surgery-specific risks. A sudden change in level of consciousness requires immediate action to determine the cause. Tingling in the mouth is a sign of a possibly serious allergic reaction and may occur if the client receives a new medication for the first time. This client is at high risk of anaphylactic shock. A client who is ready to transfer to the floor is stable and therefore not a priority situation. The client with diabetes who has a blood sugar of 90 is within a safe range and does not require emergent treatment or monitoring.

32. Number 3 is correct.

Rationale: The nurse is responsible for knowing which tasks can and cannot be delegated. Ultimately, the nurse is responsible for the outcome of all delegated tasks. Only the licensed nurse can call and receive report on clients. UAPs may perform tasks with stable clients who will have predictable outcomes. Assisting stable clients set up meal trays or sit on a bedpan is within the realm of tasks that UAPs may perform. The client who had a cardiac stent placed is two days post-op, and there are no complications mentioned that would indicate this client is unstable.

33. Number 5 is correct.

Rationale: Quality improvement is the process by which a nurse identifies a need for practice improvement and develops policies and/or procedures to improve practice. Identifying and minimizing fall risk for clients who are high risk for falls is an example of the quality improvement process. Delegation is the process by which an RN assigns other tasks to assistive personnel or to an LPN. Peer review is part of the review process when a scientific paper is presented to a medical or nursing journal for publication. Consultation is the process in which other health care providers, specialists, or social workers are involved in client care as the need arises. Client referral involves directing the client to a case worker or community service to assist in client needs. Referrals may be made to other health care facilities or rehabilitation facilities.

34. Numbers 1, 3, 4, and 5 are correct.

Rationale: West Nile virus is reportable due to the fact that it can easily be spread by mosquitoes over a large area. City and county municipalities are able to spray to prevent the spread of certain mosquito-borne diseases. Gunshot wounds must be reported to local police or sheriff departments. Elder abuse and neglect, along with child abuse or neglect, must be reported to local authorities for follow-up investigation and to ensure client safety. Bites from unknown dogs must be reported due to the risk of rabies, especially in stray dogs. Herpes simplex is not a reportable condition. The ED nurse must be knowledgeable of facility policies and procedures for carrying out reporting required conditions.

35. Number 4 is correct.

Rationale: Nursing students learn by doing, and educating clients about their medications is one of the most important skills in nursing. The student nurse should answer only when the precepting nurse is in the room. If any information is incorrect, the RN can gently offer the correct information and use it as a teaching moment for the student nurse. There is no reason to ask the family to step out of the room unless the client specifically requests it. Passing off medication questions to the health care provider is inappropriate, unless the client is receiving a medication that is unfamiliar to the nurse or is an experimental drug. It is incorrect to tell the client that the student nurse cannot answer questions about medication. A student nurse precepting in the ICU has already passed several medication tests.

36. Number 4 is correct.

Rationale: The client has made his wishes known to the nurse by refusing to sign the consent for blood. Upon admission to the facility, all clients are asked about special religious beliefs that affect care. A power of attorney completed before the client arrives at the facility allows the client to personalize what he does not wish to have done, so he may refuse blood on the power of attorney and allow his daughter to make choices regarding artificial hydration or food, for example. The nurse has an ethical duty based on the principle of client autonomy to not knowingly act against client wishes, even if she does not agree with them. Notifying the charge nurse to let the night shift nurse address the issue does not solve the problem and is irresponsible. Getting a consent for the daughter to sign goes against client wishes, which were recorded upon admission. There is no need to notify the surgeon or to order a type and cross. To give blood to the client against his wishes is considered assault and battery and may result in legal action involving the health care providers, including the surgeon, nurse, and facility. Although the client presents himself as a Jehovah's Witness, the nurse should still ask questions regarding transfusions, preferably out of the presence of friends or family members who may influence the client's true wishes. HIPAA allows the nurse to ask others to leave the room during the questioning process if the client is able to communicate, thereby preserving his privacy.

37. Numbers 4 and 5 are correct.

Rationale: In most states, LPNs may transcribe written (but not verbal or telephone) orders and sign off. The RN normally signs off the orders after ensuring accuracy and whether they are completed. The RN is responsible for LPN orders she signs off on during her shift. LPNs can perform finger-prick blood glucose testing, and so can UAPs who have been trained and checked off on how to use the equipment. In most states drawing blood from a PICC line may only be performed by an RN. Accessing a port may only be performed by an RN who has been certified competent in this skill. Hemodynamic monitoring is another advanced skill limited to RNs working in ICUs where they have demonstrated competency. Nurse practice acts vary slightly among the states. In some states, LPNs may perform limited activities with peripheral IVs after training and certification.

38. Number 1 is correct.

Rationale: The nurse has a legal and ethical duty to report any caregivers who may be impaired, whether it is a physician or an unlicensed assistive personnel. The nurse should immediately notify the nurse manager and/or the charge nurse. Facility policies will guide them on the proper response and whether to notify risk management or security. Since the physician may be impaired, any orders written may require review by another health care provider before implementing. Confronting the physician may result in escalating a potentially volatile situation and is inappropriate. The client should not be informed at this time of the physician's possible impairment until the situation has been followed up per facility guidelines. Another physician should not be consulted by the nurse, as this is a situation requiring intervention by management. The nurse should not enter orders that were written while the ordering physician was possibly impaired, even if it is a routine lab and seems to be an appropriate choice. The nurse assumes liability for entering any such orders and could be held liable if the order caused any harm to the client.

39. Number 4 is correct.

Rationale: If the client is stable, the nurse should accept the assignment and ask for another nurse with knowledge of chest tubes to educate him on chest tube management. The licensed nurse should be open to learning new skills when there is someone on staff who can assist him. The nurse should learn how to position the tube, mark drainage, chart output, and understand troubleshooting, such as what to do if an air leak develops. Chest tube management is an expected skill set in critical care settings. Stable clients may be on medical floors; training on equipment common to a care area of the facility should be readily available for new nurses. Asking for a different group of clients prevents the nurse from learning a valuable new skill set. Asking to be floated may disrupt staffing in other areas of the facility if no additional staff is needed. Refusing the assignment should be reserved for situations such as performing hemodialysis, which is not something quickly learned at the bedside. If the nurse is in an area where no other nurses have chest tube experience, the nurse manager should be notified. In cases like this, a nurse may be able to come from the ICU every 2 hours or so to round on the client, check the chest tube, and show the new nurse how to manage the tube.

40. Number 4 is correct.

Rationale: Injections on infants less than 18 months old should be done in the vastus lateralis, not the dorsogluteal area. The dorsogluteal area is not recommended for children less than 3 years of age. The correct needle length for this client is 7/8 inch to 1 inch in length. The injection should be given at a 90-degree angle. A 27-gauge needle is appropriate for injecting in the vastus lateralis.

41. Number 3 is correct.

Rationale: The nurse should inform the client that it is not safe to keep valuables in the room, and that security can bring a form stating which items the client would like to have locked up. The nurse cannot force the client to place items with security, but should inform the client of the option. The charge nurse's office is not a place to store client valuables. The client should not be encouraged to leave valuables in a drawer when he leaves the room. Insisting that the client call someone when the client has no one to call is counterproductive and may be interpreted as confrontational.

42. Numbers 2 and 4 are correct.

Rationale: A UAP can obtain a pulse oximeter reading on a client once he has demonstrated competency in using the device, which clips onto the finger similar to a clothespin. In many facilities, this is part of taking routine vital signs. The UAP can also prompt the client to do coughing and deep breathing once the nurse has shown the client how to perform it; however, the nurse must be the one to initially educate the client on the technique. UAPs cannot teach or assess clients; this is an activity reserved for the nurse. Only the nurse can assess lung sounds. Administering oxygen must be done only by the nurse. If the client is already on nasal cannula and gets up to use the restroom, the UAP may assist the client back to bed and place the nasal cannula back on the client once the UAP has demonstrated the proper technique. In no instance may the UAP be the one to initiate oxygen therapy, nor may he adjust the flow rate. The nurse should educate the client on incentive spirometer use. Depending on the facility, the nurse or respiratory therapist should assess and chart the client's number of attempts, the highest reading obtained, and gauge the work of breathing on a scale.

43. Number 2 is correct.

Rationale: Fever, a shrill cry, diarrhea, and nuchal rigidity indicate meningitis, which is a medical emergency. The infant must be placed on respiratory isolation immediately, monitored for seizures, and prepared for a lumbar puncture. Those in close contact with the infant may need prophylactic treatment as well. The client with abdominal pain and nausea is stable at this moment and can be seen later. The jogger is not the top priority because she has a good pedal pulse and no deformity in the ankle, which indicates that she is stable. The client who was working outside and presents with tachypnea, diaphoresis, and fatigue is at risk for heat syncope and should rest in a cool area and be taught to limit exposure in extreme heat, take frequent breaks, and drink plenty of water. This client is also stable. The child who fell off a bicycle onto grass while wearing a helmet is ambulatory, wore protection, and landed on a soft surface. Although he should still have an assessment to check for head injuries, he is not currently in a life-threatening situation like the infant.

44. Number 1 is correct.

Rationale: The best roommate for this client is a client with gout in the large toe. Necrotizing fasciitis is worse in immunocompromised clients, and this client has a history of diabetes and hepatitis. This leaves the client vulnerable to worsening the infection or developing a new infection on top of the necrotizing fasciitis. Gout is not a communicable illness, so this is the best roommate choice for this client. A client with fever, vomiting, and diarrhea may potentially have a contagious condition that can worsen the outcome for the client. The client with MRSA is not a good choice because there is a chance that the MRSA could infect the client with necrotizing fasciitis. The client with severe dementia and the tendency to wander is at risk of cross-contamination and further infecting the client with necrotizing fasciitis because of her inability to perform hand hygiene. Clients with necrotizing fasciitis are generally not contagious to healthy persons, but contact and universal precautions, along with hand hygiene, prevents them from further colonization by bacteria.

45. Numbers 1, 2, 3, and 4 are correct.

Rationale: The nurse understands that continuity of care only occurs when all people involved in client care maintain open, two-way communication so that nothing is overlooked or forgotten. Using standardized handoff reports ensures that all important data is conveyed to each following shift, without any omissions. Daily chart checks involve reviewing all orders written during the previous shift and ensuring that they have been completed or ordered, such as a series of daily labs. The nurse should follow up on incomplete orders or outstanding labs before the end of shift so that the next shift does not have to assume responsibility. Knowing proper procedures and forms needed to transfer clients helps to ensure that all orders "follow" the client to the next area. Telling the next shift that they need to draw labs that were due on the current shift is poor nursing practice and may affect treatments and medications ordered by the health care provider. The nurse must ensure that all orders on clients are carried out, even if that means staying over to finish that shift's work. Unless informed otherwise by the charge nurse or facility policy regarding overtime, the nurse is expected to finish all work for his shift before leaving.

46. Number 3 is correct.

Rationale: Even though the nurse cared for the client the previous day, she is no longer assigned to the client. Accessing the chart, even if she cared for the client previously, is a HIPAA violation in this instance. The nurse may not realize it, since she cared for the client previously. It is important to not become complacent about HIPAA compliance. The nurse should not go to the client's room unless she is called in there to help turn or perform another action. She does not legally have access at this time to view the chart. The nurse should not ask the current nurse about the client's condition, since this is still illegally sharing information that she is not privy to. HIPAA violations are not limited to viewing charts; any sharing of information about a client that the nurse is not caring for violates HIPAA regulations.

47. Numbers 1, 2, 5, and 6 are correct.

Rationale: Nurse-sensitive indicators in a quality improvement program consist of measurements of client care that are directly impacted by nursing care. Fall injury rates, restraint utilization rates, pressure ulcer prevalence and incidence, and client satisfaction with pain management are just a few. These are areas in which nurses assess diligently and know when to intervene. While staying within the unit budget is always a goal, it is not a nurse-sensitive indicator. Upgrading computer charting programs is not a nurse-sensitive indicator.

48. Numbers 3, 4, and 5 are correct.

Rationale: Charting should always contain only objective facts regarding what the nurse sees, hears, or feels. Noting that the client tolerated 80% of the lunch tray with no complaints of nausea or stomach cramping is an objective observation. It is important to note how well the client tolerated the meal. If the client complained of nausea while eating, this observation would be noted, preferably in the client's own words, such as "I started to get nauseated when I tried to eat." The observation about the abdominal dressing is factual and objective, noting the size of the area of light staining. When a client ambulates in the hall, it is important to chart the distance, whether assistive devices were used, and how well the client tolerated it. The nurse states that no dyspnea or syncope was noted. Statements that the client appeared anxious when family came to visit infers that the client was anxious due to the family's visit. This is presumptive on the nurse's part, as the client could be appearing anxious from unvoiced thoughts. Likewise, the nurse makes it sound as if the client is angry because her medications were changed, when there is no evidence that this is the case. The nurse should avoid charting that a client "appears" to have a certain type of reaction to an event, and chart only those objective facts without speculation.

49. Number 1 is correct.

Rationale: In an emergency situation where the client is suffering a potentially life-threatening event, it is not necessary to obtain consent. Trying to obtain consent from a family member wastes valuable time, since the client's identity is unknown. The client may not gain consciousness, so waiting until he can be roused is not the correct action. Asking the police to run the tag number wastes precious time that the client needs to be prepped for surgery, and is not a feasible option. Informing the health care provider that consent cannot be obtained does not apply in an emergency situation. The client is at high risk for death from internal bleeding.

50. Number 4 is correct.

Rationale: The nurse is using evidence-based decision-making to improve performance. Methods within performance improvement include collaboration and consultation. Informatics addresses processing data in an organized method to allow for storage and retrieval.

51. Number 1 is correct.

Rationale: A mid-shaft clavicle fracture needs to be immobilized to prevent further damage to the joint. Weight-bearing exercise is associated with a fracture in the lower extremities. An intake of 1,900 cc/day is the recommended amount for a healthy individual, making 1,500 cc/day suboptimal. Surgical repair for a fractured mid-shaft fracture is typically not required.

52. Number 1 is correct.

53. Number 2 is correct.

Rationale: While celiac disease is incurable, persons with the disease typically are able to control their symptoms when they follow a gluten-free diet. A chef salad with oil and vinegar dressing is the best option as it contains no gluten protein.

54. Number 4 is correct.

Rationale: Nurses work with patients and their families along with a variety of relevant health care team members and third-party persons. Evaluation of both positive and negative outcomes of patient advocacy should be addressed by the nurse. Providing physical, emotional, and spiritual support is within the scope of the nurse as an advocate. Advocacy practices may extend outside health care settings.

55. Number 2 is correct.

Rationale: A married minor may give informed consent. The remaining statements are true.

56. Correct answer: prone

57. Correct answer: supine

58. Correct answer: Fowler's

59. Correct answer: right lateral recumbent

60. Correct answer: left lateral recumbent

61. Correct answer: Trendelenburg's

62. Numbers 1, 2, 5, and 6 are correct.

Rationale: Primary prevention is focused on using strategies to prevent the actual occurrence of cancer. Secondary prevention uses screening to detect cancer in the early stages when it is most curable.

63. Number 4 is correct.

Rationale: Effective stress management techniques and debriefing can help team members use counseling and other resources to help prevent PTSD. Nurses play key roles before, during, and after a disaster. The critical incident stress debriefing team meets with team members to provide coping strategies. The administrative review analyzes what went wrong and what went right with the plan.

64. Numbers 2 and 3 are correct.

Rationale: In addition to immunocompromised clients and older adults, clients with infection in the head or neck are also at increased risk. Tooth abscess, otitis media, and sinusitis have been linked to meningitis. CDC recommendations include an initial vaccine between ages 11 and 12 years with a booster at 16 years. Booster shots are recommended for adults living in cramped quarters (dorms, military barracks, group homes) or traveling to areas where outbreaks are common.

65. Number 3 is correct.

Rationale: Although the nurse does not touch the sterile field with the clean gloves, there is still contamination because clean gloves were used to remove a sterile object. The syringe is now contaminated, and the close proximity of the clean gloves to the sterile field poses a transmission risk. Any time there is even a suspicion of contamination, the sterile field must be reestablished. Options 1, 2, and 4 reflect safe practice for sterile technique.

66. Number 4 is correct.

Rationale: Pulling the client up in bed is always a two-person task, or more if client is obese. The bed position may be flat or Trendelenburg as the client tolerates. Each person grasps the draw sheet and on the count of three, pulls the client up smoothly while taking care not to hit his head on the bed. Options 1, 2, and 3 are incorrect techniques and may harm the client or the nurse.

67. Number 4 is correct.

Rationale: Remember the mnemonic PASS to guide you: Pull pin, Aim at base of the fire, Squeeze the handles, and Sweep from side to side to ensure even and complete coverage. Options 1, 2, and 3 do not demonstrate proper use of a fire extinguisher.

68. Number 3 is correct.

Rationale: The nurse cannot give a medication via a route other than what was ordered without contacting the health care provider and obtaining a new order. The nurse should notify the pharmacy so that the missing medication can be replaced. Options 1, 2, 4, 5, and 6 do not address the route of administration.

69. Number 2 is correct.

Rationale: Droplet precautions focus on diseases that are spread by large droplets (greater than 5 microns) expelled into the air and by being within 3 feet of a client. Contact precautions are used for direct and indirect contact with clients and their environments. Airborne precautions are used with diseases that are transmitted by droplets smaller than 5 microns. These smaller droplets remain in the air longer and necessitate the use of an N95 respirator. These clients require a negative pressure or negative airflow room. Protective environments focus on a very limited client population that require a room with positive airflow greater than 12 exchanges per hour through HEPA filters.

70. Number 4 is correct.

Rationale: Blood must be given within a certain time frame, and delaying the administration may cause the blood to expire. Most facilities allow a 30-minute to 1-hour time frame for "on time" medication administration. Option 1 is incorrect because a 30-minute delay will not be too late. Option 2 is incorrect because IV medications are *never* given in tubing that is infusing blood, blood products, or TPN. Option 3 is incorrect because it involves stopping blood and infusing medication through the same tubing as the blood.

71. Numbers 1, 4, and 5 are correct.

Rationale: A bed missing a rail is a possible safety hazard and should not be used, even if it is otherwise serviceable. Extension cords pose a fall risk, and outside equipment that has not been inspected for safety may not be used in a health care facility, especially items typically purchased for home use. Equipment with a frayed cord is an electrical hazard and should not be used regardless of its safety inspection label.

72. Number 1 is correct.

Rationale: Placing dirty linen on the floor can transfer microorganisms and increase the risk of spreading infection. Dirty or clean linen should never be placed on the floor. Hand washing and using gloves help lower the spread of infection and are part of universal or standard precautions. Draping the client shows respect for the client's modesty and helps prevent the client from becoming too cold. Asking about toileting needs before the bath allows for removal of soiled linen if the client has an accident with the bedpan before clean linen is placed on the bed.

73. Numbers 3 and 4 are correct.

Rationale: The client is hyperoxygenated before suctioning to decrease suction-induced hypoxemia. Inserting the catheter upon inspiration minimizes oxygen loss from suctioning while the client is exhaling. When resistance is met or the client coughs, the nurse should pull the catheter back 1 cm to avoid trauma to the tracheal mucosa. Pulling back prevents the catheter tip from resting against the mucosal wall and stimulates cough. Normal saline is no longer used routinely in tracheal suctioning unless ordered by the health care provider due to the risk of bronchospasm or introducing organisms to the respiratory tract. Intermittent suctioning should be performed for no more than 10 seconds to avoid hypoxemia. Rotating the catheter upon removal helps avoid injury to the mucosal lining.

74. Number 1 is correct.

Rationale: The full container should be replaced with a new one. Sharps should never be placed on top of the container or forced into it, as this increases the risk of a needlestick injury. A dirty sharp should never be placed in a pocket because it is now contaminated from the client, even if the safety device is covering the needle.

75. Numbers 2 and 4 are correct.

Rationale: A client with a chest tube should not be placed in a Trendelenburg's position as this will prevent drainage from going into the chest tube drainage device. Constant bubbling in the water seal after clamping off suction indicates an air leak. The nurse should check and tighten all connections and check the tubing for a leak. If a leak is noted in the tubing, replace the drainage device. Check the insertion site by removing the dressing and verifying that the chest tube eyelets are not visible. If no leaks can be seen or heard at the insertion site, the lung is the source of the leak. If the leak persists after troubleshooting, notify the health care provider. A semi-Fowler's position is appropriate and facilitates drainage into the drainage system. Constant gentle bubbling in the suction control chamber and tidaling in the water seal chamber that corresponds to respiration are expected findings.

76. Numbers 1 and 4 are correct.

Rationale: The head of the bed should be elevated 30 degrees to promote venous drainage and prevent hemorrhage caused by excessive blood flow to the brain. The client should be monitored for signs of increased intracranial pressure such as increased blood pressure with widening pulse pressure and altered level of consciousness. Elevating the head of the bed 90 degrees is incorrect as increased hip flexion should be avoided. Neurological status should be monitored more frequently in the client immediately post-op, often every 15 minutes during the first hour, then every 30 minutes for the second hour, or according to health care provider orders. Antiembolism stockings should be in place either when the client returns to the room or immediately upon arrival. The client should not be positioned on the operative side due to the risk of brain shift.

77. Number 3 is correct.

Rationale: The nurse caring for the client with a radioactive implant should don a lead gown before performing any client care; therefore, the nurse only needs to retrieve the implant with long-handled forceps and place it into a lead container. Clients with implants should have a lead container and long-handled forceps available in the room in case of dislodgement. Once the implant is retrieved, the health care provider should be notified. Attempting to reinsert the implant is beyond the scope of nursing practice and should be performed only by the health care provider.

78. Number 4 is correct.

Rationale: Soiled linen should remain in the room until the source of radiation is removed; the linen may then be disposed of as usual. Setting up the meal tray is part of client care and should not be overlooked, and all personnel caring for the client should wear dosimeter badges to measure the amount of radiation exposure. Closing the door upon entering and exiting and keeping the door closed minimizes the risk of radiation exposure to other clients and staff.

79. Numbers 2, 3, and 4 are correct.

Rationale: Before giving metoprolol, the nurse should check the blood pressure and apical pulse. If the apical pulse is less than 60, the nurse should hold the medication and contact the health care provider. The nurse should always check for allergies before administering any medications. Joint Commission safety guidelines require that at least two patient identifiers are used before administering medications. The client's name, date of birth, and medical record number on the bracelet should match the chart. The nurse would not hold metoprolol for a heart rate greater than 80 bpm. There are no indications that grapefruit juice should be avoided when taking this medication.

80. Number 4 is correct.

Rationale: Special call light adapters are available for clients with limited mobility of the hands. Clients with Guillain-Barre syndrome tend to maintain the ability to turn the neck. Call light adapters can be placed on the pillow so that the client can turn his head and press the call light. A client should never be left without alternatives to call for help, so options 1 and 3 are incorrect. Often families cannot stay around the clock, so this may not be a reasonable request; even if someone stays with the client, having the ability to call for help on his own adds a layer of security and comfort for the client.

81. Number 2 is correct.

Rationale: When carrying heavy objects, the weight should be held as close to the body as possible to avoid back strain. When bending over to pick something up, the nurse should bend her knees to avoid back injury. When pulling clients up in bed, the bed should be at a comfortable height so that no one has to bend over to lift the client. Safety is a priority, and the nurse should utilize as many nurses as needed for safe lifting. Whenever possible, mechanical lift devices should be used to minimize back strain for the nurse and ensure client safety.

82. Number 3 is correct.

Rationale: Securing pieces of tape to a tray table or bed rail introduces pathogens from contaminated surfaces to the client's skin when applied. This increases the risk of pathogens entering the puncture site and causing infection in the client. If additional tape needs to be applied after the clear dressing, it should be removed from the roll just prior to application, without touching it to other surfaces. Washing the hands before and after placing an IV helps minimize the risk of infection. Use of alcohol or other approved skin cleanser helps remove pathogens and minimize the risk of infection. These products should dry completely before attempting to place the IV.

83. Numbers 2, 3, and 4 are correct.

Rationale: Vomiting should never be induced in an unconscious person. The Poison Control Center should be called before inducing vomiting. The number should be posted on or near each phone in households with small children. Placing chemicals on a high shelf does not prevent access; many toddlers become adept climbers and can reach dangerous items anyway. Chemicals should be locked in a cabinet with child-proof locks for maximum safety. Vomiting should never be induced in persons who have consumed lye, household cleaners, or grease.

84. Number 2 is correct.

Rationale: The client may not be aware of the danger of keeping chemicals so close to food, so the nurse should gently explain to the client in a respectful manner. The nurse can then say that a home safety inspection for other hazards is free and ask if the client would like one. The nurse can point out fall hazards, such as slippery rugs, or a frayed cord on a lamp that may start a fire. The nurse should always be on the lookout for environmental hazards to the client so that corrective action may be taken. There is no need to notify the health care provider or social services in this instance. The nurse should never keep quiet about situations that may place the client in jeopardy.

85. Numbers 2, 3, and 5 are correct.

Rationale: If the person vomits, saving the vomitus may help identify the substance ingested, especially in younger children. Quickly identifying the poisonous substance is key to intervention with an antidote. All homes with small children should post the number of the Poison Control Center near the telephone for quick access in an emergency, or the number should be programed into cell phones. Older adults may forget that they have already taken their medication or not be able to clearly read medication labels, which can lead to accidental overdose. Vomiting should never be induced unless instructed to do so by Poison Control. If the person needs to be transported to the hospital, emergency services should be called for an ambulance. The ambulance can get to the hospital quicker, and EMTs can start an IV and begin supportive treatment immediately. The nurse should never advise a client to drive quickly to the hospital, as this puts the client at risk for an accident.

86. Number 2 is correct.

Rationale: Activating the emergency response plan is the first priority and the most critical. Once the plan is activated, the appropriate person will call in extra staff. Restocking items that will most likely be needed would be addressed by the response plan and delivered from central supply by support staff. The charge nurse or other designated personnel would then move noncritical clients to a safe area and open up beds for incoming clients. Each facility's response plan may vary slightly, but it will address all protocols needed to ensure quick, efficient distribution of personnel and resources. Mock disasters and drills help facilities stay current and update the emergency response plan as needed.

87. Number 3 is correct.

Rationale: Droplet precautions, along with standard precautions, are used with clients infected with meningitis. Measles requires airborne precautions, while adenovirus requires droplet precautions. Barrier protection calls for either a private room or a cohort client with the same infection. Disseminated varicella zoster requires airborne precautions.

88. Number 1 is correct.

Rationale: The skin cannot be sterilized, according to the principles of surgical asepsis. The edges of a sterile field are considered unsterile. If a sterile object touches an unsterile object, the sterile object is considered contaminated. Sterile objects that are out of view or below waist level are considered unsterile. Sterile objects can become contaminated by airborne microorganisms.

89. Number 2 is correct.

Rationale: When removing PPE, gloves are removed first, then eye protection, followed by the mask, and then the gown. Hand hygiene is performed last. PPE should be applied preferably before entering the client's room. When donning PPE, hand hygiene is first, followed by the gown, mask, eye protection, and lastly, gloves.

90. Number 1 is correct.

Rationale: The priority nursing diagnosis is risk for injury. Client safety is always the priority, especially with a client who has a history of falls and Alzheimer's or confusion. Impaired skin integrity is an important nursing diagnosis but is not the priority for this client. There is nothing to indicate that this client has altered body image; risk for injury would take priority over altered body image. Impaired physical mobility due to dementia with Lewy bodies is a medical diagnosis, not a nursing diagnosis.

91. Number 5 is correct.

Rationale: The nurse should verify the client's identity by comparing the name, date of birth, and medical record number on the armband with the medication order. The 2012 National Patient Safety Goals require using at least two identifiers to avoid medication errors. Verifying the client's allergies should be done after correctly identify the client. Verifying the client's name and room number is not as accurate. Asking the client to state her name and date of birth is not reliable in persons with altered mental status or in a nonresponsive client. Scanning the wristband and barcode should be done only after the two identifiers are completed, just prior to administering the medications.

92. Number 1 is correct.

Rationale: Infants should be placed on their backs for sleeping. Placing an infant on her stomach for sleep increases the risk of sudden infant death syndrome (SIDS). The American Academy of Pediatrics recommends that newborns have the first checkup 3 to 5 days after birth. Infants should use an approved car seat when riding in a car, and never use car seats that have been in a crash or bought secondhand, as their safety status is unknown. Keeping important numbers such as the pediatrician and poison control center handy saves time in an emergency.

93. Answers:

Disease	Precaution
1. measles	airborne
2. shingles	airborne
3. tuberculosis	airborne
4. mumps	droplet
5. diphtheria	droplet
6. influenza	droplet
7. herpes simplex	contact
8. C. diff	contact
9. MRSA	contact

94. Number 2 is correct.

Rationale: E-cigarettes may contain nicotine and other toxins and are not approved for smoking cessation. Although social smoking is intermittent, it can still have an adverse effect on overall health. Option 3 states the correct method to calculate pack years. Nicotine replacement therapy has a success rate of 50 percent to 70 percent and is highest when used in conjunction with a smoking cessation program.

95. Number 3 is correct.

Rationale: When curative treatments or life-prolonging therapies have stopped, hospice may begin. Hospice clients have a prognosis of 6 months or less to live. Care may extend beyond the 60- and 90-day periods if the client meets eligibility requirements. Palliative care does not follow specific time periods. Palliative care consults can be provided concurrent with curative therapies.

96. Number 2 is correct.

Rationale: Processed foods such as baked ham are among the highest in sodium, along with preserved and pickled foods. Most fresh fruits and vegetables are low in sodium. Condiments tend to be high in sodium, and learning to read labels helps the client identify appropriate diet choices. Frozen pizza and many other frozen prepared foods are high in sodium because they are processed.

97. Number 1 is correct.

Rationale: From gestational weeks (GW) 18 to 30, the height of the fundus in centimeters is approximately the same as the number of weeks of gestation ±2 GW if the client's bladder is empty. With a full bladder, as much as a 3 cm variation is possible.

98. Number 3 is correct.

Rationale: At 6 months of age the baby should be aware of her surroundings and, when appropriate, laugh and make squealing sounds. The other stated behaviors are considered normal for a 6 month old.

99. Number 1 is correct.

Rationale: The current goal of antiviral therapy is to reduce the viral load for undetectable levels. At this time there is no indication that antiviral therapy cures HIV. There is a low risk of transferring HIV from the infant to other household members. HIV-positive mothers should not breastfeed but instead purchase formula based on the health care provider's guidance. Many secondary infections are common to HIV-positive infants, including pneumonia and herpes simplex. The infant should be closely monitored for these developments.

100. Number 4 is correct.

Rationale: The client should brush the teeth immediately after eating. While omelets contain protein, they are often prepared in butter or grease. Fried and high-fat foods should be avoided. Cool foods with little aroma and no spices are preferable. Large fluid intake should be avoided early in the morning and when nauseated, and consumed at other times instead.

101. Number 2 is correct.

Rationale: Naegele's Rule is based on accurate recall of the client's last menstrual period. It assumes a regular 28-day cycle. The estimated date of birth is calculated by taking the first day of the last period, subtracting 3 months, and adding 7 days.

102. Number 2 is correct.

Rationale: The primary stage of syphilis is characterized by a primary lesion, the chancre, that appears 5 to 90 days after infection. Secondary syphilis occurs 6 weeks to 6 months after the chancre appears and is characterized by a widespread, symmetric maculopapular rash on the palms and soles. An early latent infection is one that was acquired in the preceding year. The latent phase is asymptomatic for most individuals and occurs if left untreated.

103. Numbers 1, 3, and 4 are correct.

Rationale: Risk factors for AFE include diabetes, placenta previa or abruption, preeclampsia, eclampsia, advanced age, labor induction, forceps-assisted or cesarean birth, and uterine rupture or cervical laceration.

104. Number 3 is correct.

Rationale: The kidneys are in position at 16 weeks with typical shape and plan. Testes descend to the scrotum at 24 weeks. The bladder and urethra separate from the rectum at 8 weeks. Primitive respiratory responses begin at 20 weeks.

105. Number 3 is correct.

Rationale: A FHR of greater than 160 bpm lasting more than 10 minutes may indicate early fetal hypoxemia, fetal cardiac arrhythmias, infection, or fetal anemia. A normal FHR is from 110 to 160 bpm. Moderate variability is considered a normal finding. Minimal variability may occur with prematurity.

106. Number 4 is correct.

Rationale: Comfort measures such as side positioning during breastfeeding can help minimize fatigue. There is no evidence that supports PPF as being more common in cesarean births; it is, however, associated with long labor and cesarean births. Fatigue tends to worsen over the first 6 weeks after birth. Symptoms of PPF can be interrelated with postpartum depression.

107. Number 4 is correct.

Rationale: Most women with MG tolerate labor well as it does not affect smooth muscle. Approximately 10 percent to 15 percent of neonates born to women with MG develop neonatal myasthenia. The response of women with MG is unpredictable and can range from remission to exacerbation to continued stability throughout pregnancy. Clients with MG are already at risk for respiratory muscle weakness; regional anesthesia is preferred.

108. Numbers 3 and 4 are correct.

Rationale: The Rinne test compares bone conduction of sound with air. The Weber test uses a tuning fork to provide lateralization of the sound. Allen's test evaluates the patency of the ulnar and radial arteries by compressing them with the thumbs. Phalen's test involves 90-degree flexion to the wrists and tests for carpal tunnel syndrome.

109. Number 1 is correct.

Rationale: Clients older than 65 years and those with dense breasts are at the highest increased risk of developing breast cancer. Women who have their first child after age 30 or who are obese are at a low increased risk. A family history of two first-degree relatives with breast cancer is a moderate increase in risk.

110. Numbers 1, 2, 4, and 5 are correct.

Rationale: The health care provider should be consulted before receiving any vaccinations, and live vaccines should not be given. Avoiding aspirin and using electric razors and soft toothbrushes will help minimize the risk of bleeding. Mouth rinses may be prescribed for thrush and ulcers. Low-grade fever, sore throat, or chills indicate infection and should be reported to the health care provider.

111. Numbers 2 and 3 are correct.

    Rationale: Holding the cane on the unaffected side allows the cane to work with the weaker leg. The cane should move in tandem with the affected leg. Holding the cane on the affected side is incorrect technique. Moving the cane at the same time as the unaffected leg will not offer stability. The cane should be held 4 to 6 inches from the side of the foot; holding the cane too far away will not provide stability and may cause the client to fall.

112. Number 3 is correct.

    Rationale: The prescribed diet for dumping syndrome is high in fat and protein and low in carbohydrates. Lying down after meals prevents dumping syndrome. Weakness and dizziness, along with perspiration and tachycardia, are common assessment findings. Eating small meals and avoiding fluid intake with meals helps minimize symptoms.

113. Number 4 is correct.

    Rationale: The T-tube should be clamped before meals and the client observed for nausea, chills, abdominal distention, or discomfort. If nausea or vomiting occurs, the tube should be unclamped. A sudden increase in bile output should be reported to the health care provider. The semi-Fowler's position promotes drainage into the tube, along with keeping the drainage system below the level of the gallbladder.

114. Number 3 is correct.

    Rationale: If the reservoir bag kinks or twists, the client can suffocate. The mask should fit snugly on the face to avoid loss of oxygen. The flow rate should be adjusted to keep the bag inflated. A properly working mask will have valves opening upon expiration and closing on inhalation.

115. Number 2 is correct.

    Rationale: Clients age 65 – 85 are in the ego integrity versus despair stage. This is a time of reflection on life. Successful clients can look back with satisfaction, while unsuccessful clients may feel as if their lives were wasted. Young adults aged 19 – 34 years are in the intimacy versus isolation stage. Adolescents aged 12 – 18 years are in the identity versus role confusion stage. Adults aged 35 – 64 are in the generativity versus stagnation stage.

116. Number 4 is correct.

    In the 15 – 24 age group, unintentional injuries are the most common cause of death. This age group is at high risk for drinking and driving, motor vehicle accidents, and other unintentional injuries. Prevention and awareness of alcohol and drug abuse should be included in teaching. Suicide is the second most common cause of death in this age group, with homicide being the third most common. The nurse should inform the audience about suicide prevention and give the number of a hotline to call if needed. Personal safety should be covered as well, since many college students tend to consume alcohol and walk around campus, night clubs, and other areas late at night when they are vulnerable. Females especially should be taught to not go out alone at night and to never let their drink out of their sight at a party to avoid someone slipping a date-rape drug into their drink.

117. Numbers 1, 4, and 5 are correct.

    Rationale: Hypertension is often called the silent killer because one-third of people with high blood pressure are unaware of it. Hypertension has few signs or symptoms until it causes a stroke or heart attack. Few people experience facial flushing, sweating, and headaches that indicate hypertension until it has progressed to a serious, life-threatening condition. The southeastern United States is often called the "stroke belt" due to the higher incidence of hypertension and stroke in the region. Lack of physical activity also increases the risk of hypertension. Clients over age 60 are at greatest risk, and hypertension is higher in African Americans, especially those living in the southeast.

118. Number 3 is correct.

Rationale: This child is now due for the third round of hepatitis B and DTaP. Hib is given at 2, 4, and 12 months. MMR and varicella are not given until 12 months of age at the earliest. Hepatitis A is also not given until 12 months of age.

119. Number 1 is correct.

Rationale: This client is in the anger stage of grief. During the anger phase, the client may ask questions such as "Why me?" The client feels cheated out of life too early and knows that pancreatic cancer is a harder cancer to treat successfully. In the denial stage, the client refuses to accept the reality of the diagnosis. Denial is a defense mechanism at this stage. In the bargaining stage, the client may pray that if he is healed, he will become a faithful church-goer or be a better spouse. Acceptance is the final stage, in which the client comes to terms with reality. The client may exhibit signs of emotional detachment. In the depression stage, the client accepts the reality but may feel sadness or fear.

120. Number 4 is correct.

Rationale: HRT increases the risk of coronary artery disease, stroke, deep vein thrombosis, and breast cancer. It lowers the risk of osteoporosis-related fractures. The risks and benefits of HRT must be evaluated by the prescriber, based on the client's medical history.

121. Number 2 is correct.

Rationale: Most women of average weight should gain about 25 to 35 pounds during pregnancy. If they are overweight, they should gain a little less, whereas underweight women should gain a little more. Excessive weight gain increases the risk of preeclampsia. Failure to lose extra weight after the baby is born increases the risk of hypertension and diabetes. For most women, 15 to 20 pounds is inadequate weight gain, while a gain of 35 or more pounds is excessive. The client should work with her health care provider to monitor her weight gain and maintain an appropriate weight.

122. Number 1 is correct.

Rationale: Apgar scores measure five areas: appearance, pulse, grimace, activity, and respiration. The highest score for each item is 2. Therefore, the optimum score is 10. A score of 1 in an area indicates the infant is okay but diminished in that area. The lowest score for an area is 0. Poor activity would rate as 0. Apgar scores are obtained one minute after birth.

123. Number 3 is correct.

Rationale: Infants should roll from the tummy to the side by 10 months. By age 15 months, infants should be able to walk alone. Waving good-bye should be accomplished by 7 months. Transferring a toy from one hand to the other occurs by 9 months. New parents should be aware of general time frames for achieving motor skills so that they can notify the health care provider if the infant does not achieve milestones.

124. Number 4 is correct.

Rationale: The best time to perform testicular self-examination is just after bathing because the scrotum is more relaxed. Testicular cancer is one of the most curable cancers. It is most common in men ages 15 to 35. Any lump or swelling regardless of size should be reported to the health care provider.

125. Number 4 is correct.

Rationale: A pack year is one pack of cigarettes smoked daily for one year. This client smokes two packs per day. The calculation is 2 (packs per day) × 20 (years smoking) = 40 pack years. The other calculations are incorrect for this client.

126. Number 2 is correct.

Rationale: Clients with hypertension should avoid a high-sodium diet. Baked chicken with fresh green beans is the lowest sodium option listed. Frozen foods and processed foods are among the highest in sodium. While a spinach salad is healthy, the frozen pizza contains far too much sodium. Ham is processed meat, which is very high in sodium. Canned foods, especially soups, are high in sodium unless specifically labeled "low sodium" or "lower in sodium." The nurse should teach the client hidden sources of sodium in the everyday diet.

127. Number 2 is correct.

Rationale: Men should have a prostate-specific antigen test starting at age 50, not 55. Colorectal cancer screening should begin at age 50. High-density lipoprotein should be greater than 50 mg/dL for women. Risk factors for hypertension include being over age 60 and leading a sedentary lifestyle. Depending on the client's family medical history, the health care provider may recommend screening at an earlier age.

128. Numbers 1, 3, and 5 are correct.

Rationale: Language barriers, lack of a support system, and cognitive dysfunction are some of the barriers to learning. Low levels of literacy, environment, and cultural or background considerations may impede learning. Motivation to learn and adequate financial resources make it easier for the client to learn.

129. Numbers 1 and 2 are correct.

Rationale: Unintentional injuries are the leading cause of death for teenagers. Wearing seatbelts, even on short trips, and using approved helmets when bike riding can help prevent injuries. One hour after the last drink of alcohol is not a safe window for driving, especially when multiple drinks have been consumed. Condoms are not 100 percent effective against sexually transmitted infections, even when used correctly. Abstinence is the only method guaranteed to avoid sexually transmitted infections. Never dive into untested waters, even with the arms over the head to "break" the fall. If the bottom of a body of water is not visible, it should not be considered safe for diving.

130. Number 1 is correct.

Rationale: By 2 years of age, a child may use one hand more than the other. The remaining activities are consistent with achievement by a child 18 months of age.

131. Number 3 is correct.

Rationale: Clients who are tactile or kinesthetic learners prefer to learn by touching and doing. If they are learning how to administer insulin injections, they learn better by holding the syringe in their hand as opposed to simply watching a video or reading a handout. A client's living situation can affect his readiness and ability to learn. A client who has visual deficits will have a harder time reading a medication bottle and may be embarrassed about verbalizing his needs. The age and developmental stage must be considered; teaching a school-age child is much different from teaching a grown adult. Clients should be allowed to demonstrate their understanding of teaching, ask questions, and practice skills if necessary. There are many barriers to learning, including financial resources, lack of support systems, and a low level of literacy.

132. Number 4 is correct.

Rationale: Simvastatin is a Category X medication, meaning it has been proven to have a harmful effect on the human fetus and is contraindicated in pregnancy. The risks outweigh the benefits in Category X drugs. Metformin and amoxicillin are Category B drugs, meaning that animal studies do not demonstrate a risk to the fetus, and no well-controlled studies have been done in pregnant women. Gabapentin is a Category C drug, meaning that animal studies demonstrate a risk to the fetus, but it is possible that the benefits outweigh the risks in pregnant women. Very few drugs are tested in pregnant women due to ethical concerns of conducting clinical trials that may expose the fetus to harm.

133. Number 3 is correct.

Rationale: Suicide, unintentional injuries, and homicide are the three main causes of death for college-age young adults. HIV is one of the top 10 causes of death in people ages 25 – 34. Cancer is the leading cause of death for people ages 45 – 64. Heart disease is the second-leading cause of death for people ages 45 – 64.

134. Numbers 1, 2, and 3 are correct.

Rationale: Breast massage, frequent breastfeeding, and pumping breasts between feedings stimulate lactation in the postpartum client. Vigorous exercise should not be done one week after birth; the client should follow the health care provider's guidelines regarding when vigorous exercise can be resumed. Applying warm, not cold, compresses to the breasts stimulates lactation.

135. Number 3 is correct.

Rationale: HRT lowers the risk of bone fractures caused by osteoporosis but increases the risk of breast cancer and stroke. HRT increases the risk of coronary artery disease in all women, especially smokers, who already increase their risk of CAD by smoking.

136. Number 2 is correct.

Rationale: Signs of colic include pulling the legs up and crying after feedings. To determine if this condition needs further investigation, a diary of symptoms should be compiled by the mother and reviewed by the nurse. A baby who looks yellow may be experiencing hyperbilirubinemia. During their first 3 months of life, babies can cry up to 2 hours per day. A quiet child may be experiencing hypothyroidism. Being alert for brief periods of 10 – 20 minutes at a time is expected of normal babies at 2 weeks of age.

137. Number 1 is correct.

Rationale: Located between the first and second interspaces in the anterior chest are bronchovesicular sounds. Normally heard throughout the lung fields are vesicular sounds. Located between the second and third intercostal spaces of the anterior chest are bronchial sounds. Heard over the trachea are tracheal breath sounds.

138. Number 3 is correct.

Rationale: Within 12 hours of birth, children born to HBV-infected mothers should receive the hepatitis B vaccine, making breastfeeding a viable option. The second vaccine should be given to the child at 1 – 2 months and the third dose at 6 months of age. By age 9 – 18 months the infant should be tested for the presence of HBV. Optimal nutrition for newborns consists of exclusive breastfeeding for the first 6 months of age.

139. Number 4 is correct.

Rationale: Telling the client that everything will be okay or not to worry is an example of giving reassurance. Options 1 and 2 are examples of giving advice instead of asking the client what she thinks she should do. The nurse should never offer solutions that she has tried, as it takes focus off the client. Agreeing or disagreeing with the client implies that the nurse has the right to judge the client's ideas as right or wrong.

140. Number 4 is correct.

Rationale: Clang association often involves rhyming words. Echolalia speech is characterized by repeating the other person's words or phrases repeatedly. Mimicry is a technique used to try and identify with the speaker. Word salad is a jumble of random, unrelated words that do not express a complete thought. Neologisms are made-up words that have meaning only to the speaker.

141. Number 4 is correct.

Rationale: The client with delusion of control or influence believes that her behavior is controlled by certain people or objects. With somatic delusion, the client has false ideas about the functioning of his body. For example, a man may believe he is pregnant and will give birth. Delusions of grandeur involve feelings of superiority of power, knowledge, or importance. A client with delusions of grandeur may believe that he is God. The client suffering delusions of persecution feels that people are out to get her, for example, that a neighbor is plotting to kill her.

142. Number 1 is correct.

Rationale: Nonhealing ulcers and the presence of a stage 2 ulcer indicate a situation that has been going on more than just a few days; the client's limited mobility makes her more vulnerable to decubitus than someone more mobile. No specific findings indicate intentional physical violence. Emotional violence involves inflicting mental anguish or making threats. Economic exploitation involves illegally using one's assets and other funds for personal gain instead of ensuring that the funds are used to care for the client. The son is worried about treatment cost, and this is not an unreasonable concern for family members who care for elderly family members on limited incomes. He may be unaware of assistive programs available for his mother. The home health nurse should seek social services to assist the client in getting proper medical help and notify the client's health care provider.

143. Number 1 is correct.

Rationale: While all actions are an important part of client care during ECT, airway is always the priority. The nurse should be prepared to suction if needed and assist the anesthesiologist with oxygenation as required.

144. Number 3 is correct.

Rationale: Options 1 and 2 reflect the beliefs of people of many backgrounds and should be considered when caring for clients of different cultures and religions. Option 4 may be true of any patient regardless of background; furthermore, level of education has no bearing on the ability to provide basic personal information, and well-educated patients may still have limited English language skills. However, option 3 reveals sensitivity about the complex life circumstances of a client. Depending on the setting in which the nurse is working, social workers or other liaisons may be available and appropriate for consultation in caring for clients of varying backgrounds.

145. Number 4 is correct.

Rationale: Orienting the client to reality is the best therapeutic communication tool to use with this client. Presenting reality does not belittle the client or disregard her feelings, but provides an alternative line of thought to consider. Asking what the voices are saying encourages the behavior and may further confuse the client. Offering to move the patient to another room implies agreement that the voices are real. Notifying the physician is important with new-onset symptoms but is not a therapeutic response for this client as it fails to reorient to reality.

146. Numbers 4 and 5 are correct.

Rationale: White males over 80 are at the greatest risk among age, race, and gender groups, with 84% of elderly suicide victims being male. All threats of suicide should be taken seriously and immediate care should be sought out with the appropriate professionals. Chronic pain and serious illnesses such as cancer increase the risk of suicide. Whites are at the greatest risk of suicide among all ethnic groups. The risk of suicide may increase once antidepressants are effective because they may give the client the energy to formulate and carry out a suicide plan.

147. Number 2 is correct.

Rationale: Improvement in mood and an interest in outside activities or hobbies indicate that the client is responding positively to the medication. Depressed individuals often sleep a lot and skip work or school because they don't feel like doing anything. Tachycardia is a side effect of the medication and should be followed up to determine if another medication or dose is more suitable for this client.

148. Numbers 2, 3, and 4 are correct.

Rationale: All evidence must be preserved and collected following a strict chain of custody in order to be admissible in court, should the client pursue legal action. Rape kits are available in the ED that utilize a standard format of what information and items to collect. Some EDs have SANE (sexual assault nurse examiner) nurses who perform forensic nursing functions with specialized training. Photographing injuries provides further evidence for the medical record. Reassuring the client that she did what was needed to survive offers comfort. Before beginning any assessments or treatments, the client's mental condition should be evaluated. If the client is in extreme distress, it may be necessary to delay certain treatments or provide medication per the health care provider. The nurse should remain with the client at all times, as the pelvic examination may be painful and/or trigger flashbacks. If possible, ask the client if she would prefer a female physician. Advising the client on clothing choices implies that the client is to blame for the assault and may make the client defensive or less compliant with treatment. The client should receive information on rape crisis groups or other forms of support and counseling once she is able to comprehend and process the information.

149. Number 2 is correct.

Rationale: The safest option for the client is one-on-one observation by a staff member trained to work with potentially volatile clients. Distracting the client with a task may be helpful, but it is not the best choice here. Also, access to towels or sheets may allow the client to try and hang himself. Chemical and physical restraints should be used only as a last resort; physical restraints can escalate some clients to more violent behavior. Keeping the client in the day room is not an option because it is not the responsibility of other clients to watch out for one another and it shifts responsibility away from staff. Placing the client in isolation, even after removing potentially dangerous articles, is not the safest option and should not be used as a priority treatment. Clients have died in seemingly safe conditions in isolation, and this creates issues with risk management. Client safety is always the first priority.

150. Numbers 1, 3, and 4 are correct.

Rationale: Risk factors for domestic violence include being under age 30 and growing up in a home where child and spousal abuse occurred. Victims tend to have multiple abusive relationships over their lifetime. Many abusers severely restrict the victim's movement, so social isolation from friends and family is common. If the client is employed, she typically works in a low-paying field or goes through multiple jobs. Economic factors such as low income and lack of education are common in domestic violence, although it can occur in any environment.

151. Numbers 1, 5, and 6 are correct.

Rationale: Clients with delirium develop fever and other manifestations of delirium within 48 to 72 hours after the last drink. Disorientation and fluctuating levels of consciousness are common. Other signs in the delirium stage include anorexia and insomnia.

152. Numbers 1, 4, and 5 are correct.

Rationale: The prodromal phase may be brief, only a few weeks or months, but the average length according to most studies is 2 to 5 years. The residual phase usually follows the active schizophrenic stage, during which time negative symptoms can remain. Clients usually experience impaired role functioning and a flat affect. Treatment during the prodromal phase is focused on family coping, cognitive therapy, and support for identified problems. Clients in the premorbid phase tend to do poorly in school, have few or no friends, and avoid social activities. During the active phase, schizophrenia is not caused by drug abuse, medication interactions, or medical conditions.

153. Number 3 is correct.

Rationale: This client is suffering from sundowning syndrome, in which some clients become increasingly confused and irritated late in the afternoon. It is common in clients with dementia or Alzheimer's, but can occur outside those diagnoses. Reorienting and reassuring the client in a soft voice can help calm agitation. Distraction can help the client focus on something else and may calm the client. While asking a family member to stay may help, many clients do not have family that can stay around the clock due to work and other obligations. Xanax can help decrease anxiety and allow the client to rest, but less invasive measures are always preferable. Dosing a client simply to make her sleep or rest for the nurse's convenience is a form of restraint (chemical). Threatening the client with restraints is more likely to escalate the situation, and the client may become physically violent. Some clients with sundowning syndrome may suffer hallucinations or mood swings. Being in the hospital interrupts normal patterns of sleep and rest, and certain medications or medical conditions may make the client more likely to have an episode.

154. Numbers 2, 3, 4, and 5 are correct.

Rationale: Clients with bulimia can develop erosion of the tooth enamel from repeated vomiting due to the acid in the vomitus. Binging and purging can occur with both anorexia nervosa and bulimia. Anorexics tend to eat very low-calorie diets, restrict certain food groups, or exercise compulsively in order to lose weight. Many clients with eating disorders feel that the only thing they can control is their weight, and often feel pressured by family to achieve perfection. Clients with anorexia are obsessed with fear of obesity.

155. Number 1 is correct.

Rationale: Current recommendations regarding oral health suggest beginning dental care for a child by the first birthday. Age 2 is past the recommended age range for first dental visits. Age 3 is also past the recommended age range for first dental visits. Waiting until the child starts kindergarten increases the risk of cavities and the buildup of tartar.

156. Numbers 2, 4, and 5 are correct.

Rationale: Inadequate coping can manifest with physical symptoms, general irritability, and destructive behavior toward self or others. The client may or may not be able to verbalize the inability to cope. When coping mechanisms fail, anxiety can trigger defense mechanisms to protect the self. Inadequate coping can be caused by a number of factors. Lack of a family or social support system, serious medical diagnoses, crisis situations, and lack of psychological resources contribute to the inability to cope. Coping mechanisms are not always destructive; many coping mechanisms are positive and allow the individual to effectively manage stress. The nurse should not criticize the client's defense mechanisms that are not effective. Instead, the nurse should suggest ways to develop better defense mechanisms and work with the client to enhance and reinforce those skills. The nurse must be aware of which coping and defense mechanisms the client uses in order to develop a suitable plan of care.

157. Number 4 is correct.

Rationale: This client clearly has the means (a gun) with easy access (within reach of the bed) to commit suicide. The client is at high risk and should be placed on suicide precautions, including 24-hour observation. All possible hazards should be removed from the environment. Plastic utensils should be used with all meals, and the client should not wear or have a belt or shoestrings in the room. The health care provider should be notified of the findings. Options 1 and 3 express despair and frustration, but not necessarily suicidal intentions. Option 2 indicates that the client has an adequate family support system and is a positive response without suicidal ideations.

158. Numbers 1 and 5 are correct.

Rationale: During an active hallucination, safety is the first priority. The nurse should administer medications as ordered to manage the hallucinations. Asking the client if he hears voices telling him to harm himself or others is important for both client and nurse safety, as well as others in the area. A client having hallucinations should not be touched. The nurse should not tell the client that others are experiencing the same thing as this only reinforces the hallucination and false beliefs. The client should be moved to an area with decreased stimuli, not taken to the dayroom with others. The nurse should gently attempt to reorient the client to reality. Going along with what the client says he is experiencing reinforces false beliefs and interferes with reorienting the client to reality.

159. Number 4 is correct.

Rationale: The nurse is presenting reality while acknowledging that the client's perception is real to her. This response shows respect for the client's feelings. Suggesting that the client take a nap diverts attention away from the topic and does not present a solution to the problem. This response may lead to agitation in the client. Options 2 and 3 acknowledge that the client's misperception is real, and do not help reorient the client to reality. The nurse should never "play along" when clients are experiencing visual or auditory hallucinations.

160. Number 4 is correct.

Rationale: Pulling out hair or eyelashes, picking compulsively at the skin, and rocking back and forth are signs of unaddressed anxiety or stress. The nurse should intervene and ask the client what is bothering her. Open-ended questions allow the client to verbalize her feelings without a simple yes-or-no answer. Options 1 and 3 show clients engaging in healthy outlets. Two clients arguing over the TV does not necessarily indicate inadequate coping. In a group environment, clients will have different tastes in entertainment. As long as a compromise is reached without physical or verbal violence, this situation does not reflect anxious behavior like self-harm does. While pulling out one's hair or other "picking" behavior does not constitute suicidal behavior, it is still considered self-harm.

161. Number 1 is correct.

Rationale: The termination stage begins with the initial group meeting. Members' feeling about their accomplishments are explored during the termination stage. Members may be unclear about the group's purpose during the initial stage. Group roles and responsibilities are established in the initial stage of group therapy.

162. Number 4 is correct.

Rationale: Characteristics of disorganized schizophrenia include extreme social withdrawal, inability to perform activities of daily living, inappropriate affect, and grimacing mannerisms. Residual schizophrenia is characterized by being diagnosed with schizophrenia in the past, extreme social isolation, and impaired role functioning. Several years may pass between episodes. Paranoid schizophrenia includes hostility, delusions, violence, persecutory themes, and suspiciousness. Clients with catatonic schizophrenia experience waxy flexibility, psychomotor disturbances, stupor, and excessive purposeless motor activity. They may also be automatically obedient to directions and exhibit stereotypical or repetitive behaviors. Undifferentiated schizophrenia does not meet the definition of paranoid, disorganized, or catatonic schizophrenia. It is characterized by disorganized speech, delusions and hallucinations, flat affect, social withdrawal, and catatonic or disorganized behavior.

163. Number 3 is correct.

Rationale: The nurse can change the client's physiologic response by directing him to take deep breaths. This directive will shift the client's focus to the present. During a panic attack the client will be unable to move his focus to a long-term memory. Providing the client with a glass of water could prove harmful as he may be unable to physically perform the acting of drinking. The client most likely will not be able to identify the source of his anxiety.

164. Numbers 2, 3, and 4 are correct.

Rationale: Interventions for schizophrenia include reassuring the client that the environment is safe and engaging in simple, concrete activities such as puzzles or word games. Art, writing, and music can help the client safely express his feelings. A neutral approach is less threatening than an overly warm and friendly approach. The nurse should inform the client when she is leaving to orient the client to reality and reassure him.

165. Numbers 3 and 4 are correct.

Rationale: Clients who are easily bored, have poor and shallow interpersonal relationships, and enjoy being the center of attention have histrionic personality disorder, which is one of the four types of Cluster B personality disorders. Clients who are impulsive, exhibit unpredictable behavior, experience extreme mood shifts, are easily angered, and play people against each other exhibit borderline personality disorder, which is a Cluster B personality disorder. Other Cluster B personality disorders include narcissistic and antisocial personality disorders. Preoccupation with rules and details, hoarding, ritualistic behavior, and extreme devotion to work are characteristics of obsessive-compulsive personality disorder, which is one of the Cluster C personality disorders. Other Cluster C personality disorders include dependent and avoidant personality disorders. Clients who are suspicious of others and engage in magical thinking, eccentric behavior, paranoia, and relationship deficits exhibit schizoid personality disorder, which is a Cluster A personality disorder. Clients who are suspicious and untrusting of others, are argumentative, are controlling of others, and have thoughts of grandiosity have paranoid personality disorder, which is a Cluster A disorder. The other Cluster A disorder is schizotypal personality disorder.

166. Number 4 is correct.

Rationale: In applying the nursing process, the most appropriate action is to assess the situation by interviewing the client. Recording suspicions in the medical record without further assessment would be premature. Obtaining information from the client, rather than his family, is most appropriate. Notifying the physician should occur after assessment.

167. Number 3 is correct.

Rationale: Suicide and other violent behaviors are high risk for clients who experience posttraumatic stress disorder and pose the most significant of the problems listed. While panic attacks and short-term memory loss may occur with posttraumatic stress disorder, suicide is the most important problem. Anorexia is not seen in clients with posttraumatic stress disorder, though anorexia nervosa may present as a co-occurring disorder.

168. Number 3 is correct.

Rationale: Response 3 is consistent with being culturally sensitive to the client's needs. Death is understood differently based on one's culture. Dietary habits vary in importance between cultures. Explaining the nurse's cultural beliefs to the client is unnecessary as the client's needs are what is important.

169. Number 1 is correct.

Rationale: In response 1, the nurse expresses sympathy, acknowledges the family's loss, and leaves the decision to view their loved one with the family. The second and third responses assume the family wants to view their loved one. In the last response, the nurse makes the decision about the family viewing the body.

170. Number 2 is correct.

Rationale: Attendance at all therapy sessions should be an expectation established within the confines of the therapeutic relationship. Requirement of attendance places the client in a position where failure to attend all sessions, rather than being a point for learning, becomes a mechanism for punishment. Using this approach will not assist the client in achieving the desired outcome of abstinence from drugs.

Establishing a therapeutic relationship with a client who is addicted to drugs requires open, supportive communication consistent with options 1 and 3. Determining the presence of a concurrent psychiatric disorder is necessary to provide a comprehensive therapeutic approach.

171. Numbers 1 and 4 are correct.

Rationale: Agoraphobia is the fear of being in open spaces. Panic attacks and the fear of leaving home are symptoms associated with the disorder. Neither short-term memory nor auditory hallucinations are associated with agoraphobia.

172. Number 4 is correct.

Rationale: The nurse can explain to the client and the family the signs that indicate death is near. The nurse should allow the client and family to discuss goals for care, such as pain relief. The client may wish to have heroic measures taken, or he may prefer to be kept comfortable without heroic interventions. The nurse should respect the client's wishes, even if they differ from what she thinks is right. Telling the family that she will have the doctor come talk to them passes off responsibility, and may make the family more anxious if they have to wait to talk to the doctor. The nurse knows the information to share, and should take the opportunity to establish rapport with the family and reassure them that their wishes will be respected. Telling the family not to worry and that other treatments may be effective belittles their feelings and offers false hope.

173. Number 4 is correct.

Rationale: A perceived loss is one that is not obvious to those around the person experiencing the loss. Disappointment over the birth of a child of the "wrong" sex would not be obvious to those around her unless she verbalized it. Losing a job, failing a class, and losing a spouse are events that would obviously be perceived as a loss.

174. Numbers 1, 2, and 6 are correct.

Rationale: Risk factors for spousal abuse include alcohol or drug use by either partner and low income or living at the poverty level. An unplanned pregnancy may trigger violence in the spouse, especially if the couple has any of the other risk factors. The more risk factors a couple has, the greater the potential for abuse. The risk is greater for those under the age of 30. A higher level of education lessens the risk of abuse, but does not guarantee it will not occur. Having a large circle of friends is less risky than being socially isolated from friends or family. Many abusers control their spouses by keeping them from family and friends and limiting their freedom. The nurse must understand that simply living at a low income level or having less education does not automatically mean that the relationship is abusive, because abuse can occur in any environment for any number of reasons.

175. Number 4 is correct.

Rationale: Physical signs and symptoms of opioid addiction can be physical, psychological, and behavioral. Physical signs and symptoms include runny nose, bloodshot eyes, sleep disturbance, slurred speech, impaired coordination, and change in appetite. Psychological signs and symptoms include irritability, paranoia, unusual breathing, anxiety/irritability, mood swings, outbursts of anger, and unusual fear. Behavioral signs and symptoms include lack of personal hygiene, neglect of responsibilities, secretive spending, and foregoing social connections. Hypotension, diaphoresis, and shallow respirations are not characteristic of opioid abuse.

176. Number 4 is correct.

Rationale: Phenytoin (Dilantin) may be given to a person experiencing seizures while undergoing withdrawal from alcohol. For a disturbed heart rate, lidocaine (Xylocaine) may be given. For hallucinations, Haldol (haloperidol) may be given. For drowsiness, the nurse would lessen the dosage of diazepam.

177. Number 2 is correct.

Rationale: A common physiological symptom of fentanyl intoxication is nausea. Constipation, rather than diarrhea, is a common symptom of fentanyl intoxication. Urinary function is not affected by fentanyl. Drowsiness, rather than anxiety, is a common symptom of fentanyl intoxication.

178. Number 1 is correct.

Rationale: Bipolar disorder results in dramatic changes in a person's mood and energy. In the mania phase, people feel energized, even euphoric. When in the depressed stage, people have low energy and resist engaging with the world. The need to repeat a given behavior is consistent with obsessive-compulsive disorder. Hallucinations—believing/seeing/smelling/hearing things that do not exist—is associated with schizophrenia. Intense feelings about the need to protect oneself is associated with post-traumatic stress disorder.

179. Number 2 is correct.

Rationale: Carbohydrates help maintain postmeal glucose levels, and proper carbohydrate intake helps achieve glucose regulation and glycemic control. Balancing cholesterol intake with protein intake follows current ADA dietary recommendations. Fiber also helps stabilize carbohydrate metabolism and lower cholesterol.

180. Number 1 is correct.

Rationale: Elevating the head of the bed with blocks or a large, wedge pillow can prevent reflux. Large meals should be avoided; instead the diet should consist of 4 to 6 small meals throughout the day. Lying on the right side, not the left, helps promote oxygenation and frequent swallowing to help clear the esophagus. Liquid antacids should be taken 1 hour before and 2 to 3 hours after meals.

181. Number 4 is correct.

Rationale: Lacto-vegetarians eat milk, cheese, and dairy but no meat, fish, poultry, or eggs. The lacto-ovo-vegetarian includes eggs in the diet; option 3 reflects this diet choice. Vegans eat only plant-based foods and would choose option 2. Option 1 contains poultry and would not fall under vegetarian diet guidelines.

182. Number 3 is correct.

Rationale: The affected limb is elevated to decrease edema and promote venous return for the first 24 hours. After this time, the client is normally positioned supine with the affected limb flat on the bed to prevent hip contracture. Wedging a pillow between the thighs causes abduction at the hips and can cause contracture. The client would not be placed on the left side due to increased pressure on the operative site, which could cause bleeding and impede blood flow.

183. Number 2 is correct.

Rationale: A high Fowler's position facilitates insertion of the tube and prevents aspiration should the client vomit. The other positions do not facilitate insertion and greatly increase the risk of pulmonary aspiration.

184. Numbers 2 and 4 are correct.

Rationale: Positioning the client supine with the right upper abdomen exposed allows the best access to the right intercostal spaces. Raising the right arm and extending it behind the head opens up the intercostal area and keeps the arm out of the way. The liver is located on the right side; positioning the client with the left upper abdomen exposed does not allow access to the site. The client should be placed supine, never in a low Fowler's or other elevated position. The client's right arm should not be positioned across the front of the chest as this does not provide maximum access to the site.

185. Numbers 1 and 5 are correct.

Rationale: Clients should never be lifted onto a bedpan, as this can cause muscle strain for both the client and nurse. If the client cannot raise up for bedpan placement, the client should be rolled onto the bedpan. The fracture bedpan differs from a regular bedpan in that it is smaller and has a shallow upper end. The shallow end should go under the buttocks, and the deeper end where the handle is should be placed under the upper thighs. Unless contraindicated, the bed should not be placed flat as this causes the client to hyperextend the back while hips are elevated on the bedpan. Placing the call light within reach and stepping out for a few minutes preserves client privacy and dignity. If the client has not called within 5 minutes, the nurse should check back on the client. A confused client may forget that the bedpan is in place and remain on it too long, which can increase the risk of decubitus and/or skin shear.

186. Number 2 is correct.

Rationale: Asking clients what works for them shows respect for their practices and beliefs. Some low-risk therapies that the client might try include music therapy, meditation, prayer, and relaxation techniques. For mild pain, distraction may be helpful to remove the focus from the pain. Once the nurse knows the client's preferences, the health care provider can be consulted as to which therapies may be ordered. The nurse should not recommend any herbs or supplements for pain. This constitutes practicing medicine without a license. Any medication the client takes, including over-the-counter medicines or supplements, must be ordered by the provider. Some herbal mixtures or supplements can be toxic, and there is no consistent standard for such products. The client has had anesthesia for the procedure, therefore increasing the risk of an interaction between anesthesia and an unknown substance. Telling the client that they only use "real" medicine in the hospital shows a lack of respect for the client and her beliefs and is insulting. The nurse should not insist on opioids or other medications if the client states that she does not want to take them. While yoga may help relieve stress and pain, a client who is newly post-op will not be able to perform such activities. The nurse is also pushing his own agenda by telling the client what works for him. The focus is on therapies that help the client, not the nurse.

187. Number 1 is correct.

Rationale: Clearing the pump ensures that IV fluid intake will be accurate. A client on strict I's and O's is not necessarily on fluid restriction, and may receive IV fluids, blood, or antibiotics and other medications. Options 2 and 3 shift responsibility from the nurse to the client, which is not acceptable. The nurse monitors all intake and output. Option 4 is rude and not appropriate; the client may ask for other fluids in between meals.

188. Number 4 is correct.

Rationale: In the immediate post-catheterization phase, the client remains on bed rest for 4 to 6 hours with the accessed extremity kept straight until hemostasis is achieved. The client would not have bathroom privileges during this period and should be offered the bedpan or urinal as needed. Keeping the head of the bed at 45 degrees would place too much pressure on the access site. Ambulation to prevent clot formation occurs only after bed rest time is up and hemostasis is achieved. Frequent inspection of the femoral site for hematoma, oozing, or frank bleeding is a priority throughout the recovery process.

189. Answers:

Pulmonary Disorder	Nursing Intervention
1. emphysema	teach diaphragmatic, pursed-lip breathing
2. asthma	identify and minimize pulmonary irritants
3. cystic fibrosis	provide frequent mouth care to reduce chances of infection from mucus being present
4. chronic bronchitis	teach controlled coughing

Pulmonary Disorder	Nursing Intervention
5. pneumonia	hydration of at least 2L/day to thin and loosen pulmonary secretions
6. influenza	prevent spread of infection to others
7. pulmonary embolus	monitor for right-sided heart failure
8. pneumothorax	monitor drainage from chest-tube system

190. Answers:

Endocrine Disorder	Endocrine Disorder
1. tumor posterior pituitary gland	instruct on high-sodium, low-potassium diet
2. hypoparathyroidism	instruct on low-sodium, high-potassium diet
3. Addison's disease	measure urine specific gravity
4. Cushing's disease	monitor airway

191. Answers:

Injured Brain Area	Nursing Intervention
1. frontal lobe	give simple instructions; reorient as needed
2. temporal lobe	speak clearly due to impaired hearing
3. occipital lobe	assist with ADL due to visual disturbances
4. brain stem	monitor vital signs
5. parietal lobe	provide simple, one-step instructions
6. cerebellum	assist with walking

192. Numbers 2, 3, and 5 are correct.

Rationale: Older clients are more susceptible to CNS side effects of cimetidine, including agitation, confusion, and disorientation. Tetany is a neuromuscular side effect of hypomagnesemia. Constipation is a side effect of cimetidine in the GI system.

193. Number 4 is correct.

Rationale: Cyclopentolate HCl is a mydriatic medication used to dilate the pupils preoperatively and for eye examinations. Use of mydriatics is contraindicated in clients with cardiac dysrhythmias, as this increases the risk of serious side effects such as tachycardia and hypertension due to systemic absorption. This can lead to stroke, myocardial infarction, and cardiac ischemia, especially in the elderly or those with pre-existing myocardial disease. Osteoporosis, hypothyroidism, and renal insufficiency are not conditions that would contraindicate use of mydriatics.

194. Number 2 is correct.

Rationale: Side effects of prednisone include hypokalemia. Anxiety, confusion, and lethargy are signs of hypokalemia and should be reported. Increased appetite and slight weight gain are common side effects that do not need to be reported; weight gain greater than 5 pounds per week or continued weight gain should be reported. A strong, bounding pulse would not be an expected finding in hypokalemia.

195. Number 4 is correct.

Rationale: Terbutaline is contraindicated with coronary artery disease. It may increase blood glucose levels and should be used with caution in diabetes. Migraines and osteoarthritis are not contraindications for this medication.

196. Number 2 is correct.

Rationale: Nitroglycerin and dopamine are compatible. The other drug combinations listed are not compatible.

197. Numbers 1, 3, and 4 are correct.

Rationale: The client should tilt the head back and look up. The nurse then gently pulls the lower lid down and places the drop into the conjunctival sac without touching the applicator to the eye or any other surface. The nurse should wait 3 to 5 minutes between drops to allow maximum absorption. Pulling the upper lid up and placing drops just above the pupil is not correct technique. The client should not squeeze the eyes or rub them after the drops have been administered.

198. Number 1 is correct.

Rationale: Fosamax should be taken with water at least 30 minutes before breakfast or other medications. Clients should report fever and not lie down for at least 30 minutes after taking Fosamax. Food, especially dairy, interferes with absorption.

199. Number 3 is correct.

Rationale: The Parkland formula calls for crystalloid only (Lactated Ringer's) solution for initial fluid replacement. D5W and colloid solutions are not used in the Parkland formula. The Modified Brooke formula prescribes 5% albumin in isotonic saline for the first 24 hours.

200. Number 2 is correct.

Rationale: Seizures are a serious, adverse drug effect that may occur when taking Adderall. Nausea and constipation are common side effects but are not considered adverse drug effects. Adderall normally decreases appetite, causing weight loss instead of weight gain.

201. Numbers 3 and 5 are correct.

Rationale: Vitamin C toxicity causes occult rectal bleeding and increased estrogen levels. Muscle weakness is a sign of vitamin D toxicity. Halos around objects do not occur with vitamin C toxicity. Dry mucous membranes may occur with vitamin A toxicity.

202. Number 1 is correct.

Rationale: Atypical antipsychotics can cause tachycardia, not bradycardia. Diabetes can occur due to changes in glucose metabolism. These drugs can cause weight gain and obesity. Although rare, neuroleptic malignant syndrome can occur and cause death. Signs and symptoms include muscle rigidity, fever, confusion, and elevated creatinine levels.

203. Number 2 is correct.

Rationale: Calcium channel blockers cause vasodilation and decrease total peripheral resistance, which leads to a decrease in blood pressure. The other options do not correctly describe the mechanism of action of calcium channel blockers. Vasoconstriction coupled with increased total peripheral resistance would raise, not lower, blood pressure. Increasing the pressure on one component results in overall blood pressure increase, even if the other component is decreased.

204. Number 4 is correct.

Rationale: Upper body flushing, often called "red man syndrome," is a side effect of vancomycin that can occur especially if the drug is infused too rapidly. Side effects of cephalexin include diarrhea, easy bruising, dark urine, and joint pain. Side effects of amoxicillin include black or "hairy" tongue, stomach pain, nausea and vomiting, and pale or yellowed skin. Side effects of gentamicin include loss of appetite, rash, increased thirst, and muscle twitching. Side effects of antibiotics may be minor, severe, or life-threatening.

205. Number 3 is correct.

Rationale: Nitroglycerin should be taken one tablet at a time, sublingually every 5 minutes up to three doses over 15 minutes as needed for chest pain. If pain relief does not occur, 9-1-1 should be called. It is not safe to take nitroglycerin if taking sildenafil unless approved by the health care provider. Nitroglycerin should be taken one tablet at a time and never chewed or crushed. The pills must be kept in a dark container to prevent loss of effectiveness of the medication.

206. Number 3 is correct.

Solution:

amount of solution (mL)/time (in minutes) × drop factor (gtt/ml) = flow rate (gtt/min).	Determine flow rate by multiplying rate of infusion and number of drops per milliliter of the fluid being administered.
1,000 ml/360 min (6 hrs × 60 min/hr) × 10 gtt/mL	Substitute and solve.
= 27.7 gtt/min	
28 gtt/min	Round up to find the flow rate.

207. Number 1 is correct.

Rationale: Lactulose is a laxative given to lower ammonia levels in clients with hepatic encephalopathy. Elevated BUN indicates a dysfunction in the body's ability to convert protein to nitrogen; this coupled with elevated ammonia levels would present as confusion. Sucralfate is an anti-ulcer medication used in the management of GI ulcers. Lamotrigine is an antiepileptic medication used to control seizures. Gabapentin is an anticonvulsant and mood stabilizer.

208. Number 2 is correct.

Rationale: Oral thrush (candidiasis) occurs when the fungus Candida albicans accumulates on the lining of the mouth. While more likely to occur in babies, this condition also appears in persons with a suppressed immune system. The medication should be swished in the mouth, then either spit out or swallowed. To make the best contact with the oral mucosa, the medication should be taken after meals. The solution should not be diluted with other liquids. The standard frequency of nystatin is four times a day.

209. Number 4 is correct.

Rationale: Metabolism of acetaminophen occurs primarily in the liver, causing an elevation of liver enzyme levels. Metabolic alkalosis is not associated with acetaminophen overdose. Blood urea nitrogen level results from metabolism of protein by the liver and is not associated with acetaminophen overdose. A decrease of hemoglobin and hematocrit is consistent with anemia.

210. Number 3 is correct.

Rationale: Assessment of the therapeutic level of lithium in the blood is required to determine the next course of action. An extra dose of lithium carbonate may make the symptoms more pronounced. The client's behavior does not warrant a trip to the emergency department, although he should seek medical attention. There is not enough information yet to determine whether hemodialysis is necessary.

211. Number 3 is correct.

Rationale: Ibuprofen will alter the effect of lithium and should be avoided. Breastfeeding is not recommended as lithium passes into breast milk and may have undesirable effects on a nursing infant. Driving, using machinery, or performing any activity that requires alertness or clear vision should be avoided until the patient is sure she can perform such activities safely. The patient should also drink extra fluids to prevent dehydration, a common side effect of taking lithium.

212. Number 3 is correct.

Rationale: Risperidone is the only atypical antipsychotic medication listed. Atypical antipsychotics treat the negative symptoms of schizophrenia, such as alogia (poverty of speech). Loxapine, thioridazine, and haloperidol are used to treat the positive symptoms of schizophrenia, such as hallucinations.

213. Number 2 is correct.

Rationale: A baked chicken breast with green beans is an acceptable diet choice for the client on MAOI. Clients on MAOI should avoid all foods containing tyramine, which can cause hypertensive crisis. Yogurt, sausage, and sauerkraut are high in tyramine.

214. Number 3 is correct.

Rationale: Uncontrolled narrow-angle glaucoma is a contraindication for duloxetine hydrochloride therapy, as it can further increase pressure in the eye. The nurse should notify the health care provider so that an alternative medication may be considered, along with treatment of glaucoma. Insomnia is a common side effect of duloxetine hydrochloride. The nurse can educate the client about nonpharmacologic methods to improve sleep. Decreased appetite and weight loss are side effects of the medication. If the weight loss is too fast or too much, the health care provider should be notified; otherwise, small fluctuations in weight over a long period of time should not be a concern. Removal of a skin cancer, while important, is not an anticipated side effect of duloxetine hydrochloride.

215. Numbers 1, 2, 4, and 6 are correct.

Rationale: Signs and symptoms of overdose with tricyclic antidepressants include confusion, dry mouth, dysrhythmias, and flushing of the skin. Tachycardia and dilated pupils are other signs. Cardiac rhythm may progress to intraventricular blocks, complete atrioventricular blocks, and ventricular fibrillation. The nurse should prepare for gastric lavage to avoid further absorption of the medication.

216. Numbers 3 and 4 are correct.

Rationale: A single dose starts to wear off within 30 minutes and is essentially gone after 90 minutes. Bystanders, with education and training, are able to successfully administer naloxone (Narcan) to persons experiencing an opioid overdose. Naloxone (Narcan) is administered by intramuscular (IM) injection in the muscle of the arm, thigh, or buttocks. Alternately, the medication may be administered by nasal spray. The medication typically works within 5 minutes.

217. Number 2 is correct.

Rationale: Oxygen and suctioning are key to maintain the client's airway. Forcing a tongue blade into someone's mouth may chip teeth and cause aspiration of tooth fragments. Improper placement of a tongue blade can block the airway. Padding the bed rails may embarrass the client and family, and bed rails may be considered restraint in some facilities. A safer option would be to place a mattress on the floor. Restraint mitts should not be used on this client as there is no other indicated need for the mitts, and clients should be treated using the least restrictive means possible.

218. Number 3 is correct.

Rationale: As COPD worsens, blood oxygen levels decrease (hypoxemia) and carbon dioxide increases (hypercarbia). Options 1, 2, and 4 do not reflect the expected ABG results.

219. Number 2 is correct.

Rationale: Eschar on at least part of the wound indicates a stage 4 wound. Partial-thickness skin loss is found in stage 2 wounds. Areas that are red and do not blanch with external pressure are stage 1 wounds.

220. Number 2 is correct.

Rationale: The client should be positioned with the legs abducted using a pillow or splint. Floating the client's heels is appropriate to prevent skin breakdown. Application of SCDs reduces the risk of venous thromboembolism. Deep breathing and incentive spirometer use help prevent respiratory complications.

221. Numbers 1, 2, and 5 are correct.

Rationale: Clients with heat stroke have a body temperature of greater than 104°F. Tachycardia, hypotension, and tachypnea are other expected findings in heat stroke.

222. Numbers 1, 5, and 6 are correct.

Rationale: Late signs of increased ICP include seizures, severe headache, and nausea and vomiting (often projectile). Irritability, restlessness, and disorientation are early signs of increased ICP.

223. Number 3 is correct.

Rationale: Spermicides can increase the risk of cystitis and another form of birth control should be used if possible. Voiding before and after intercourse minimizes the risk of bacteria being introduced into the urethra. Loose-fitting cotton underwear helps prevent irritation to the area. Burning upon urination may indicate another infection and should be assessed by the health care provider for diagnosis and treatment.

224. Number 4 is correct.

Rationale: Abdominal pain that increases with cough or movement and is relieved by bending the right hip or knees indicates perforation and peritonitis. Untreated peritonitis can be life-threatening. Pain is a common finding in appendicitis and other inflammatory bowel problems. Family history can play a part in the risk of abdominal alterations. Nausea and vomiting are common findings.

225. Number 1 is correct.

Rationale: The correct order is inspection, auscultation, palpation, percussion. Abdominal assessment varies slightly from other assessments in that auscultation is performed before palpation or percussion in order to avoid changing the intensity and frequency of bowel sounds.

226. Numbers 1, 3, 4, and 5 are correct.

Rationale: Chest pain, hematoma formation, and decreased pulses are signs of cardiac ischemia. The nurse should call the Rapid Response Team or health care provider immediately. Difficulty swallowing may indicate possible stroke. A decreased appetite is not a complication of cardiac catheterization and does not require emergent care.

227. Number 2 is correct.

Rationale: Before touching the client, the nurse should wash her hands and don gloves for protection from blood or other body fluids. While all of the other steps are part of the procedure, safety against blood-borne pathogens is the priority.

228. Number 4 is correct.

Rationale: A client with severe weakness on one side will have difficulty turning and repositioning without assistance and will require turning and skin assessment every 2 hours. Neuropathy affects the client's ability to feel pain and causes damage to the skin to be less apparent to the client. An elderly client who can get up with assistance has more mobility than one with weakness and neuropathy. Younger clients tend to be at lower risk of skin breakdown, and although this client has diabetes, his hemoglobin A1C reflects well-controlled blood sugars. Being blind is not necessarily a risk factor for skin breakdown, especially in the client who is able to live independently. Although the client with the chest tube may have diminished mobility, the ability to reposition independently minimizes the risk of skin breakdown from lying in one position too long.

229. Number 3 is correct.

Rationale: Swimming should be avoided and care should be taken when shaving or showering. A Medic-Alert bracelet is useful in life-threatening situations. Loose-fitting, high-neck sweaters and shirts may be worn to cover the stoma or tracheostomy tube. Green houseplants help increase humidity. Clients may also increase the humidity by using saline in the stoma as ordered, sitting pans of water around the house, or using a humidifier. Low humidity may make it more difficult to breathe and cause crusting around the stoma.

230. Number 1 is correct.

Rationale: Rapid weight gain is the best indicator of fluid excess, because visible signs of fluid overload may not be present. Fluid overload often results in distended veins in the hands and neck and moist crackles in the lungs. A combination of diuretics and nutrition therapy, including fluid and sodium restrictions, is the treatment for fluid overload.

231. Numbers 1, 2, and 5 are correct.

Rationale: Keeping personal articles within reach minimizes the risk of the client leaning out of bed to retrieve items. The client must understand how to use the call button, and the nurse should secure it to the bed within easy reach. The nurse should remind the client to call for assistance when he needs to get up and before he has an urgent need to go to the restroom. Some clients wait until they need to use the restroom and then try to hurry out of bed, increasing the risk of falls. Use of all four bed rails is a form of restraint, and agency policy should be followed regarding their use. Dimming the room lights makes it more difficult to see and increases the fall risk. Use of safety lights under the bed or nightlights reduces the risk of falls.

232. Number 2 is correct.

Rationale: The priority with any dysrhythmia is to check the client and the leads first to ensure that the client is truly having a rhythm change. Improperly placed or loose leads can mimic dysrhythmias; coughing or movement can create artifacts. Ventricular fibrillation is a life-threatening emergency; once the client is checked, the nurse should immediately call a code and initiate CPR when the backboard arrives. While waiting on the crash cart, the client should be positioned flat with the rails down for access. If the client is not intubated, pull the bed away from the wall for the anesthetist. The room should be cleared of furniture or other items that will crowd the room. Diltiazem is given in cases of supraventricular tachycardia and is not part of the ACLS protocol for treatment of ventricular fibrillation. Drugs are given only after shocking the client to stabilize the rhythm and improve cardiac output.

233. Numbers 2 and 3 are correct.

Rationale: Clients undergoing brachytherapy have radioactive isotopes inside the body and are radioactive and potentially hazardous to others. Their bodily wastes are radioactive and require special handling until the isotope is completely eliminated from the body. Teletherapy uses a source of radiation outside the body; therefore, these clients are not radioactive. The dose is always less than the exposure because of energy loss on the way to the target tissue. Gamma rays are most commonly used for radiation due to their ability to deeply penetrate tissues.

234. Number 4 is correct.

Rationale: Greater-than-expected head circumference and bulging fontanels are a finding of shaken baby syndrome due to subdural brain hemorrhage. An infant at 2 months does not yet track with the eyes.

Crying is not a typical sign of shaken baby syndrome. External signs of abuse are usually absent; retinal hemorrhage is revealed on ophthalmoscopic examination. The nurse is legally obligated to report all cases of suspected child abuse or neglect.

235. Number 3 is correct.

Rationale: Increased risk factors for HIT include being female and heparin use as postsurgical thromboprophylaxis. HIT is more common in clients who have been on unfractionated heparin or who have used heparin for longer than 1 week. Enoxaparin is a low-molecular weight heparin, which carries a lower risk of developing HIT. It is often prescribed for clients with unstable angina to help increase blood flow through the heart.

236. Number 3 is correct.

Rationale: The client who responds quickly, but only to commands has a Ramsay score of 3. The client with an RSS of 1 is restless, anxious, or agitated. Clients with an RSS of 2 are alert, oriented, and cooperative. Clients with an RSS of 4 respond briskly to stimulus. A client with a sluggish response to stimulus is scored as a 5. A client with an RSS of 6 is deeply sedated and does not respond to stimulus.

237. Numbers 1, 2, and 5 are correct.

Rationale: Lithium has a narrow therapeutic range of 0.6 to 1.2 mEq/L. A level of 2.2 mEq/L indicates moderate toxicity. The nurse should notify the health care provider immediately, as severe toxicity can cause tonic-clonic seizures, coma, or death. Treatment typically involves administering IV fluids to dilute the concentration of the medication, holding the medication, and possible hemodialysis in severe cases. The client may exhibit signs of toxicity such as confusion, slurred speech, and severe diarrhea. A mechanical soft diet will not treat the toxicity. The nurse would hold the next dose and prepare to draw lab work, including lithium and electrolyte levels, BUN and creatinine, and a CBC.

238. Number 1 is correct.

Rationale: This client is exhibiting signs of an air embolism, which is a complication of hemodialysis. The nurse should stop the dialysis immediately and turn the client on the left side in the Trendelenburg's position. The health care provider should be notified immediately. The nurse should administer oxygen and assess vital signs and pulse oximetry. Positioning the client in this manner helps to trap the air in the right side of the heart so it cannot travel to the lungs. Clotting at the graft site would be present when there is no thrill to palpate or a bruit to auscultate. A clotted graft site would not produce this client's signs. Dialysis encephalopathy is caused by aluminum toxicity from dialysate water that contains aluminum. Signs include mental cloudiness, speech disturbances, bone pain, and seizures. Disequilibrium syndrome is characterized by nausea and vomiting, headache, hypertension, muscle cramps, and confusion.

239. Number 4 is correct.

Rationale: Clients having a renal mass removed should be placed in a prone position with a pillow under the shoulders and abdomen. Options 1, 2, and 3 are incorrect positions for this procedure.

240. Number 2 is correct.

Rationale: BNP, or B-type natriuretic peptide, is a hormone released by the heart in response to pressure changes within the heart. It is used to gauge the severity of congestive heart failure. A normal range in a client with heart failure is 0 to 100 pg/mL. A BNP of 760 pg/mL indicates severe heart failure. ALT (alanine aminotransferase) tests liver enzymes. The normal range of ALT is 7 – 56 units per liter, so a value of 33 units/L is within normal limits. WBC (white blood cell) count normally ranges from 4,500 to 11,000 mcL, so a value of 10,450 is within normal limits. Direct bilirubin is a by-product of RBC breakdown. Normal lab values for direct bilirubin range from 0 to 0.3 mg/dL, so a value of 0.2 mg/dL falls within normal limits.

241. Numbers 1, 2, and 3 are correct.

Rationale: This is an elevated total bilirubin level. Signs and symptoms include itchy skin, nausea, and pale stools. Dark urine, not colorless urine, would be present. Normal total bilirubin levels range from 0.3 to 1.9 mg/dL.

242. Number 4 is correct.

Rationale: Clients with hypoparathyroidism have low parathyroid hormone levels on blood tests. Hypocalcemia, not hypercalcemia, is also present. Magnesium levels are decreased, while phosphorus levels are increased.

243. Numbers 1, 2, and 3 are correct.

Rationale: Clients with thrombocytopenia have decreased platelets. The nurse would expect to see signs of bleeding such as epistaxis, petechiae, and vomiting blood. Hematocrit and platelet count would both be decreased in this client.

244. Number 2 is correct.

Rationale: Tuna, along with sardines, scallops, and organ meats, is high in purine and should be avoided by clients with gout. Green peas are a medium-purine food and should be limited to a half cup per day. Low-purine foods include fruit and fruit juices, corn bread, pasta, bread, nuts, and peanut butter. Tea, 1 percent or skim milk, low-fat cheese, and low-fat ice cream are suitable diet choices on a low-purine diet.

245. Number 1 is correct.

Rationale: Shellfish allergy is a possible contraindication to IV contrast medium. Depending on the severity of the allergy, IV diphenhydramine may be given. A history of schizophrenia and allergy to cephalosporins is not a contraindication to contrast dye. The presence of a pacemaker does not affect the use of contrast dye.

246. Numbers 2, 3, and 5 are correct.

Rationale: Serious complications of electroconvulsive therapy (ECT) include airway compromise, cardiac dysrhythmias, and neurological complications. The nurse should monitor vital signs and assess for the return of the gag reflex. Telemetry can detect changes in heart rhythm. Neurological complications include numbness and tingling and memory loss. Orienting the client and performing neurological assessments are part of the recovery process. Skin burns are rare and mild side effects most commonly caused by improper lead placement. Loss of bladder control is not a serious complication. The client should be offered toileting before the procedure.

247. Number 2 is correct.

Rationale: The normal pH is 7.35 – 7.45. A pH of 7.67 is highly alkalotic and should be reported immediately to the health care provider. The normal range for hCO3 is 22 – 26 mEq/L. The normal range for paCO2 is 35 – 45 mmHg. ABGs are used to assess how well the lungs move oxygen into the blood and remove carbon dioxide. They are used to guide ventilator settings in clients who require mechanical ventilation.

248. Number 1 is correct.

Rationale: Following a liver biopsy, the client should avoid lifting, straining, and coughing for 1 to 2 weeks. The client must lay on the right side following the procedure and may experience some pain or discomfort throughout. The client should expect some pain in the right shoulder as anesthesia wears off. Generally a small bandage is required to cover the incision.

249. Number 2 is correct.

Rationale: The therapeutic INR is generally 2.0 to 3.0, so the nurse should expect an order to decrease the warfarin dose. Increasing the warfarin dose increases the risk of bleeding. Protamine sulfate is the antidote for heparin, not warfarin. The client should be observed closely for signs of bleeding until the INR stabilizes in a therapeutic range.

250. Number 1 is correct.

Rationale: The Holter monitor cannot be worn while swimming or bathing and should be kept dry. The monitor stays in place for the entire time monitoring is performed, including sleep. Metal detectors, electric razors, microwaves, and other electrical devices may interfere with the signal and should be avoided. Cell phones should be kept at least 6 inches away from the monitor. Clients should keep a log and note any chest pain, shortness of breath, or skipped heart beats while wearing the monitor.

251. Number 1 is correct.

Rationale: An A1C level below 7 is the target goal for most clients with diabetes, as it indicates good glycemic control. Given the A1C level of 6.9, there is no indication to increase or decrease medications. Since the client's A1C is within the goal, there is no indication that the client needs an insulin pump.

252. Number 4 is correct.

Rationale: Clients with AV fistulas should avoid wearing tight sleeves or jewelry over the access area because restricting the blood flow may lead to clotting. A watch should be switched to the opposite arm. Fistulas take several weeks to mature to the point where they may be used. Blood pressures should not be taken in the arm with the fistula. The client should also not have needle sticks in the access arm.

253. Numbers 1, 4, and 5 are correct.

Rationale: Adverse effects of adenosine include nausea, chest pain, and facial flushing. The nurse should stop the infusion and monitor the client for abatement of symptoms. Adenosine has a half-life of 10 seconds, so symptoms should resolve shortly. A respiratory rate of 18 and heart rate of 97 are within normal limits and do not require any intervention.

254. Numbers 1, 3, 4, and 5 are correct.

Rationale: Based on the confusion and drop in systolic blood pressure, the client may be becoming septic. The nurse should obtain blood cultures to determine if bacterial infection is triggering the response; this will also indicate which antibiotics would be effective. Fever can decrease oxygenation, so the client should be placed on oxygen. Antipyretics should be administered, and the nurse should follow up and recheck the temperature in 30 minutes or so to see if it is decreasing. The client should rest and avoid physical activity. There is no need to make the client NPO; fluids help with hydration and should be encouraged if the client can drink. Although the client may want a blanket if experiencing chills, the room temperature should be decreased and excess blankets removed.

255. Answers:

Laboratory Test	Normal Value
calcium	8.5 – 10.9 mg/L (serum)
pH	7.35 – 7.45 (arterial blood gases)
specific gravity	1.010 – 1.030 (urine)
potassium	3.5 – 5.1
LDL	Less than 100 mg/dL (serum)
HDL	40 – 59 mg/dL (serum)

256. Number 3 is correct.

Rationale: Many clients with dementia pull out an IV because they see it and know that they don't normally have one. Placing the IV in an inconspicuous place, such as where it can be covered by the gown or wrapped up in gauze, prevents the client from pulling it out, because he cannot see it. Restraints should not be the first-line intervention for this client, as this may increase confusion and agitation. If the family can stay with the client, they can help watch, but many clients do not have family close by that can stay with them around the clock. Threatening the client with a more invasive procedure should never be used as a means of obtaining cooperation.

257. The correct order is:

2.	explain the procedure to the client
8.	set up the prescribed oxygen delivery system and bring in equipment for emergency reintubation
1.	hyperoxygenate the client
5.	thoroughly suction the ET tube and the oral cavity
7.	rapidly deflate the ET tube cuff and remove tube at peak inspiration
3.	immediately instruct the client to cough
4.	apply oxygen by nasal cannula or face mask
6.	teach the client how to use an incentive spirometer every 2 hours

Rationale: Explaining the procedure to the client first helps minimize fear. Equipment should be set up before performing the procedure. Hyperoxygenation should be performed before suctioning to avoid dropping the client's oxygen saturation levels. Deflating the tube cuff aids in removal and prevents injury to client. Coughing helps clear any remaining secretions. The nurse should apply oxygen to the client and ensure it is in place before teaching. The client should demonstrate use of incentive spirometer to verify proper technique and lower risk of respiratory complications.

258. Number 4 is correct.

Rationale: The normal pH in adults ranges from 7.35 to 7.45. Albumin values range from 3.5 to 5.0 g/dL. Normal hemoglobin ranges from 12 to 16 g/dL for women and 14 to 18 g/dL for men. Normal potassium levels are 3.5 – 5.0 mEq/L. Potassium levels become elevated in burns due to disruption of the sodium-potassium pump, red blood cell hemolysis, and tissue damage.

259. Numbers 3, 4, and 5 are correct.

Rationale: Males develop GBS slightly more often than females. The acute or initial period lasts from 1 to 4 weeks, beginning with the onset of symptoms and ending when no further deterioration occurs. GBS tends to be self-limiting with muscle weakness and temporary paralysis. Infections are commonly associated with GBS, with Campylobacter jejuni one of the more common bacterial infections.

260. Number 3 is correct.

Rationale: The priority after this procedure is monitoring the client for excessive bleeding. The nurse should observe the dressing for 24 hours for signs of bleeding or infection. It is not necessary to keep the client NPO after this procedure. Contact sports should be avoided for 48 hours. No further site care is required other than observing the dressing for 24 hours, unless signs of infection are noted.

261. Number 2 is correct.

Rationale: Foods high in purines should be avoided as they can trigger an exacerbation. All forms of aspirin and diuretics should be avoided. Excessive alcohol intake and fad "starvation" diets can trigger a flare-up.

262. Number 1 is correct.

Rationale: Upper GI bleeding causes an increased heart rate, decreased hematocrit and hemoglobin, and weak peripheral pulses.

263. Number 4 is correct.

Rationale: FAS is characterized by microcephaly, small eyes or short palpebral fissures, thin upper lip, and flat midface. Syphilis presents with maculopapular dermal rash on palms and soles. TORCH syndrome is a group of infections that produce various congenital malformations. The acronym stands for toxoplasmosis, other infections, rubella, cytomegalovirus, and herpes simplex. Brachial plexus injury describes a type of paralysis associated with a difficult birth.

264. Number 1 is correct.

Rationale: Gluten avoidance is the key focus of managing celiac disease. Rice, millet, and corn are suitable dietary choices for this client. All rye, oats, wheat, and barley should be eliminated from the client's diet to avoid exacerbating the condition.

265. Numbers 2, 4, and 5 are correct.

Rationale: Foul odor and purulent drainage should be reported, along with sudden increases in output. The T-tube should not be irrigated, clamped, or aspirated without an order. The tube should be clamped prior to meals. If nausea or vomiting occur, unclamp the tube. The drainage system should be kept below gallbladder level. The tube should not be removed without an order. The nurse should chart the amount, consistency, color, and odor of any drainage.

266. Number 2 is correct.

Rationale: Chronic myelogenous leukemia contains mostly granulocytes, not lymphocytes, in the bone marrow, with a typical age of onset in the 40s. Acute lymphocytic leukemia presents with mostly lymphoblasts in the bone marrow. It is the earliest-onset leukemia, appearing before age 15 years. Acute myelogenous leukemia appears after age 50 years, with mostly lymphocytes present in the bone marrow.

267. Number 4 is correct.

Rationale: *Pneumocystis jiroveci* pneumonia is the most common opportunistic infection in children with HIV. Hepatitis C and strep throat are not commonly opportunistic infections limited to children with HIV. Although cytomegalovirus may be present in HIV, it is not the most common opportunistic infection.

268. Number 3 is correct.

Rationale: Following a mastectomy, the client should be positioned with the head of the bed at 30 degrees or more, with a pillow supporting the arm on the affected side to allow lymphatic fluid return. The other options describe either incorrect bed positioning or incorrect placement of the pillow.

269. Number 1 is correct.

Rationale: The transducer must be at the level of the right atrium in order to accurately measure arterial blood pressure and other hemodynamic pressures. Options 2, 3, and 4 are incorrect positions for the transducer and will not give accurate results.

270. Number 3 is correct.

Rationale: This client is experiencing acute adrenal insufficiency, or Addisonian crisis. This is a life-threatening event if left untreated. Treatment consists of IV saline, dextrose, or hydrocortisone. IV spironolactone would not be given, since it is a potassium-sparing diuretic. Boluses of normal saline or dextrose 5% in normal saline are the fluids of choice to deliver medications and restore fluid balance. Since the client is hyperkalemic, fluids containing potassium would not be given. Also, potassium is never given as a bolus due to the risk of cardiac dysrhythmias.

271. Number 4 is correct.

Rationale: Intake includes everything the client took in liquid form, including IV fluids, flushes, and antibiotics; drinks; and soups. Output measurement includes wound drainage, diarrhea, urine, gastric suction, and emesis. All output, no matter how small or seemingly insignificant, is counted.

272. Number 2 is correct.

Rationale: Oxygen delivery at 2 L/minute via nasal cannula is equivalent to 28% FiO2. A flow rate of 1 L/minute is equal to 24% FiO2. A flow rate of 3 L/minute is equal to 32% FiO2. A flow rate of 4 L/minute is equivalent to 36% FiO2.

273. Number 4 is correct.

Rationale: Nasal cannulas, non-rebreather masks, simple face masks, and partial rebreather masks are examples of low-flow oxygen delivery systems. A tracheostomy collar requires a flow rate of at least 10 L/minute to maintain the proper FiO2. High-flow oxygen delivery systems include the venturi mask, face tent, T-piece, tracheostomy collar, and aerosol mask. Non-rebreather masks should have a flow rate sufficient to keep the reservoir bag two-thirds full.

274. Numbers 1, 4, and 5 are correct.

Rationale: The client will be on different medications following surgery. The nurse should demonstrate to the client how to splint the incision when coughing or breathing deeply to minimize pain and lessen pressure on the incision site. After surgery, the client will be on the ventilator and have one or more chest tubes. The client will be encouraged to ambulate as early as possible to prevent complications from pneumonia. The client will have a urinary catheter following surgery and will not need to void in a bedpan.

275. Number 1 is correct.

Rationale: Glossitis, or a smooth tongue, is a sign of vitamin B12 deficiency anemia. Inflammation causes the tongue to appear smooth. Paresthesias are found in pernicious anemia. Weakness and pallor are found in iron deficiency anemia. Dark purple or cyanotic skin on the face and mucous membranes are signs of polycythemia vera.

276. Number 4 is correct.

Rationale: A systolic murmur occurs between the S1 and S2 heart sounds. A diastolic murmur will be heard between S2 and S1. Options 1 and 2 are incorrect for hearing a systolic murmur. A murmur can occur during any phase of the cardiac cycle.

277. Number 1 is correct.

Rationale: The mitral and tricuspid valves produce the S1 sound when they close. Option 3 describes the action that produces the S2 sound. Options 2 and 4 do not describe the mechanism of the S1 heart sound.

278. Numbers 1, 3, and 5 are correct.

Rationale: Gargling with warm saline can decrease discomfort caused by a sore throat. Many people think that an antibiotic is what they need for a sore throat, when most sore throats are actually caused by a virus. Antibiotics are ineffective on viruses. Overuse of antibiotics for sore throats can lead to antibiotic resistance. Increased fluid intake with water and warm beverages or soups can help with the pain. A humidifier should be used to add moisture to the air. The doctor will not prescribe an antibiotic if it is determined that the client's sore throat is caused by a virus.

279. Number 4 is correct.

Rationale: Severe edema can occur in areas that were not burned, due to the leakage of electrolytes and fluids from the vascular space. The fluid shift causes hyperkalemia and hypovolemia.

Hemoconcentration is caused by vascular dehydration, which increases blood viscosity. Excessive weight gain can occur during the first 12 hours following the burn and may continue for 24 – 36 hours due to the fluid shift.

280. Number 1 is correct.

Rationale: Anemia is a prime concern after a total knee replacement. A hemoglobin level of 10.2 g/L is low (normal is 13.5 – 17.5 for men, 12.0 – 15.5 for women) and might require a blood transfusion. Bleeding on the dressing of 2 cm is not of concern. Circle, date, and time the bleeding initially and monitor closely for changes. Recheck the temperature in 30 minutes; if above 100.6, report finding to the doctor. Complaint of pain at the incision site is routine, and pain medication should be administered as prescribed.

281. Number 3 is correct.

Rationale: A medical condition such as a seizure or stroke may have been the underlying cause of the drowning event and would require further treatment once the client's respiratory status is stabilized. Drowning in very cold water appears to have a protective effect by causing a reduction in cardiac output and reducing the cerebral metabolic rate, even with prolonged arrest. Aspiration of both salt and fresh water decreases surfactant to the lungs and leads to decreased lung compliance. Contaminants in the water such as microbes, mud, chemicals, and algae may play a significant role in how much damage to the lungs is sustained.

282. Numbers 1, 3, 4, and 6 are correct.

Rationale: Rabies causes encephalitis, which causes paralysis and difficulty swallowing water. This manifests as an apparent fear of water, which can cause the client to become adversely irritated when he or she sees water or hears running water. Nuchal rigidity, convulsions, and tonic or clonic muscle contractions can occur during the neurological phase. In the prodromal phase, the client can have irritability, extreme salivation, sore throat, fever, and hyperexcitability. During the paralytic phase, the client becomes unconscious, has loss of bowel and urinary control, and has irregular or labored breathing. Current treatment includes one dose of immunoglobulin and five doses of rabies vaccine over a period of 28 days. Aches and pains in different parts of the body and light sensitivity occur during the prodromal phase.

283. Number 3 is correct.

Rationale: Impaired consciousness, visual loss, bilateral sensory and motor dysfunction, and pupil abnormalities are seen with basilar artery strokes. Memory problems, visual hallucinations, visual deficits, and hemisensory disturbances occur with posterior cerebral artery strokes. Weakness in the foot and leg, sensory loss in the foot and leg, incontinence, ataxia, and lack of spontaneity occurs with anterior cerebral artery strokes. Ataxia, contralateral facial weakness, contralateral hemiplegia, visual deficits, speech impairments, and perceptual impairments occur with middle cerebral artery strokes.

284. Number 4 is correct.

Rationale: Dumping syndrome signs and symptoms include sweating, heart palpitations, vertigo, and the urge to lay down shortly after eating. Onset of symptoms occurs within 5 to 30 minutes after eating. Signs and symptoms of appendicitis include rebound tenderness and abdominal rigidity, pain in the lower right quadrant, nausea and vomiting, and low-grade fever. Cholecystitis manifests with pain to the right upper quadrant that radiates to the right scapula, Murphy's sign, belching, indigestion, and nausea and vomiting. Signs and symptoms of ulcerative colitis include abdominal cramping and tenderness, severe diarrhea that may present with mucus and blood, weight loss, anorexia, and malaise.

285. Numbers 4, 5, and 6 are correct.

Rationale: Cancer of the tongue causes difficulty swallowing due to enlarged lymph nodes in the neck. Sores that bleed or do not heal over time are another sign of tongue cancer. Chewing may be difficult or painful for clients with cancer of the tongue. Weight loss, not weight gain, can occur due to difficulty chewing and swallowing. Poor-fitting dentures or loose teeth are another sign. A black, hairy tongue is caused by overgrowth of yeast and bacteria and is a benign condition unrelated to cancer of the tongue.

286. Number 4 is correct.

Rationale: ACE inhibitors alone are less effective in African American clients unless they are combined with a calcium channel blocker or a thiazide diuretic. Therefore, the client would not be given an ACE inhibitor by itself. Amiloride can cause hyperkalemia in clients with impaired renal function, especially if given in conjunction with ACE inhibitors. Atenolol can increase the incidence of diabetes and mask symptoms of hypoglycemia, as well as delay recovery from hypoglycemic episodes.

287. Numbers 1 and 4 are correct.

Rationale: Home management of chronic pancreatitis includes eating small meals throughout the day and avoiding heavy meals. Nicotine and caffeine can worsen symptoms. Alcohol contributes to flare-ups and should be avoided. The client should rest frequently until full strength has returned and the health care provider has approved of vigorous activity. Spicy foods stimulate the GI tract and should be avoided. Bland, high-protein, low-fat, and moderate-carbohydrate meals and snacks are the best for the client.

288. Number 3 is correct.

Rationale: Chronic back pain, weight loss, joint pain and itching, and visual disturbances describe signs and symptoms of ankylosing spondylitis. Reiter syndrome is characterized by burning upon urination, joint pain, and eye infection with pain, redness, and drainage. Marfan syndrome presents with excessive height, elongated hands and feet, scoliosis, and cardiovascular problems. Signs and symptoms of systemic necrotizing vasculitis include peripheral arterial disease with severe pain and necrosis of fingers or toes, kidney or heart failure, and stroke-like symptoms.

289. Number 2 is correct.

Rationale: Oliguria, the production of an abnormally small amount of urine, is indicative of stage 5 chronic kidney disease. Symptoms of stage 3 chronic kidney disease include shortness of breath, tea-colored urine, and edema in the lower extremities.

290. Numbers 3, 4, and 6 are correct.

Rationale: The client's level of consciousness must be assessed as part of a standard admission assessment, as it will determine treatments needed. The client is placed supine to avoid orthostatic alterations in blood pressure due to cardiac instability. The client should be handled gently to prevent ventricular fibrillation. The nurse should administer CPR if the client does not have spontaneous circulation. Heating blankets are contraindicated in severe hypothermia; the treatment of choice is extracorporeal rewarming via cardiopulmonary bypass or hemodialysis. A rectal temperature is the most accurate in the hypothermic client. Massaging the extremities may injure frostbitten extremities and should not be performed.

291. Number 4 is correct.

Rationale: The purpose of ECT is to trigger a short-term seizure of 30 – 90 seconds. As such, administration of an anticonvulsant prior to the procedure is contraindicated. An anticholinergic agent is administered prior to ECT to lessen secretions that could be aspirated. Cleansing the body prior to an ECT promotes effective transmission of the electrical current. Fasting after midnight prevents aspiration of stomach contents during the procedure. As an intrusive medical procedure, an informed consent in writing is required.

292. Number 4 is correct.

Rationale: The American Red Cross advises to complete the following if you encounter a conscious, choking person who is unable to cough, speak, or breathe: send someone to call 9-1-1, lean the person forward, and give five back blows with the heel of your hand. If ineffective, perform the Heimlich maneuver to remove the obstruction. The other stated actions are performed on unconscious persons.

293. Number 4 is correct.

Rationale: Applying ice to a recent soft tissue injury will decrease blood flow and decrease swelling; it should be done first. Administration of an OTC medication is effective, yet it is not the most appropriate nursing action to be done initially. Heat will increase blood flow and swelling. Massage promotes blood flow and can increase swelling, causing further damage.

294. Number 2 is correct.

Rationale: Indoor swimming is recommended as an exercise as it takes place in a warm, moist environment. Bronchoconstriction associated with asthma may occur with exercises that require prolonged rapid breathing, including distance running, soccer, and basketball.

295. Number 3 is correct.

Rationale: Metabolic (nonrespiratory) alkalosis is consistent with the stated values. The stated pH of 7.58 is alkalotic. The value of PaCO2, 48 mm Hg is within normal range indicating a nonrespiratory (metabolic) origin. The value of HCO3 of 44 mEq/L is indicative of metabolic alkalosis. A Base Excess of +13 mEq/L is consistent with severe metabolic alkalosis.

296. Number 1 is correct.

Rationale: A resting tremor is a primary motor symptom of Parkinson's disease seen in either the hand or the foot on one side of the body. Sleep disturbance, constipation, and fatigue are nonmotor symptoms of Parkinson's disease.

297. Number 4 is correct.

Rationale: The normal serum calcium level is 8.5 – 10.2 mg/dL, making the client's results extremely high (hypercalcemia). The condition typically results from hyperparathyroidism. The priority treatment of choice is intravenous bisphosphonates. Calcitonin is the secondary medical treatment of choice followed by corticosteroids. Renal dialysis is not considered an acceptable treatment.

298. Number 2 is correct.

Rationale: Seizures are associated with meningiomas along with headache, weakness in an arm or leg, and personality changes. Other stated symptoms are not seen with this type of cancer.

299. Number 2 is correct.

Rationale: Assessment of the client is a priority in the nursing process; therefore, obtaining vital signs would be a priority. The nurse must assess before performing interventions such as relief of pain, administration of IV fluids, and preparation for surgery.

300. Number 3 is correct.

Rationale: Cefazolin can cause a reaction in clients allergic to penicillin. The nurse should hold the medication and notify the health care provider. Administering the cefazolin is likely to trigger another allergic reaction, which potentially may worsen. The pharmacy cannot change health care provider orders. The nurse should consult the health care provider before giving diphenhydramine in order to give the cefazolin, as the provider will more than likely order another medication from a different drug family.

301. Numbers 2, 4, and 5 are correct.

Rationale: Furosemide increases urine output, which removes excess fluid from the body. Pitting edema of +1 indicates an improvement due to the fluid loss. Urine output of 250 mL/hr is an expected finding in this client. Crackles in the lungs should be decreased or absent. Pitting edema of +3 indicates an increase in edema. Shortness of breath should be resolved, not merely decreased.

302. Numbers 1, 5, and 6 are correct.

Rationale: Left-side heart failure manifestations include dyspnea, weak peripheral pulses, and crackles or wheezes in the lungs. Left-sided heart failure causes pulmonary congestion and decreased cardiac output. Right-sided heart failure causes systemic congestion, leading to an engorged spleen, dependent edema, and jugular vein distention.

303. Number 1 is correct.

Rationale: Diabetics should check the feet daily for injury since diabetes causes a loss of sensation in the feet over time. A cut that goes unnoticed may become infected and progress to amputation. Eye examinations should be done on a yearly basis. Heating pads should be avoided on the feet due to the risk of injury caused by loss of sensation. The client should be encouraged to adhere to a diabetic diet and not to take extra insulin just to be able to eat off-limits food.

304. Numbers 1 and 2 are correct.

Rationale: Following an inguinal hernia repair, the nurse should encourage fluid intake to prevent constipation and straining during bowel movements. If the client cannot void, intermittent catheterization should be performed. Ice, not heat, should be applied to the scrotum to minimize swelling. The client should turn and deep breathe, but avoid coughing. The client should be encouraged to ambulate as soon as possible after surgery. Lifting more than 10 pounds should be avoided until approved by the health care provider.

305. Numbers 2, 4, and 6 are correct.

Rationale: An NG tube is placed to avoid complications from nausea, vomiting, and abdominal distention. IV fluids correct dehydration. Monitoring stools for bleeding is important because blood loss may lead to a drop in blood pressure or, in severe cases, progress to hypovolemic shock. A client in the acute phase of diverticular disease should have a low-fiber diet if she is able to eat. A high-fiber diet should be introduced gradually once the acute phase has resolved. Enemas are contraindicated because they cause an increase in intestinal motility. Coughing should be avoided because it increases intra-abdominal pressure.

306. Numbers 1, 3, 5, and 6 are correct.

Rationale: This client is exhibiting signs of intussusception. The nurse should monitor for and report respiratory distress immediately. Respiratory distress can be caused by pressing the knees up to the abdomen. Passage of a normal, brown stool indicates reduction of the intussusception. An NG tube is placed to decompress the stomach. Fever and changes in blood pressure can indicate perforation and shock. The client should be kept NPO until the intussusception is resolved. A barium enema is contraindicated for any client at risk of bowel perforation.

307. Answer: The correct order follows:

5.   Turn on AED. Follow visual and/or audio prompts.

2.   Open the person's shirt and wipe the chest dry. Remove any visible patches.

3.   Attach the AED pads and plug in the connector.

1.   Make sure no one is touching the client. Tell everyone to "stand clear."

4.   Push the "analyze" button to analyze the client's heart rhythm.

7.   As prompted, press the "shock" button after clearing the client.

6.   Begin CPR.

308. Number 2 is correct.

Rationale: Dry wheat toast with water is the best menu option for this client. Clients with gastric ulcers should avoid foods that contain caffeine since they trigger the release of gastrin. Although milk and dairy products may initially have a soothing effect because they coat the stomach, they also trigger the release of gastric acid and should be avoided. Dietary management of gastric ulcers is controversial, but the client should avoid foods that may trigger symptoms.

309. Numbers 1, 3, and 6 are correct.

Rationale: Veno-occlusive disease is the blockage of blood vessels in the liver and is a complication of bone marrow transplant, also known as hematopoietic stem cell transplant. Manifestations include jaundice, weight gain, and right upper quadrant pain. Liver enlargement is another sign of veno-occlusive disease.

310. Number 3 is correct.

Rationale: Removing stitches is a sterile procedure. The nurse should wash her hands and use sterile technique when removing stitches. Soap and water is not sufficient for cleaning the stitches prior to removal. Washing the hands and using regular gloves is not sterile. The sterile field must be maintained during the procedure, which contraindicates the use of regular gloves. It is not necessary to wear a gown, a mask, gloves, an eye shield, and shoe covers unless the client is on contact precautions. Nothing in this question indicates that the client is on contact precautions.

311. Number 2 is correct.

Rationale: In an emergency situation, type O blood can be given because it is the universal donor. There is not enough time to draw a type and match before the client bleeds out. Type AB+ blood is the universal recipient. There is not enough time to ask the family to donate blood for the client.